1999
YEAR BOOK OF
NEUROLOGY AND NEUROSURGERY®

Statement of Purpose

The YEAR BOOK Service

The YEAR BOOK series was devised in 1901 by practicing health professionals who observed that the literature of medicine and related disciplines had become so voluminous that no one individual could read and place in perspective every potential advance in a major specialty. In the final decade of the 20th century, this recognition is more acutely true than it was in 1901.

More than merely a series of books, YEAR BOOK volumes are the tangible results of a unique service designed to accomplish the following:

- to *survey* a wide range of journals of proven value
- to *select* from those journals papers representing significant advances and statements of important clinical principles
- to provide *abstracts* of those articles that are readable, convenient summaries of their key points
- to provide *commentary* about those articles to place them in perspective.

These publications grow out of a unique process that calls on the talents of outstanding authorities in clinical and fundamental disciplines, trained literature specialists, and professional writers, all supported by the resources of Mosby, the world's preeminent publisher for the health professions.

The Literature Base

Mosby and its editors survey approximately 500 journals published worldwide, covering the full range of the health professions. On an annual basis, the publisher examines usage patterns and polls its expert authorities to add new journals to the literature base and to delete journals that are no longer useful as potential YEAR BOOK sources.

The Literature Survey

The publisher's team of literature specialists, all of whom are trained and experienced health professionals, examines every original, peer-reviewed article in each journal issue. More than 250,000 articles per year are scanned systematically, including title, text, illustrations, tables, and references. Each scan is compared, article by article, to the search strategies that the publisher has developed in consultation with the 270 outside experts who form the pool of YEAR BOOK editors. A given article may be reviewed by any number of editors, from one to a dozen or more, regardless of the discipline for which the paper was originally published. In turn, each editor who receives the article reviews it to determine whether or not the article should be included in the YEAR BOOK. This decision is based on the article's inherent quality, its probable usefulness to readers of that YEAR BOOK, and the editor's goal to represent a balanced picture of a given field in each volume of the YEAR BOOK. In addition, the editor indicates when to include figures and tables from the article to help the YEAR BOOK reader better understand the information.

Of the quarter million articles scanned each year, only 5% are selected for detailed analysis within the YEAR BOOK series, thereby assuring readers of the high value of every selection.

The Abstract

The publisher's abstracting staff is headed by a seasoned health care professional and includes individuals with training in the life sciences, medicine, and other areas, plus extensive experience in writing for the health professions and related industries. Each selected article is assigned to a specific writer on this abstracting staff. The abstracter, guided in many cases by notations supplied by the expert editor, writes a structured, condensed summary designed so that the reader can rapidly acquire the essential information contained in the article.

The Commentary

The YEAR BOOK editorial boards, sometimes assisted by guest commentators, write comments that place each article in perspective for the reader. This provides the reader with the equivalent of a personal consultation with a leading international authority—an opportunity to better understand the value of the article and to benefit from the authority's thought processes in assessing the article.

Additional Editorial Features

The editorial boards of each YEAR BOOK organize the abstracts and comments to provide a logical and satisfying sequence of information. To enhance the organization, editors also provide introductions to sections or individual chapters, comments linking a number of abstracts, citations to additional literature, and other features.

The published YEAR BOOK contains enhanced bibliographic citations for each selected article, including extended listings of multiple authors and identification of author affiliations. Each YEAR BOOK contains a Table of Contents specific to that year's volume. From year to year, the Table of Contents for a given YEAR BOOK will vary, depending on developments within the field.

Every YEAR BOOK contains a list of the journals from which papers have been selected. This list represents a subset of the approximately 500 journals surveyed by the publisher and occasionally reflects a particularly pertinent article from a journal that is not surveyed on a routine basis.

Finally, each volume contains a comprehensive subject index and an index to authors of each selected paper.

The 1999 Year Book Series

Year Book of Allergy, Asthma, and Clinical Immunology: Drs. Rosenwasser, Boguniewicz, Borish, Nelson, Routes, and Spahn

Year Book of Anesthesiology and Pain Management®: Drs. Tinker, Abram, Chestnut, Roizen, Rothenberg, and Wood

Year Book of Cardiology®: Drs. Schlant, Collins, Gersh, Graham, Kaplan, and Waldo

Year Book of Chiropractic®: Dr. Lawrence

Year Book of Critical Care Medicine®: Drs. Parrillo, Balk, Calvin, Franklin, and Shapiro

Year Book of Dentistry®: Drs. Meskin, Berry, Jeffcoat, Leinfelder, Roser, Summitt, and Zakariasen

Year Book of Dermatology and Dermatologic Surgery™: Drs. Thiers and Lang

Year Book of Diagnostic Radiology®: Drs. Osborn, Dalinka, Groskin, Maynard, Pentecost, Ros, Smirniotopoulos, and Young

Year Book of Emergency Medicine®: Drs. Wagner, Dronen, Davidson, King, Niemann, and Hamilton

Year Book of Endocrinology®: Drs. Bagdade, Braverman, Horton, Kannan, Landsberg, Molitch, Morley, Odell, Poehlman, Rogol, and Fitzpatrick

Year Book of Family Practice®: Drs. Berg, Bowman, Davidson, Dexter, and Scherger

Year Book of Gastroenterology: Drs. Aliperti and Fleshman

Year Book of Hand Surgery®: Drs. Amadio and Hentz

Year Book of Medicine®: Drs. Klahr, Frishman, Malawista, Mandell, Jett, Young, Barkin, and Bagdade

Year Book of Neonatal and Perinatal Medicine®: Drs. Fanaroff, Maisels, and Stevenson

Year Book of Nephrology, Hypertension, and Mineral Metabolism: Drs. Schwab, Bennett, Emmett, Hostetter, and Moe

Year Book of Neurology and Neurosurgery®: Drs. Bradley and Gibbs

Year Book of Nuclear Medicine®: Drs. Gottschalk, Blaufox, Coleman, Strauss, and Zubal

Year Book of Obstetrics, Gynecology, and Women's Health: Drs. Mishell, Herbst, and Kirschbaum

Year Book of Oncology®: Drs. Ozols, Eisenberg, Glatstein, Loehrer, and Urba

Year Book of Ophthalmology®: Drs. Wilson, Augsburger, Cohen, Eagle, Grossman, Laibson, Maguire, Nelson, Penne, Rapuano, Sergott, Spaeth, Tipperman, Ms. Gosfield, and Ms. Salmon

Year Book of Orthopedics®: Drs. Morrey, Beauchamp, Currier, Tolo, Trigg, and Swiontkowski

Year Book of Otolaryngology–Head and Neck Surgery®: Drs. Paparella, Holt, and Otto

Year Book of Pathology and Laboratory Medicine®: Drs. Raab, Cohen, Dabbs, Olson, and Stanley

Year Book of Pediatrics®: Dr. Stockman

Year Book of Plastic, Reconstructive, and Aesthetic Surgery®: Drs. Miller, Bartlett, Garner, McKinney, Ruberg, Salisbury, and Smith

Year Book of Psychiatry and Applied Mental Health®: Drs. Talbott, Ballenger, Frances, Lydiard, Meltzer, Jensen, and Tasman

Year Book of Pulmonary Disease®: Drs. Jett, Castro, Maurer, Peters, Phillips, and Ryu

Year Book of Rheumatology, Arthritis, and Musculoskeletal Disease™: Drs. Panush, Hadler, Hellman, LeRoy, Pisetsky, and Simon

Year Book of Sports Medicine®: Drs. Shephard, Drinkwater, Eichner, Torg, Alexander, and Mr. George

Year Book of Surgery®: Drs. Copeland, Bland, Deitch, Eberlein, Howard, Luce, Seeger, Souba, and Sugarbaker

Year Book of Urology®: Drs. Andriole and Coplen

Year Book of Vascular Surgery®: Dr. Porter

1999

The Year Book of NEUROLOGY AND NEUROSURGERY®

"Published without interruption since 1902"

Neurology

Editor
Walter G. Bradley, D.M., F.R.C.P.
Professor and Chairman, Department of Neurology, University of Miami School of Medicine, Florida

Neurosurgery

Editor
Scott R. Gibbs, M.A., M.D.
Director of Brain and Neuro-Spine Center, Division of Neurosurgery, Southeast Missouri Hospital; Staff Neurosurgeon, St. Francis Medical Center, Cape Girardeau, Missouri

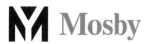 Mosby

St. Louis Baltimore Boston Carlsbad Naples New York Philadelphia Portland London
Madrid Mexico City Singapore Sydney Tokyo Toronto Wiesbaden

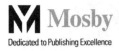
Mosby
Dedicated to Publishing Excellence

Publisher: Theresa Van Schaik
Associate Publisher: Gretchen Murphy
Developmental Editor: Jaime Pendill
Manager, Periodical Editing: Kirk Swearingen
Production Editor: Amanda Maguire
Project Supervisor, Production: Joy Moore
Production Assistant: Laura Bayless
Manager, Literature Services: Idelle L. Winer
Illustrations and Permissions Coordinator: Chidi C. Ukabam

1999 EDITION
Copyright © February 1999 by Mosby, Inc.

Printed in the United States of America
Composition by Reed Technology and Information Services, Inc.
Printing/binding by Maple-Vail

Mosby, Inc.
11830 Westline Industrial Drive
St. Louis, MO 63146
Customer Service: customer.support@mosby.com
www.mosby.com/Mosby/CustomerSupport/index.html

International Standard Serial Number: 0513–5117
International Standard Book Number: 0–8151–9649–0

Cont 4/18/99

APR 1 4 1999

Nina Felice Schor, M.D., Ph.D.

Professor, Departments of Pediatrics, Neurology, and Pharmacology, University of Pittsburgh; Attending Physician, Children's Hospital, Pittsburgh, Pennsylvania

Julio Sotelo, M.D.

Professor of Neurological Sciences, Universidad Autonoma de Mexico; General Director, Instituto Nacional de Neurologia y Neurocirugia, Mexico, D.F.

David A. Stumpf, M.D., Ph.D.

Professor and Chairman, Department of Neurology; Professor of Pediatric Neurology, Northwestern University Medical School; Professor and Chairman of Neurology, Northwestern Memorial Hospital, Chicago, Illinois

Vincent C. Traynelis, M.D.

Associate Professor of Neurosurgery, The University of Iowa Hospitals and Clinics, Iowa City, Iowa

Nicolas de Tribolet, M.D.

Professor and Chairman, Hôpital Cantonal Universitaire de Genève, Genève, Switzerland

Ronald J. Tusa, M.D., Ph.D.

Professor of Neurology and Otolaryngology; Bascom Palmer Eye Institute, University of Miami School of Medicine, Anne Bates Leech Hospital, Miami, Florida

Olivier Vernet, M.D.

Maître d'ensiegnement et de recherche, Université de Lausanne; Médecin Associé, Centre Hospitalier Universitaire Vaudois, Lausanne, Switzerland

Clark Watts, M.D., J.D.

Clinical Professor of Neurosurgery, University of Texas Health Science Center, San Antonio, Texas

Table of Contents

Journals Represented

Mosby and its Editors survey approximately 500 journals for its abstract and commentary publications. From these journals, the Editors select the articles to be abstracted. Journals represented in this YEAR BOOK are listed below.

Academic Emergency Medicine
Acta Neurochirurgica
Acta Radiologica
American Journal of Emergency Medicine
American Journal of Medicine
American Journal of Neuroradiology
American Journal of Physical Medicine & Rehabilitation
American Journal of Respiratory and Critical Care Medicine
Annals of Internal Medicine
Annals of Neurology
Annals of Otology, Rhinology and Laryngology
Annals of Thoracic Surgery
Archives of Disease in Childhood
Archives of Neurology
Archives of Physical Medicine and Rehabilitation
Archives of Surgery
Bone Marrow Transplantation
Brain
British Journal of Psychiatry
British Journal of Radiology
British Medical Journal
Canadian Journal of Anaesthesia
Canadian Journal of Surgery
Cancer
Cephalalgia
Childs Nervous System
Clinical Journal of Pain
Clinical Pediatrics
Critical Care Medicine
Developmental Medicine and Child Neurology
Epilepsia
European Journal of Endocrinology
Gastroenterology
Headache
Human Pathology
International Journal of Radiation, Oncology, Biology, and Physics
Journal of Bone and Joint Surgery (British Volume)
Journal of Human Hypertension
Journal of Infectious Diseases
Journal of Neurological, Surgical Nursing
Journal of Neurology, Neurosurgery and Psychiatry
Journal of Neuropathology and Experimental Neurology
Journal of Neurosurgery
Journal of Nuclear Medicine
Journal of Orthopaedic Research
Journal of Orthopaedic Trauma
Journal of Pediatrics

Journal of Spinal Disorders
Journal of Vascular Surgery
Journal of the American College of Cardiology
Journal of the Neurological Sciences
Lancet
Mayo Clinic Proceedings
Neurology
Neurosurgery
New England Journal of Medicine
Obstetrics and Gynecology
Orthopedics
Pain
Pediatric Emergency Care
Pediatric Neurology
Pediatric Research
Plastic Surgical Nursing
Prenatal Diagnosis
Radiology
Regional Anesthesia
Science
Sleep
Spinal Cord
Spine
Stroke
Surgical Neurology
The Laryngoscope Journal

STANDARD ABBREVIATIONS

The following terms are abbreviated in this edition: acquired immunodeficiency syndrome (AIDS), cardiopulmonary resuscitation (CPR), central nervous system (CNS), cerebrospinal fluid (CSF), computed tomography (CT), deoxyribonucleic acid (DNA), electrocardiography (ECG), health maintenance organization (HMO), human immunodeficiency virus (HIV), intensive care unit (ICU), intramuscular (IM), intravenous (IV), magnetic resonance (MR) imaging (MRI), and ribonucleic acid (RNA).

NOTE

The YEAR BOOK OF NEUROLOGY AND NEUROSURGERY is a literature survey service providing abstracts of articles published in the professional literature. Every effort is made to assure the accuracy of the information presented in these pages. Neither the editors nor the publisher of the YEAR BOOK OF NEUROLOGY AND NEUROSURGERY can be responsible for errors in the original materials. The editors' comments are their own opinions. Mention of specific products within this publication does not constitute endorsement.

To facilitate the use of the YEAR BOOK OF NEUROLOGY AND NEUROSURGERY as a reference tool, all illustrations and tables included in this publication are now identified as they appear in the original article. This change is meant to help the reader recognize that any illustration or table appearing in the YEAR BOOK OF NEUROLOGY AND NEUROSURGERY may be only one of many in the original article. For this reason, figure and table numbers will often appear to be out of sequence within the YEAR BOOK OF NEUROLOGY AND NEUROSURGERY.

NEUROLOGY

WALTER G. BRADLEY, D.M., F.R.C.P.

Highlights of a Year's Advances in Neurology

I have just returned from attending the 50th anniversary meeting of the American Academy of Neurology in Minneapolis. This meeting was highly successful, particularly for the depth of the presentations on advances in neurological sciences. Perhaps most fascinating were the Plenary Symposia—in the Decade of the Brain Symposium, Dr. Fred Gage presented information about stem cells in the adult central nervous system. It is becoming clear that our old concept of the brain's formation before birth with all the neurons that it will ever have is not correct. Rather, neurons continue to be produced and incorporated into the olfactory bulb. New neurons are formed in certain other areas of the adult brain in a variety of different disease states. If this capacity can be harnessed and amplified, there may be hope for reconstitution of the central nervous system. If so, the happy day may dawn that neurological degenerations such as amyotrophic lateral sclerosis, Alzheimer's disease and Parkinson's disease can be arrested. The meeting also celebrated the award of the Nobel prize to Dr. Stanley Prusiner for his work on protein conformational changes and their role in prion diseases.

I had the honor of presenting the Scientific Session Plenary Highlights, which allowed me to review the wide range of topics presented at the annual meeting. I will summarize some of these studies because they broaden the scope of the selections in this edition of the *Yearbook of Neurology and Neurosurgery*.

Many papers were presented this year on the topic of advances in movement disorders, particularly deep brain stimulation (DBS). A series of papers demonstrated the major benefit of DBS in the thalamus for essential tremor and the tremor of Parkinson's disease. Globus pallidus (especially the externa) and subthalamic nucleus DBS proved to be very effective for end-stage parkinsonism.

The restless legs syndrome can be due to may different conditions, including peripheral neuropathies. However, the more florid cases are probably due to basal ganglia dysfunction. A number of studies demonstrated significant improvement following treatment with the newer dopamine agonists.

As befits the fact that stroke is one of the major neurological killers and producers of disability, a good number of presentations dealt with cerebrovascular disease. An interesting study from Rochester, Minnesota, evaluated the role of neurologists in outcome measures for patients suffering acute strokes. In patients without atrial fibrillation, when correction was applied for all co-morbidity factors in patients on a neurological service or on a general medical service with neurological consultations, the death rate was one third that of the death rate for patients on a general medical ward without neurological assistance. However, for patients with atrial fibrillation on a neurology ward there was a three-fold increase in death rate compared with those on a general medical ward.

Several papers demonstrated that cerebral blood flow measures, determined using both PET and Xenon CT scans, are significantly better than CT brain imaging studies for separating patients with stroke syndrome who have critical ischemia of the brain requiring urgent treatment from those with transient ischemic attack who do not require, for example, tissue plasminogen activator therapy.

Endovascular invasive procedures with the implantation of carotid stents for internal carotid stenosis is proving to be safe and effective.

Several studies of spinal cord injury offer hope in a number of fields. Treatment with 4–aminopyridine in a 3–6 month trial significantly improved sensorimotor function in patients with apparently complete spinal cord injury. This indicates not only the therapeutic potential for 4–aminopyride and for 3, 4-diaminopyridine, but also that many such lesions are in fact not complete. Sildenafil (Viagra) proved effective in patients with erectile dysfunction from spinal cord injury.

Epidemiological studies of risk factors for Alzheimer's disease and dementia continue to produce a good deal of important information. At last year's Annual Meeting of the American Academy of Neurology, studies presented demonstrated that hormonal replacement in postmenopausal women and a moderate intake of wine in both sexes can reduce the risk of dementia by two thirds.

This year, a study demonstrates that current smoking increases the risk of developing dementia eight-fold compared with a population of patients who had never smoked. Another study showed that long-term hypertension significantly increases the risk of dementia and the amount of periventricular white matter changes on T2-weighted MRI scans.

A very interesting study from Germany shows that sports scuba divers with a patent foramen ovale are at significant risk of cerebral damage. This study demonstrates by transcranial Doppler that bubbles of air remain in the middle cerebral artery for up to 1 hour, and also shows that the number of white matter lesions on T2-weighted MRIs increase in proportion to the size of the patent foramen ovale.

The field of molecular genetics continues to advance rapidly. A series of papers demonstrates that several, but not all, mutant proteins in the dominantly inherited spinocerebellar ataxias become fixed in the nucleus. The role of the polyglutamine tract expansions and the binding of mutant proteins to nucleosomes and other intranuclear bodies will undoubtedly be of key importance to our understanding of these diseases.

The mental retardation of Duchenne's muscular dystrophy may be explained by the discovery that apo-dystrophin DP140, a partial transcript of the whole dystrophin gene, may play a major role in brain development. Patients with deletions involving domain 3 [exon 45–60] that impair the transcription of DP140 are particularly likely to have mental retardation.

A new gene locus for familial amyotrophic lateral sclerosis was reported, adding to the already known chromosome 21q SOD1 gene mutations and chromosomes 2q and 15q, which are linked to autosomal-recessive loci on familial amyotrophic lateral sclerosis, although the gene product is not known. The new gene reported at the 50th Annual Meeting of the American Academy of Neurology is present on the X chromosome. We await with excitement the investigation of candidate genes.

The phenotypic variability of human prion diseases, from spongiform encephalopathy with myoclonus and dementia (Creutzfeldt-Jakob disease), to cerebellar, motor neuron disease and other variants, may now be understood on the grounds of a polymorphism at codon 129 in the prion gene, and in the size of the protease-resistant fragment of the prion protein that accumulates in brain.

Peripheral nerve disease continues to give rise to a number of new discoveries each year. A further series of cases of pure axonal polyneuropathy responding to intravenous immunoglobulin was presented. It was also demonstrated that chronic inflammatory demyelinating polyneuropathy may be responsible for a major part of the neuropathy in many severe diabetic patients.

The seizure field has quieted somewhat after the flurry of the development of new drugs in the last 3 or 4 years. A study of vagal nerve stimulation showed that this continued to be an effective treatment in about two thirds of cases for at least 3 years.

In the field of migraine, a host of new triptan derivatives appear likely to improve the efficacy/side effect profile currently available with sumatriptan succinate.

In summary, these presentations, as well as the articles reviewed in the body of this volume of the *Year Book of Neurology and Neurosurgery*, continue to demonstrate the fact that the 1990s truly are the decade of the brain. Because it looks as if this rate of progress in understanding the brain and, eventually, mind function, will continue to increase exponentially in the coming decades, perhaps we should look to the year 2000 for declaration of the millennium of the brain and mind.

Walter G. Bradley, D.M., F.R.C.P.

1 Cerebral Vascular Disease

Genetics of Stroke
Carter ND (St George's Hosp, London)
J Hum Hypertens 11:553–554, 1997   1–1

Introduction.—The clinical phenotype of stroke is complicated. It can be broadly divided into infarct and hemorrhage. Previous and future stroke research is described.

Background.—Current research strategies focus on infarct-related ischemic stroke because this is the cause of 80% of strokes. Several trials have reported that stroke is a polygenic condition. Genes have been identified in a series of mendelian stroke phenotypes (Table 1). Identified genes provide pathophysiologic phenotypes and linkage information, which may provide clues to candidates for polygenic stroke. Rat models of stroke have yielded useful paradigms for the human trait. Recent trials have contributed to the ability to identify candidate genes for susceptibility or severity of ischemic stroke. These trials have identified quantitative trait loci for susceptibility to stroke. One trial identified 3 loci by genome scanning; 1 mapped to the atrial natriuretic peptides (ANP) locus. Another trial independently detected the ANP locus as a linked marker to ischemic stroke.

Future Strategies for Mapping Polygenic Stroke.—Two approaches are used for mapping polygenic stroke: association trials with polymorphisms in identified candidate genes and a positional cloning strategy. Loci for association investigations include fibrinogen, plasminogen activator inhibitor-1, factor VII, von Willebrand factor, and platelet IIb/IIa receptor. These trials necessitate accurate phenotype and genetic evaluation and comparison of polymorphism frequency with age-matched controls without stroke. The strategy for a genome-based search uses allele sharing by sib pairs or other close relatives. Polymorphic microsatellite markers can be scanned over the genome to show linkage. About 3,000 polymorphic markers are required to perform a systematic search by gene scanning.

Conclusion.—Scanning for stroke-prone mutations is now possible with advances in the genome mapping program. Treatment protocols may be

TABLE 1.—Examples of Human Mendelian Traits Associated With Stroke

Disease	Type of stroke	Gene/chromosome location
CADASIL	Ischaemic	19q12
Mitochondrial encephalopathy, lactic acidosis and stroke-like episodes (Melas)	Ischaemic	Mitochondrial tRNA-leu
Hereditary haemorrhagic telangiectasia-1	Intracerebral haemorrhage	Endoglin
Hereditary haemorrhagic telangiectasia-2	Intracerebral haemorrhage	Activin receptor-like kinase 1
Hereditary cerebral haemorrhage with amyloidosis-Dutch type	Intracerebral haemorrhage	Amyloid precursor protein
Hereditary cerebral haemorrhage with amyloidosis-Icelandic type	Intracerebral haemorrhage	Cystatin C
Ehlers-Danlos type IV	Subarachnoid haemorrhage	Collagen 3A1
Polycystic kidney disease	Subarachnoid haemorrhage	Polycystin
Marfan syndrome	Subarachnoid haemorrhage	Fibrillin

(Courtesy of Carter ND: Genetics of stroke. *J Hum Hypertens* 11:553–554, 1997.)

based on molecular processes associated with individual genes or groups of genes in patients susceptible to stroke.

▶ This overview, although quite brief, is useful for its table, which summarizes examples of human mendelian traits associated with stroke, and for its general perspective. With advances in molecular genetics now coming at an accelerating pace, our means of screening patients at risk of stroke for potentially injurious gene products emerges as an intriguing possibility in the not-so-distant future.

M.D. Ginsberg, M.D.

Knowledge of Risk Among Patients at Increased Risk for Stroke
Samsa GP, Cohen SJ, Goldstein LB, et al (Duke Univ, Durham, NC; Bowman Gray School of Medicine, Winston-Salem, NC; Research Triangle Inst, Research Triangle Park; et al)
Stroke 28:916–921, 1997 1–2

Background.—When patients recognize that they have an increased risk for a stroke, they are more likely to engage in and comply with stroke prevention methods. The perceived risk of having a stroke in a diverse group of patients at increased risk was studied.

Methods.—The study population included 621 patients from the Academic Medical Center Consortium, 321 from the Cardiovascular Health Study, and 319 from United HealthCare plans. Awareness of stroke risk was the primary outcome.

Findings.—Only 41% of the patients were aware of their increased stroke risk, including less than half of those who had previously had minor strokes. About 74% of patients who recalled a physician informing them of their increased stroke risk were aware of this risk compared with 28% of those who did not recall a physician informing them of this risk. Those most likely to be aware of their stroke risk were younger, depressed, in poor current health, or with a history of transient ischemic attacks.

Conclusions.—Less than half of patients at increased risk for strokes are aware of this risk. Health care providers play an important role in educating patients about an increased risk for strokes. Information should be targeted toward patients least likely to be aware of their risk.

▶ Because awareness of an increased stroke risk makes it more likely that patients at risk will adopt preventive measures, the findings fo this study should give physicians and others who care for patients with strokes considerable pause. The authors cite 2 possible explanations for the fact that relatively few patients are aware of their increased stroke risk: (1) inadequate transmission of information by providers and (2) suboptimal retention or disbelief of this information by patients. These results stress the importance of effective communication about risk and stroke prevention by physicians and health care providers. This factor appears, on the basis of this and other studies, to be the rate-limiting step in making patients aware of their increased risk—a necessary first step in stroke prevention. This important article deserves widespread attention.

M.D. Ginsberg, M.D.

Stroke Patients' Knowledge of Stroke: Influence on Time to Presentation

Williams LS, Bruno A, Rouch D, et al (Indiana Univ, Indianapolis; Regenstrief Inst for Health Care, Indianapolis, Ind)
Stroke 28:912–915, 1997   1–3

Background.—To be effective, new treatments for acute strokes will probably need to be given shortly after the onset of the stroke. Little information is available on patients' general knowledge about their strokes, their interpretation of stroke symptoms, and how these factors affect the timing of their decision to seek medical care.

Methods.—Sixty-seven consecutive patients with strokes were interviewed within 72 hours of stroke onset. Ninety-six percent of the patients had ischemic strokes, and 4% had cerebral hemorrhages. Early arrival was defined as being within 3 hours of the patients' awareness of symptoms.

Findings.—Thirty-eight percent of the patients said they knew the warning signs of a stroke, but only 25% interpreted their symptoms correctly. Those who had previously had strokes were more likely to interpret their symptoms correctly but were not more likely to seek medical attention early. Eighty-six percent of the patients arriving more than 3 hours after the onset of the stroke believed that their symptoms were not serious. Patients arriving early were more likely to arrive by ambulance and to have more severe strokes than those arriving late. Arrival by ambulance and early arrival were independently correlated.

Conclusions.—About one fourth of patients experiencing strokes correctly interpreted their symptoms. However, in the current series, this knowledge was not associated with early arrival in the emergency department. Widespread education of individuals prone to strokes may increase the proportion of patients eligible for new acute stroke treatments.

▶ This important article deals with the theme closely related to that of Abstract 1–2, which shows that less than half of patients at increased risk for strokes are aware of this risk. In the current study of the patients interviewed within 72 hours of the onset of their strokes, only one quarter of patients correctly interpreted their symptoms as being caused by a stroke. Furthemore, there was a relationship between regarding one's symptoms as "not serious" and delaying one's arrival at a hospital after the stroke onset. Clearly, if patients with acute ischemic strokes are to benefit from such measures as the very early institution of thrombolytic therapy, it is essential that they correctly interpret their symptoms and regard them as serious. This study underscores the vital urgency of educating the population with regard to the seriousness of a stroke and the proper procedures to be followed in the event that stroke-like symptoms occur.

M.D. Ginsberg, M.D.

Time Course of the Apparent Diffusion Coefficient (ADC) Abnormality in Human Stroke

Schlaug G, Siewert B, Benfield A, et al (Beth Israel Deaconess Med Ctr, Boston; Harvard Med School, Boston)
Neurology 49:113–119, 1997

1–4

Background.—Within minutes of the onset of ischemia, diffusion-weighted MRI detects a decline in the apparent diffusion coefficient (ADC) of water in affected brain tissues. Levels of ADC eventually rebound, probably because of the loss of cell membrane integrity (which allows more movement of water molecules) and tissue death. However, the exact time course of these changes in ADC levels is unknown. These authors examined the temporal evolution of changes in ADC levels in patients with stroke.

Methods.—Acute cerebral ischemia occurred in 101 patients who underwent 157 diffusion MRI studies to characterize the region of abnormal

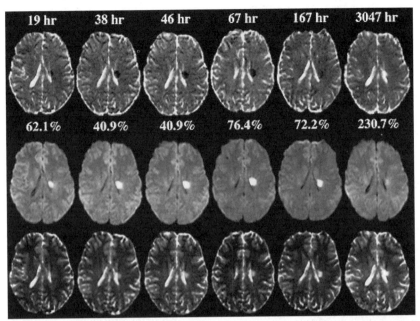

FIGURE 2.—T2-weighted images (**lower row**), diffusion-weighted MR images (**middle row**), and apparent diffusion coefficient (ADC) maps (**upper row**) with relative ADC (rADC) values in percent at several time points after the acute onset of a neurologic deficit in a 22-year-old woman, showing progression of the ischemic lesion. Note that the rADC is decreased up to the fifth time point (168 hours after stroke). Only the last MR scan at 3,047 hours showed an elevated rADC. (Reprinted from Neurology, courtesy of Schlaug G, Siewert B, Benfield A, et al. Time course of the apparent diffusion coefficient (ADC) abnormality in human stroke. *Neurology* 49:113–119, 1997, copyright American Academy of Neurology. Used with permission of Lippincott-Raven Publishers.)

diffusion. A prototype whole-body 1.5-Tesla echo planar imaging system was used in 89 MRI studies (resulting in 7 b values from 0 to 1,271 sec/mm^2), and a Siemens Vision 1.5-Tesla echo planar imaging system was used in 69 MRI studies (2 b values, 0 and 1,000 sec/mm^2). The maximum gradient amplitude was set at 35 mT/m, with 250-μsec rise times.

Findings.—Compared with the contralateral normal brain tissue, diffusion-weighted MRIs showed hyperintense areas and reduced ADC levels. The ADC values derived from either echo planar imaging system did not differ significantly. Data were expressed as the relative ADC (rADC), the ratio of lesion to control regions of interest. There was a significant effect of time on rADC values, with measurements at less than 3, 4–7, 7–12, 13–24, 25–48, and 49–96 hours averaging 0.581, 0.495, 0.465, 0.516, 0.528, and 0.638 × 10^{-3} mm^2/sec, respectively (average rADC, 58%). The rADC values up to 96 hours after stroke and more than 30 days after stroke (average, 1.472 10^{-3} mm^2/sec) differed significantly; all patients experienced a reduction in rADC levels of at least 11% in the first 24 hours and a variable but significant increase in the late subacute to chronic time points (Fig 2).

Conclusion.—The ADC levels are significantly reduced up to 96 hours after a stroke, and they increase significantly in the late subacute to chronic phases. Evaluating these changes can help clinicians in determining the time of the ischemic attack, and, thus, in managing the clinical course.

▶ Although diffusion-weighted MR has been used in a number of different clinical situations, its main use is in the evaluation of brain ischemia. In this condition, diffusion imaging can identify very early alterations in water movement when conventional spin echo MR gives normal results, and it can distinguish late (chronic) from early (acute) ischemic changes. This latter situation is important to confirming the presence of hyperacute parenchymal changes so that a patient may be triaged into a brain attack treatment protocol. In addition, this sequence is important in patients who have a history of multiple infarcts because it is often unclear clinically and radiologically as to what is new and what is old disease.

The article by Schlaug et al. contains information that allows the separation of these by virtue of differences in ADC values. While perfusion MR imaging is increasingly being evaluated to determine brain tissue at risk in stroke patients, diffusion weighted MR can, at present, be enabled on many scanners and is recommended as part of MR protocols used to assess patients with possible cerebrovascular accidents.

R.M. Quencer, M.D.

Assessment of Cerebral Perfusion and Arterial Anatomy in Hyperacute Stroke With Three-dimensional Functional CT: Early Clinical Results
Hunter GJ, Hamberg LM, Ponzo JA, et al (Harvard Med School, Boston)
AJNR 19:29–37, 1998   1–5

Introduction.—Most patients with symptoms indicative of cerebral ischemia or infarction undergo CT to exclude hemorrhage. A simple technique for rapid identification of diminished parenchymal perfusion and major-vessel compromise might enhance the rate of success of aggressive therapy. Helical CT is available in many hospitals and may be helpful in measuring intracranial vascular pathophysiology at a high spatial and temporal resolution. Quantitative 3-dimensional functional CT was evaluated to determine its feasibility in patients with hyperacute stroke.

Methods.—Of 22 patients who underwent clinically indicated CT angiography, 9 had no history of stroke or cerebral ischemia, 8 had known stroke, and 5 had hyperacute stroke. Patients with no history of stroke were assessed to obtain normal values for perfused cerebral blood volume (PBV). Patients with known disease were evaluated for the presence of major-vessel occlusion. Standard techniques were used to obtain maps of PBV and CT angiograms.

Results.—In the 9 patients with no history of stroke, the hematocrit corrected values for percent PBV were 4.6% in the gray matter, 1.75% in the white matter, 3.18% in the caudate, 2.84% in the putamen, 2.92% in the thalamus, 2.91% in the cerebellum, and 1.66% in the brain stem. In patients with mature stroke, the ischemic changes were observed on non-contrast, contrast-enhanced, and PBV scans. Before contrast administration, ischemic changes were either absent or subtle in patients with hyperacute stroke. These changes became apparent on contrast-enhanced scans. Quantitative PBV maps confirmed diminished regional perfusion. The CT angiograms in patients with hyperacute stroke indicated occlusion of vessels in locations appropriate to the PBV deficits observed.

Conclusion.—Quantitative 3-dimensional functional CT is possible in patients with hyperacute stroke. Most patients with stroke currently undergo CT to exclude hemorrhage. The addition of a helical scan during contrast infusion causes a delay of only a few minutes and produces PBV and CT angiographic data. Combined CT angiography and PBV allows simultaneous assessment of collateralization and the actual volume of brain parenchyma remaining at risk from an ischemic event.

▶ The quest for a fast and accurate means of determining the location and size of salvageable brain in the setting of an acute stroke is critical. Although advocates of MR diffusion/perfusion imaging in this setting point to the sensitivity of that technique, the frequently encountered logistical difficulties and the general paucity of MR scanners in emergency rooms speak strongly for another means of assessing the status of the brain parenchyma after an ischemic event. This article describes the use of helical CT before and after bolus contrast injection in which CT angiograms and cerebral blood volumes were obtained—the latter, in effect, giving an indication of the amount of prefused brain, the former showing sites of major vascular occlusion.

These are important pieces of information during the window of opportunity (3–4 hours) when thrombolytic therapy is being considered. This technique, although not fully refined for determining actual salvageable brain, bears consideration in patients seen with a nonhemorrhagic acute or hyperacute stroke.

R.M. Quencer, M.D.

Silent Brain Infarction on Magnetic Resonance Imaging and Neurological Abnormalities in Community-dwelling Older Adults: The Cardiovascular Health Study
Price TR, for the CHS Collaborative Research Group (Univ of Maryland, Baltimore)
Stroke 28:1158–1164, 1997   1–6

Introduction.—Lesions with an appearance typical of infarction are sometimes found incidentally at MRI. When such findings are present in older individuals without a clinical history of stroke, they are termed "silent infarcts." Participants in the Cardiovascular Health Study (CHS) underwent MRI to assess the prevalence of infarcts and the association of these lesions with demographic, cognitive, and neurologic status.

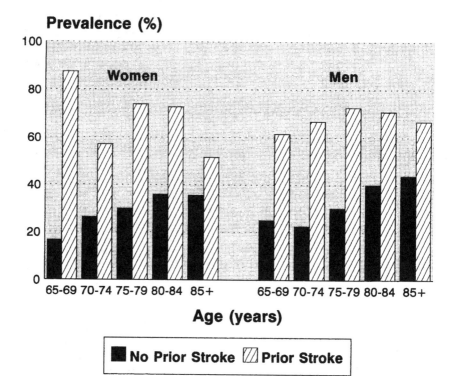

FIGURE 1.—Prevalence of MRI infarct by sex, age, and prior stroke. Association with age was significant at P less than 0.0001 in men and women without prior stroke; sex association was not significant in those without prevalent stroke (P less than 0.1). Neither sex nor age associations were significant in those with prior stroke. (Courtesy of Price TR, for the CHS Collaborative Research Group: Silent brain infarction on magnetic resonance imaging and neurological abnormalities in community-dwelling older adults: The Cardiovascular Health Study. *Stroke* 28:1158–1164. Reproduced with permission of *Stroke.* Copyright 1997, American Heart Association.)

Methods.—The CHS is a population-based observational study of 5,888 men and women aged 65 years and older from 4 communities in the United States. Three years after entry, 3,600 participants underwent cranial MRI according to a standard protocol. A short history and neurologic examination were also undertaken at this time.

Results.—Information on infarcts was obtained from 3,647 men and women. One or more MRI infarcts (lesions 3 mm or greater) were detected in 1,131 (31%) in this group. Infarcts were detected in significantly more of the 250 participants with previous, clinically recognized stroke (68%) than in those without a history of stroke (28%). There was an association between MRI infarcts and increasing age (Fig 1) among those without previous stroke. In this subgroup, silent MRI infarcts were also strongly associated with a history of migraines, lower digit symbol scores, and more abnormalities on neurologic examination. Multivariate analysis of all participants with MRI results showed that age, previous stroke, migraine history, digit symbol score, and number of neurologic abnormalities were independently associated with the presence of MRI infarcts.

Discussion.—The strong association between these MRI infarcts and abnormal neurologic and cognitive findings suggests that the lesions are not silent nor without consequences. With the high prevalence of these lesions (28%) in older men and women, population-based scanning may be of value in the investigation of cerebrovascular disease risk factors.

▶ This large population-based observational study, part of the Cardiovascular Health Study, involved MRI scanning in over 3,600 patients drawn from a population of approximately 5,800 overall participants. Despite the fact that this study population was younger and less likely to have smoked or to have had prior cardiovascular disease or hypertension than those who did not undergo scanning, 1 or more infarcts was detected in almost one third of these participants. The prevalence of MRI infarct increased with age in those patients without a prior stroke history.

The significance of these observations is that, despite the "stroke-free" clinical history, these infarcts were strongly associated with neurologic abnormalities and impaired cognitive function. This study substantiates the value of population-based MRI scanning in investigating patients at risk of cerebrovascular disease.

M.D. Ginsberg, M.D.

Predictors of Stroke Risk in Coronary Artery Bypass Patients
McKhann GM, Goldsborough MA, Borowicz LM Jr, et al (Johns Hopkins Univ, Baltimore, Md)
Ann Thorac Surg 63:516–521, 1997   1–7

Purpose.—The incidence of stroke after coronary artery bypass grafting (CABG) ranges from 0.8% to 5.2%. Previous studies have identified certain risk factors for post-CABG stroke, but these have never been combined in a predictive model. Potential predictive factors for stroke risk after CABG were analyzed.

Methods.—Factors associated with stroke were prospectively assessed in a study cohort of 456 patients undergoing initial or repeated CABG. The occurrence of postoperative stroke was assessed by the researchers, with confirmation by neurologic consultation and CT imaging. Preoperative and intraoperative factors potentially related to stroke risk were identified by means of multiple logistic regression analysis. Subsequently, the predictive factors identified were assessed in an independent validation sample of 1,298 patients.

Results.—In the logistic regression model, factors correlated with stroke were previous stroke, presence of carotid bruit, history of hypertension, older age, and history of diabetes mellitus. Just one intraoperative factor was significant: cardiopulmonary bypass time. A model was constructed to identify patients at low, medium, and high risk for stroke. With this model, most stroke patients in the validation group were correctly placed in the high-risk group. The model predicted significantly more strokes than actually occurred, however.

Conclusions.—This study identifies 5 risk factors for stroke after CABG. Distinguishing patients at high risk will promote the use of surgical modifications or pharmacologic interventions to prevent stroke, as well as enhance studies of the mechanism of stroke. The strategy used to develop the predictive model in this study might be applied to other cardiac surgical procedures as well.

▶ This is an impressively thorough study of a large patient cohort undergoing CABG. Although the risk factors identified here (previous stroke, carotid bruit, hypertension, advancing age, diabetes mellitus, and cardiopulmonary bypass time) are not surprising, the high degree of statistical significance attached to several of these factors (in particular, previous stroke, hypertension, and time on bypass) drive home the point that these factors must be taken into account in patient management. The authors suggest that high-risk patients be targeted for carotid duplex scanning and epicardial echocardiography, that consideration be given to modified surgical management; and that, in the future, pharmacologic neuroprotective strategies be considered. These are all wise recommendations.

M.D. Ginsberg, M.D.

Echocardiographic Identification of Cardiovascular Sources of Emboli to Guide Clinical Management of Stroke: A Cost-effectiveness Analysis
McNamara RL, Lima JAC, Whelton PK, et al (Johns Hopkins Univ, Baltimore, Md; Tulane Univ, New Orleans, La)
Ann Intern Med 127:775–787, 1997   1–8

Background.—There is no consensus on the use of imaging strategies to identify potential cardiovascular sources of emboli in stroke victims. The cost-effectiveness of various cardiac imaging strategies after stroke was determined.

Methods.—A Markov model decision analysis was used to determine the costs and benefits of 9 diagnostic strategies. Hypothetical patients with a first stroke and in normal sinus rhythm were included in the model.

Findings.—When visualized left atrial thrombus was used as the only indication for anticoagulation, transesophageal echocardiography done only in patients with a history of cardiac problems cost $9,000 per quality-adjusted life-year. Transesophageal echocardiography in all patients cost $13,000 per quality-adjusted life-year. Examination costs and risks of anticoagulation were markedly offset by the cost savings and reduced morbidity and mortality associated with the decrease in preventable recurrent strokes. The efficacy of anticoagulation and incidence of intracranial bleeding during anticoagulation had a moderate effect on these results. The prevalence of left atrial thrombus, rate of recurrent stroke in patients with thrombus, quality of life after stroke, cost of transesophageal echo-cardiography, and specificity of transesophageal echocardiography had a mild effect. Compared with transesophageal echocardiography, transthoracic echocardiography alone or with transesophageal echocardiography was not cost-effective.

Conclusions.—Although the initial cost is higher, transesophageal echocardiography was cost-effective when compared with other commonly used diagnostic and therapeutic techniques in patients with new-onset stroke in normal sinus rhythm. Cardiac history may be useful in determining which patients should have transesophageal echocardiography.

▶ This cost-effectiveness analysis using simulated clinical practice data in the United States reveals, not surprisingly, that transesophageal echocardiography is favorably cost-effective whereas transthoracic echocardiography, although widely used, is not. The authors reason that whereas transesophageal echo is very sensitive and rather specific for identifying left atrial thrombi, many of these thrombi in the left atrial appendage are missed on transthoracic studies.

M.D. Ginsberg, M.D.

Mobile Aortic Atheroma and Systemic Emboli: Efficacy of Anticoagulation and Influence of Plaque Morphology on Recurrent Stroke
Dressler FA, Craig WR, Castello R, et al (Saint Louis Univ)
J Am Coll Cardiol 31:134–138, 1998   1–9

Introduction.—Several reports have described the epidemiologic correlation between atheroma and systemic emboli as an index and recurrent event. Few trials have described appropriate anticoagulant choices. The influence of morphologic plaque features and antithrombotic therapy on the risk of recurrent emboli in patients with mobile aortic atheroma was examined.

Methods.—Of 1,390 patients who underwent transesophageal echocardiography (TEE) for systemic emboli since 1987, 31 had both immobile and mobile aortic atheroma. The height, width, and area of immobile and mobile portions of atheroma were quantitated in short- and long-axis views (Fig 2). The dimensions of the mobile component were used to determine three groups: small, intermediate, and large mobile atheroma. Telephone interviews and patient records were used to determine anticoagulant use and recurrent embolic or vascular events.

Results.—There was a significantly higher incidence of vascular events in patients who did not take warfarin than in those who did take it (45% vs. 5%). The incidence of stroke was 0% and 27%, respectively, in patients who did and did not take warfarin. In patients not taking warfarin, the annual incidence of stroke was 0.32. Eighteen percent of patients who did not take warfarin had myocardial infarction. Together, the risk of myocardial infarction and stroke was significantly higher in patients who

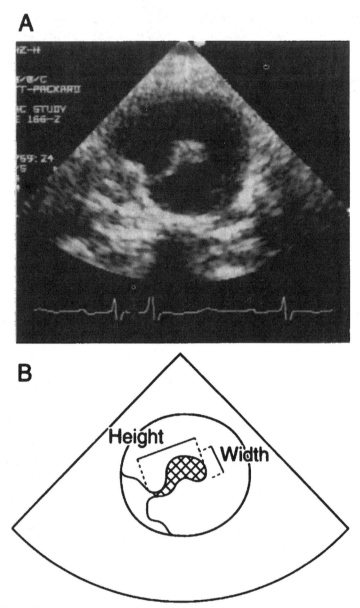

FIGURE 2.—TEE short-axis image (**A**) and schematic (**B**) demonstrating quantitation of mobile components of atheroma (*cross-hatched area*). (Courtesy of Dressler FA, Craig WR, Castello R: Mobile aortic atheroma and systemic emboli: Efficacy of anticoagulation and influence of plaque morphology on recurrent stroke. *J Am Coll Cardiol* 31:134–138, 1998. Reprinted with permission from the American College of Cardiology (Journal of the American College of Cardiology.))

took warfarin than in those who did not take it. In this cohort of 31 patients, 47% with small mobile atheroma did not receive warfarin. Thirty-eight percent of these patients had recurrent stroke, representing an annual incidence of 0.61, compared with 0% of patients treated with warfarin. No patients with intermediate or large mobile atheroma had a stroke during follow-up. Of these, only 3 were not taking warfarin.

Conclusion.—Patients with systemic emboli and mobile aortic atheroma had a high rate of recurrent vascular events. These patients should receive warfarin therapy. Need for anticoagulation should not be based on the dimensions of the mobile component of atheroma.

▶ The provocative observation that patients with mobile aortic atheromatous plaques and systemic emboli treated with warfarin have a much reduced incidence of recurrent stroke compared with untreated patients is of obvious interest, but it must be pointed out that this was a small study that was not controlled or randomized. Study patients were selected from almost 1,400 patients undergoing transesophageal echocardiography for systemic emboli, of whom 108 had high-risk aortic plaque, including 31 with mobile plaque. The study group was therefore small (31 subjects) and highly selected. In addition, there was no randomization for risk criteria. The choice of anticoagulant therapy was up to the referring physician, so the possibility of selection bias is high. Nonetheless, these data make it prudent to consider the use of warfarin in patients with evidence of embolism and mobile aortic atheromata, pending a more definitive study.

M.D. Ginsberg, M.D.

Intracranial Microembolic Signals in 500 Patients With Potential Cardiac or Carotid Embolic Source and in Normal Controls
Georgiadis D, Lindner A, Manz M, et al (Univ of Halle, Germany; Univ of Münster, Germany)
Stroke 28:1203–1207, 1997   1–10

Introduction.—The use of transcranial Doppler sonography to detect intracranial microembolic signals (MES) has been reported in several groups of patients prone to strokes. Four hundred patients with potential cardiac or carotid embolic source of stroke and 100 normal controls were monitored with transcranial Doppler sonography to evaluate the prevalence of MES, the relationship of MES to clinical parameters, and the value of MES in identifying patients with potential embolic sources.

Methods.—The study group included 300 patients with potential cardiac source (11.3% symptomatic) and 100 with potential embolic source (46% symptomatic). Eighty-nine patients with potential cardiac source had prosthetic cardiac valves and 211 had a variety of native cardioembolic lesions. The remaining 100 patients had occlusive carotid disease. Patients with a potential native cardioembolic source had transthoracic and/or transesophageal echocardiography and carotid studies; those with a potential carotid embolic source underwent continuous-wave Doppler, color-coded duplex, or intra-arterial angiography.

Results.—Patients with potential native cardioembolic source had an overall MES prevalence of 23%. The prevalence of MES ranged from 15% in the subgroup of 80 patients with valvular disease to 43% in the 70 patients with infective endocarditis. Among patients with prosthetic cardiac valves, the prevalence of MES was 55% overall; it included 58% of those with mechanical valves, 43% with porcine valves, and 20% with homografts. Few asymptomatic patients with carotid disease had MES, but the finding was common in those who were symptomatic (7% vs. 52%; 28% overall). Normal controls had an MES prevalence of 5%. There appeared to be no relationship between MES counts and patient age, sex, or medication. The specificity of MES detection in identifying patients with potential cardiac or carotid embolic sources was 95%; sensitivity was 31.3%.

Discussion.—The prevalence of MES was far higher in stroke-prone patients than in normal controls, and was highest among patients with symptomatic carotid disease and in those with prosthetic cardiac valves. Although the detection of MES had a high specificity in the identification of patients with potential embolic sources, sensitivity was low, perhaps because of a short monitoring duration, use of antihemostatic treatment, or delay in examination after the onset of neurologic symptoms.

▶ In this large series of patients monitored for MES by transcranial Doppler examination of the middle cerebral arteries, despite the fact that these patients were uncommonly examined immediately after the onset of their symptoms and that many patients were receiving antithrombotic therapy, there was, nonetheless, a high prevalence of signals observed. The prevalence was sixfold higher than in healthy subjects. Not unexpectedly, the prevalence was highest in patients with prosthetic cardiac valves and in patients with symptomatic carotid disease. Studies are needed to assess the prognostic import of these observations in terms of subsequent symptomatic embolic events.

M.D. Ginsberg, M.D.

Cerebral Microembolism in Patients With Stroke or Transient Ischaemic Attack as a Risk Factor for Early Recurrence
Valton L, Larrue V, Le Traon AP, et al (Hôpital de Rangueil, France)
J Neurol Neurosurg Psychiatry 63:784–787, 1997   1–11

Introduction.—Transcranial Doppler (TCD) can detect asymptomatic microembolic signals in patients with carotid stenosis or aortic arch atheroma. Microembolism has been related to the degree of carotid narrowing and the ulcerated appearance of the plaque in patients with carotid stenosis. The prognostic relevance of these findings is not known. The risk of early ischemic recurrence was estimated in patients with cerebral ischemia of presumed arterial origin in whom TCD monitoring showed microembolic signals.

Methods.—Thirty-two patients being treated after transient ischemic attack or stroke in the anterior circulation underwent TCD monitoring of the middle cerebral artery within 7 days of symptom onset. Monitorings were recorded on digital audiotapes and analyzed by two independent observers who were blinded to clinical data.

Results.—Six of 32 patients had microembolic signals. Five of these patients (83%) and 13 without microembolic signals (50%) had at least one potential arterial source of embolism (a nonsignificant difference). Four patients experienced early recurrence during a mean follow-up of 15 days after the initial event. Early recurrences occurred in the same arterial territory as the initial ischemic event in all 4 patients. Three of the 4 patients with early recurrence had antecedent microembolic signals. The incidence of early recurrence was 50% (3/6) and 3.8% (1/26), respectively, in patients with and without microembolic signals.

Conclusion.—A single 20-minute TCD recording of the middle cerebral artery in patients with cerebral ischemia of presumed arterial origin allowed recognition of a subset of patients with cerebral ischemia who were at high risk of early recurrence.

▶ Although this report is based on a relatively small number of patients, its results show a striking difference in stroke recurrence (50% vs. 4%) in patients with vs. those without microembolic signals on TCD monitoring of the symptomatic middle cerebral artery. If these findings are supported by a larger study, the use of TCD monitoring may come to play an important role in tailoring therapeutic approaches for prevention of secondary stroke.

M.D. Ginsberg, M.D.

Cerebral Microembolic Signals During Cardiopulmonary Bypass Surgery: Frequency, Time of Occurrence, and Association With Patient and Surgical Characteristics
Brækken SK, Russell D, Brucher R, et al (Univ of Oslo, Norway)
Stroke 28:1988–1992, 1997   1–12

Background.—Recent research has reported a positive association between the number of intraoperative cerebral microembolic signals (MES) detected by transcranial Doppler and postoperative neuropsychologic and neurologic outcomes. This suggests that the number of cerebral microemboli entering the brain during open heart surgery should be decreased. The occurrence and frequency of cerebral MES during coronary artery bypass grafting (CABG) and cardiac valve replacement (VR)—the most common types of cardiopulmonary bypass surgery—were studied. The relationship of MES with the various surgical stages and procedures and patient characteristics was determined also.

Methods.—Fifteen patients undergoing CABG and 27 undergoing VR were studied. Transcranial Doppler monitoring of the right middle cerebral artery was used to detect cerebral MES.

Findings.—All patients were found to have cerebral MES. The median number was 1048 during VR and 82 during CABG—a significant difference. In the patients undergoing VR, 85% of the MES were evident when the effective ejection was regained in the heart. In patients undergoing CABG, the greatest number was detected when the aorta was cross-clamped (18%) and when the side clamp was released (13%). The 2 groups did not differ significantly in the numbers of MES when the aorta was cross-clamped or in association with surgical procedures. The total number of MES was associated inversely with nasopharyngeal temperature.

Conclusions.—Significantly more cerebral MES were detected during VR than during CABG in the current series. Transcranial Doppler monitoring can alert the surgeon to the entrance of emboli into the cerebral circulation during CPB surgery, permitting the surgeon to take preventive measures.

▶ This interesting report further characterizes the nature of cerebral MES in patients undergoing cardiopulmonary bypass surgery. The finding of major interest is that these signals are substantially more common during valve replacement than during CABG surgery. The importance of this report, additionally, is in defining which components of these operations constitute the greatest risk: during valve replacement, the resumption of effective heart ejection; and during CABG, aortic cross-clamping. Each of these observations makes intuitive sense. This type of information should be useful in designing prophylactic strategies.

M.D. Ginsberg, M.D.

Microemboli in Patients With Vertebrobasilar Ischemia: Association With Vertebrobasilar and Cardiac Lesions
Koennecke HC, Mast H, Trocio SS Jr, et al (Columbia-Presbyterian Med Ctr, New York; Freie Universität Berlin)
Stroke 28:593–596, 1997   1–13

Background.—Previous studies using transcranial Doppler ultrasound (TCD) have demonstrated microembolic, asymptomatic high-intensity transient signals (HITS) in patients with carotid stenosis, artificial heart valves, and other cardiac conditions. However, even though about one-fourth of brain infarcts occur in the vertebrobasilar territory, only 1 case of stroke-related HITS in the posterior cerebral circulation has been reported. There have been no other studies of TCD microembolic signals in patients with posterior circulation stroke. The prevalence of asymptomatic microemboli in patients with vertebrobasilar ischemia was prospectively studied.

Methods.—The study included 52 consecutive patients with acute or recent vertebrobasilar ischemia. All were studied within 48 hours after admission, with 20-minute TCD monitoring of each posterior cerebral artery. Patients with fetal origin of the posterior cerebral artery were excluded; this finding was ruled out by carotid compression. In addition to determining the prevalence of HITS in this group of patients, the study evaluated factors potentially associated with their detection, including cardioembolic sources, vertebral or basilar occlusive disease, and infarct subtypes.

Results.—Nineteen percent of patients had detectable microembolic HITS, bilateral in 4 of 10 cases. Microemboli were detected at a mean rate of 5 per 20 minutes in HITS-positive vessels. The presence of potential cardiac sources was an independent risk factor for the detection of microembolic signals included (odds ratio [OR] 14.3). This association was particularly strong when more than 1 cardiac abnormality was present (OR 32.7) or when the patient had more than 1 high-risk source (OR 14.0). The finding of microemboli was unrelated to vertebrobasilar vessel lesions or infarct subtype.

Conclusions.—In patients with ischemia of the posterior cerebral circulation, cardiac sources of embolism are a significant risk factor for TCD detection of HITS. The risk of microembolic signals is particularly high for patients with multiple cardiac abnormalities or with cardiac findings associated with a high risk for embolism. The results suggest that cardioembolic infarcts in the posterior circulation may be more common than is generally suspected. Microemboli are less likely to become lodged in vertebrobasilar vessel abnormalities, suggesting a different set of histopathologic changes from those seen in carotid artery disease.

▶ In this studied group of 52 consecutive patients with recent vertebrobasilar ischemia, over half were studies within 2 days of symptom onset. This study establishes the important point that the HIT signals detected by transcranial Doppler were more prevalent in patients with potential cardiac embolic sources and that they were not related to the degree of vascular occlusive disease itself. This study thus reminds the clinician of the potential importance of cardioembolic events in patients with posterior circulation ischemia.

M.D. Ginsberg, M.D.

Generalized Efficacy of t-PA for Acute Stroke: Subgroup Analysis of the NINDS t-PA Stroke Trial
Brott T, for the NINDs t-PA Stroke Study Group (Univ of Cincinnati, Ohio)
Stroke 28:2119–2125, 1997   1–14

Background.—Identifying subgroups of stroke victims with an increased likelihood to benefit from or be harmed by tissue plasminogen activator (t-PA) would be useful. Final outcomes in t-PA- and in placebo-treated patients were analyzed to identify such subgroups.

Methods.—A post hoc subgroup analysis was performed of data from a randomized, double-blind, placebo-controlled clinical study of t-PA. All patients were seen within 3 hours of symptom onset. Historical, physical, and laboratory data were recorded before treatment.

Findings.—None of the pretreatment information was related to patients' response to t-PA. Outcomes were associated with t-PA treatment, age-by-deficit severity interaction, diabetes, age-by-blood pressure interaction, and early CT findings. These variables and interactions changed long-term outcomes regardless of t-PA therapy but did not change the likelihood of a favorable response to t-PA.

Conclusions.—Published guidelines should be used to select patients for t-PA thrombolysis. Selection by variables such as age or stroke severity is not supported by the current findings.

▶ The National Institute of Neurologic Disorders and Stroke (NINDS) t-PA stroke trial showed that thrombolysis carried out within 3 hours of the onset of acute ischemic stroke is efficacious in improving outcome. The authors have now conducted a post hoc analysis to attempt to identify stroke subgroups exhibiting particularly beneficial or hazardous responses to t-PA. No such subgroups could be identified. In particular, there was no statistical interaction of t-PA treatment with historical variables such as hypertension, atrial fibrillation, cardiac disease, prior stroke, thrombus on early CT, or admission blood pressure. The message to practicing clinicians is therefore clear: that it is unwarranted to assume differential responsivity of individual patients to t-PA based on any of these characteristics. Rather, the guidelines set forth in the NINDS study are sufficient, of themselves, to guide therapy.

M.D. Ginsberg, M.D.

PROACT: A Phase II Randomized Trial of Recombinant Pro-urokinase by Direct Arterial Delivery in Acute Middle Cerebral Artery Stroke
del Zoppo GJ, and the PROACT Investigators (Scripps Clinic and Research Found, La Jolla, Calif; Univ of California, San Francisco; Cleveland Clinic Found, Ohio; et al)
Stroke 29:4–11, 1998   1–15

Introduction.—Interest in recanalization of recently occluded mainstem cerebral arteries by plasminogen activators in the early moments of acute stroke has been rekindled because of the possibility that recanalization may enhance efficient neurologic recovery. The safety and recanalization efficacy of intra-arterial local delivery of plasminogen activators in acute ischemic stroke were assessed in a randomized trial of recombinant pro-urokinase (rpor-UK) vs. placebo in patients with angiographically-documented proximal middle cerebral artery occlusion.

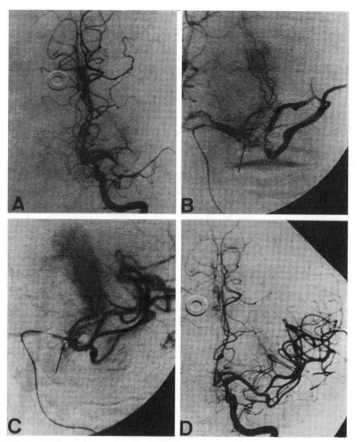

FIGURE 3.—Serial angiograms (frontal views) at baseline (**A**), baseline with initial catheter placement (**B**), 60 minutes after infusion (**C**), and 120 minutes after infusion (**D**) of rpro-UK. A, Left ICA angiogram at baseline. There is an occlusion of the midportion of the left MCA, just beyond the anterior temporal branch. **B**, Microcatheter placement at baseline. The tip of the catheter (*arrow*) has been directed into the face of the clot. During hand injection, contrast outlines a large thrombus filling the distal M1 segment and origins of the M2 (hemispheric) branches. **C**, Microcatheter injection 60 minutes after rpro-UK infusion. The tip of the catheter (*arrow*) remains in a similar location. Partial lysis is demonstrated as compared with baseline. **D**, Left ICA angiogram at 2 hours after rpro-UK infusion. Note complete lysis and normal-appearing vascular segments distal to the M1 and M2 MCA. (Courtesy of del Zoppo GJ, and the PROACT investigators: PROACT: A phase II randomized trial of recombinant pro-urokinase by direct arterial delivery in acute middle cerebral artery stroke. *Stroke* 29: 4–11, 1998.)

Methods.—Patients with symptoms of acute carotid artery territory stroke were evaluated in 37 North American clinical centers. Intracranial hemorrhage was excluded by CT scan. Patients with abrupt onset of symptoms of focal ischemia who were likely to receive treatment within 6 hours underwent carotid angiography. Those who demonstrated thrombolysis in acute myocardial infarction grade 0 or 1 occlusion of the M1 or M2 middle cerebral artery were randomized in a 2:1 ratio to receive either rpro-UK or placebo by intra-arterial infusion into the proximal thrombus face over 120 minutes. Intravenous heparin was administered to all patients. Recanalization efficacy was evaluated at completion of the 2-hour infusion. Intracerebral hemorrhage causing neurologic deterioration was appraised at 24 hours.

Results.—Forty-six of 105 patients who underwent angiography met inclusion criteria and were randomized. Of 46 patients randomized, 26 were treated with rpro-UK and 14 were treated with placebo at a median of 5½ hours from onset of symptoms. Recanalization was significantly correlated with rpro-UK (Fig 3). Hemorrhagic transformation causing neurologic deterioration within 24 hours of treatment occurred in 15.4% of patients receiving rpro-UK and 7.1% of patients who received placebo. Heparin dose influenced recanalization and hemorrhagic frequencies.

Conclusion.—There was a correlation between intra-arterial local rpro-UK infusion and superior recanalization in acute thrombotic/thromboembolic stroke, compared with placebo. These data support the clinical efficacy and safety of intra-arterial thrombolysis in patients with acute thrombotic stroke.

▶ This trial, the first to study intra-arterial administration of a plasminogen activator in a double-blinded randomized fashion, showed that although pro-urokinase is superior to saline placebo in achieving recanalization of occluded middle cerebral artery M1 or M2 segments, thrombolysis doubled the incidence of hemorrhagic transformation with neurologic deterioration. The concomitant use of heparin appears to have contributed in part to this effect. Of greater concern, however, is the fact that the median time from symptom onset to therapy was 5½ hours. In this reviewer's opinion, the window for safe thrombolysis is probably not more than 3 hours. This view is supported by the positive results of the National Institute of Neurologic Disorders and Stroke study of intravenous tissue plasminogen activator (delivered within 3 hours) in contrast to the negative outcome of the ECASS study, which had a 6-hour time window. Because the present study was designed only to test safety and recanalization efficacy, no conclusions regarding benefit can be drawn. However, the present data are of concern, and one would like to see an efficacy study designed around a narrower time window after symptom onset.

M.D. Ginsberg, M.D.

CAST: Randomised Placebo-controlled Trial of Early Aspirin Use in 20 000 Patients With Acute Ischaemic Stroke
Chen Z-M, and the CAST (Chinese Acute Stroke Trial) Collaborative Group (Radcliffe Infirmary, Oxford, England)
Lancet 349:1641–1649, 1997   1–16

Introduction.—Treatment with low-dose aspirin has been shown to prevent serious vascular events after stroke and myocardial infarction. Routine clinical practice varies considerably, however, because of a lack of reliable data on the benefits and risks of antiplatelet therapy started during the initial acute phase of ischemic stroke. Results from 2 major trials of early aspirin use suggest a small but definite net benefit.

Methods.—In the Chinese Acute Stroke Trial (CAST), eligible patients were judged to be within 48 hours of the onset of symptoms of suspected acute ischemic stroke. Randomization was to placebo or aspirin (160 mg/day) started at study entry and continued in hospital for up to 4 weeks. From a total of 413 hospitals, 10,554 patients were allocated to aspirin and 10,552 to placebo. Only comatose patients were required to have a CT scan before randomization, but scans were available for 87% of the study group. Patients were followed for the effects of treatment on mortality and recurrent stroke.

Results.—Aspirin and placebo groups were well matched in age, sex, time from stroke onset, type of stroke, and other baseline characteristics. There was a statistically significant difference between aspirin and placebo groups in the proportion of in-hospital deaths within 4 weeks (3.3% vs. 3.9%). Patients who received aspirin had significantly fewer recurrent ischemic strokes (1.6%) than those allocated to placebo (2.1%), but hemorrhagic strokes were slightly more frequent with aspirin treatment (1.1% vs. 0.9%). The combined in-hospital end point of death or nonfatal stroke was reduced with aspirin (5.3%) vs. placebo (5.9%), and fewer aspirin-treated patients were dead or dependent at discharge (30.5% vs. 31.6%).

Conclusion.—Both CAST and the parallel International Stroke Trial show that aspirin, started early after hospitalization for acute ischemic stroke, was associated with about 9 fewer deaths or nonfatal strokes per 1,000 patients treated in the first few weeks and with 13 fewer dead or dependent per 1,000 patients treated after several weeks or months of follow-up. The benefits of aspirin outweighed the small risk of hemorrhagic stroke.

▶ This huge trial complements the large International Stroke Trial in showing that aspirin therapy is beneficial in reducing death rate and the incidence of nonfatal stroke in the first few weeks after a stroke, when begun early during hospitalization. Although the proportional risk reduction is, at first glance, small (combined death and nonfatal stroke rate during first 4 weeks, 5.9% vs. 5.3%), this represents a 12% absolute risk reduction. These data justify the authors' conclusion that aspirin treatment should now be considered for almost all patients with acute ischemic stroke, provided that hemorrhagic stroke can be excluded and that there are no major contraindications.

M.D. Ginsberg, M.D.

The International Stroke Trial (IST): A Randomised Trial of Aspirin, Subcutaneous Heparin, Both, or Neither Among 19,435 Patients With Acute Ischaemic Stroke

Sandercock PAG, and the International Stroke Trial Collaborative Group (Western Gen Hosp, Edinburgh, Scotland)

Lancet 349:1569–1581, 1997   1–17

Introduction.—The International Stroke Trial (IST) was designed to provide evidence on the safety and efficacy of aspirin and of subcutaneous heparin in acute ischemic stroke. Heparin is widely used in this setting, but few randomized studies have examined the risks and benefits of the anticoagulant in a large number of patients. Although aspirin can inhibit the substantial platelet activation that occurs in acute ischemic stroke, large-scale randomized evidence of its value is lacking.

Methods.—Eligible patients had evidence of an acute stroke with onset less than 48 hours before study entry and were without clear indications for, or contraindications to, heparin or aspirin. All underwent CT to exclude intracranial hemorrhage. Half of the patients were randomly assigned to subcutaneous unfractionated heparin, either at a low dose (5,000 IU twice daily) or a medium dose (12,500 IU twice daily), while half were told to "avoid heparin." Using a factorial design, half of all patients were randomly allocated to aspirin (300 mg daily), while half were told to "avoid aspirin." Treatment continued for 14 days or until prior discharge. Clinicians were to consider giving all patients long-term aspirin at discharge. Primary outcomes were death within 14 days and death and dependency at 6 months.

Results.—The IST enrolled 19,435 patients from 467 hospitals in 36 countries. Central randomization achieved good balance between the treatment groups for prognostic factors, and compliance throughout the scheduled treatment period was good (88% to 94%). Fewer deaths occurred within 14 days in the heparin group vs. the no-heparin group (9.0% vs. 9.3%), but the difference was not significant. At 6 months, these 2 groups had an identical percentage of patients dead or dependent (62.9%). Heparin, particularly with the medium dose, was associated with a significant excess of transfused or fatal extracranial bleeds. Compared with the no-aspirin condition, aspirin treatment yielded a non-significant reduction in deaths within 14 days (9.4% vs. 9.0%). After adjustment for baseline prognosis, the benefit of aspirin was significant for death or dependency at 6 months. Patients allocated to aspirin also had significantly fewer recurrent ischemic strokes within 14 days, with no significant excess of hemorrhagic strokes.

Discussion.—Low-dose heparin yielded some modest short-term benefit for patients with acute ischemic stroke, but higher doses should be avoided. Neither low- nor medium-dose heparin offered any clinical advantage at 6 months. Immediate use of aspirin, however, should be considered in all patients without clear contraindications and especially in those without CT evidence of intracerebral hemorrhage.

▶ This huge open trial of antithrombotic therapy for acute stroke comparing medium-dose or low-dose twice-daily administration of subcutaneous heparin to aspirin, or neither therapy, establishes that neither dose of heparin confers a clinical advantage at 6 months, and the higher dose is associated with a greater number of hemorrhagic strokes, extracranial bleeds, and more deaths or nonfatal strokes within the first 2 weeks. By contrast, this trial suggests a small benefit of aspirin. Thus, the authors recommend that aspirin be begun as soon as possible after the onset of ischemic stroke. As heparin tends to be widely prescribed for patients with acute ischemic stroke, even in the absence of clear indications for anticoagulation (e.g., cardioembolic origin), the present results should stimulate a lively discussion in the field.

M.D. Ginsberg, M.D.

A Randomized Trial of Anticoagulants Versus Aspirin After Cerebral Ischemia of Presumed Arterial Origin
A Algra and the Stroke Prevention in Reversible Ischemia Trial (SPIRIT) Study Group (Univ Hosp Utrecht, The Netherlands)
Ann Neurol 42:857–865, 1997   1–18

Introduction.—Few data are available regarding the efficacy and safety of oral anticoagulation treatment in patients with cerebral ischemia. The Stroke Prevention in Reversible Ischemia Trial, an open, randomized, multicenter, controlled clinical trial undertaken to assess full-dose anticoagulation (international normalized ratio [INR], 3.0–4.5) vs. low-dose aspirin, 30 mg/day, in patients with transient ischemic attack (TIA) or nondisabling ischemic stroke of presumed arterial origin is described.

Methods.—Patients referred to a neurologist or a general physician at 1 of 58 collaborating centers were eligible if they had had a TIA or a minor ischemic stroke (grade 3 or less on the modified Rankin scale) within the preceding 6 months. Patients were randomized to open treatment with aspirin or oral anticoagulant treatment. Patients were evaluated by their neurologists every 6 months. Primary measures of outcome were "death from all vascular causes, nonfatal stroke, nonfatal myocardial infarction, or nonfatal major bleeding complication."

Results.—The trial was terminated at the first interim analysis because of a high rate of major bleeding complications, at only 17% of its predetermined number of patient-years of observation. Mean follow-up of 1,316 patients was 14 months. There was an excess of primary outcome events in the anticoagulated group (81 of 651 patients), compared with the aspirin group (36 of 651 patients). Of 15 fatal brain hemorrhages, 14 occurred in the anticoagulated group and 1 occurred in the aspirin group. Intracranial bleeding occurred in 27 and 3 patients in the anticoagulated and aspirin groups, respectively. The incidence of major bleeding complications rose sharply with the achieved intensity of anticoagulation. Bleeding incidence rose by a factor of 1.43 for each 0.5-unit increase of achieved

INR. The relative risk reduction of ischemic events was similar in both groups.

Conclusion.—Anticoagulant therapy with an INR range of 3.0–4.5 in patients with cerebral ischemia of presumed arterial origin may not be considered safe. The efficacy of a lower-intensity anticoagulation regimen needs to be assessed. There is a current United States trial comparing aspirin with anticoagulation with an INR value of 1.4 to 2.8. An observational trial of patients with atrial fibrillation indicated that the risk of stroke rose sharply at INR values lower than 2.0. A randomized trial of anticoagulation with an INR target range of 2.0 to 3.0 may safely prevent ischemic stroke in patients with atrial fibrillation. It is possible that an INR range of 2.0 to 3.0 instead of 3.0 to 4.5 may decrease the rate of major complications by two thirds.

▶ The unfortunate message of this study is that the level of oral anticoagulation used (International Normalized Ratio, 3.0–4.5) led to a 2.3-fold excess in the composite adverse outcome measure and, more alarmingly, to a 9.3–fold excess in major bleeding complications, which accounted for the composite adverse outcome. Intracerebral hemorrhage accounted for 52% of the major bleeding complications in anticoagulated patients. This dire trend forced the premature termination of this trial when only 17% of the target number of patient-years had been achieved. The very data of this study show that bleeding complications begin to rise sharply above INR values of 3 to 3.5—a range that was occupied by more than half of the person-years of the study. By contrast, the Stroke Prevention in Atrial Fibrillation Study III[1] showed that an INR range of 2.0 to 3.0 was sufficient to prevent ischemic strokes in high-risk patients with atrial fibrillation. The authors of the present study calculate that shifting the target INR range to 2.0–3.0 instead of 3.0–4.5 would have reduced the incidence of major bleeding complications by two thirds. The adverse outcome of this study therefore carries a powerful message as regards the target anticoagulation range to be chosen in patients at risk of stroke.

M.D. Ginsberg, M.D.

Reference

1. Stroke Prevention in Atrial Fibrillation Investigators: Adjusted-dose warfarin vs. low-intensity, fixed-dose warfarin plus aspirin for high-risk patients with atrial fibrillation: Stroke Prevention in Atrial Fibrillation III randomized clinical trial. *Lancet* 348:633–638, 1996.

Cerebral Protection Using Retrograde Cerebral Perfusion During Hypothermic Circulatory Arrest

Shenkman Z, Elami A, Weiss YG, et al (Hadassah Univ, Jerusalem, Israel; Hebrew Univ, Jerusalem, Israel; Harvard Med School, Boston)
Can J Anaesth 44:1096–1101, 1997   1–19

Background.—Retrograde cerebral perfusion through the superior vena cava (SVC) may protect the brain from ischemic damage during profound hypothermic circulatory arrest (PHCA). The use of the SVC perfusate as a route to administer anesthetic agents and vasodilators to the cerebral circulation in 3 patients was described.

Methods.—During repair of the ascending aorta by PHCA, the upper body was retrogradely perfused with blood cooled to 16° C through the SVC by the cardiopulmonary bypass pump. A computerized electroencephalographic monitor was used. Perfusion pressure was determined at a port in the cannula connector. Etomidate or thiopentone was injected into the SVC perfusate to stop recurring electrocephalographic activity, and nitroglycerin or nitroprusside was injected to increase retrograde flow and maintain a constant perfusion pressure.

Findings.—The retrograde administration of small boluses of etomidate (50 mg total) or thiopentone (500 mg total) eliminated recurrent electroencephalogic activity during PHCA periods of up to 61 minutes. Nitroprusside, 100 µg, and nitroglycerin, 2 µg·kg^{-1}·min^{-1}, increased retrograde flow from 220 to 550 and 660 ml·min^{-1}, respectively. Perfusion pressure was maintained at 25 to 26 mm Hg. Recovery from anesthesia and surgery was uneventful. No adverse neurologic sequelae occurred.

Conclusions.—Injecting anesthetic agents into the retrograde SVC perfusate during PHCA can suppress recurring electroencephalographic activity. Retrograde injection of vasodilators can facilitate an increase in perfusion. Both may augment brain protection.

▶ This report, although preliminary and involving only 3 patients, nonetheless describes a technique that may assume increasing importance in coming years. Retrograde cerebral perfusion is a means of delivering oxygenated blood retrogradely through the cerebral venous system. By cooling the perfusate, one may reduce brain temperature directly. Furthermore, the technique provides a means of drug delivery, as was done here by the addition of etomidate or thiopentone to the perfusate. Variants of this potential neuroprotective strategy are likely to receive further study in the future.

M.D. Ginsberg, M.D.

Brain Temperature Monitoring and Modulation in Patients With Severe MCA Infarction

Schwab S, Spranger M, Aschoff A, et al (Univ of Heidelberg, Germany)
Neurology 48:762–767, 1997   1–20

Background.—Several animal models of focal cerebral ischemia report significant reduction of infarct volumes with hypothermia and negative effects with increased brain temperature. Although deep hypothermia is used routinely during open heart surgery, little is known about temperature in the human brain during normal and pathologic conditions. To gather information on changes in brain temperature after acute stroke, brain temperature monitoring and modulation was done on 15 consecutive patients.

Methods.—The patients, 10 men and 5 women, ranged in age from 35 to 54 years. All were admitted with an acute middle-cerebral-artery (MCA)-territory stroke and treated for elevated intracranial pressure (ICP). Intracerebral temperature was recorded using 2 thermocouples, with intraventricular, epidural, and parenchymatous measurements. Simultaneous recordings of body-core temperature and jugular bulb temperature were obtained in 5 patients. Various methods were used in an attempt to control brain temperature.

Results.—The cause of stroke was cardioembolism in 10 patients, internal carotid artery dissection with secondary MCA embolization in 3, and unknown in 2. Three patients died, and all 12 survivors were discharged to rehabilitation programs. Monitoring of intracerebral temperature continued for a mean of 4.9 days. All patients showed a continuous increase in ICP values during the first 2 days after probe insertion; most had a fever greater than 39°C during the measurement period. Alcohol body washing or antipyretics were used to maintain body temperature less than 38.5°C. Brain temperature exceeded body temperature by at least 1°C in all patients, and temperature in the ventricles exceeded epidural temperature by up to 2°C. Only systemic cooling achieved sustained hypothermic brain temperatures (33–34°C), followed by a decrease in ICP. Paracetamol (1 g) or metamizol infusion (500 mg) lowered core temperature, but brain temperature reductions were small and not sustained.

Discussion.—Hypothermia may have therapeutic potential as a neuroprotective measure. Monitoring of patients with MCA stroke showed that intracerebral temperature is higher than central body-core temperature and that a temperature gradient exists within the brain. Mild hypothermia lowered critically elevated ICP in these patients.

▶ Beginning 10 years ago,[1] a very large number of experimental studies carried out in models of focal ischemic stroke, global ischemia, and head injury have shown that moderate reductions of brain temperature confer striking protection against ischemic or traumatic injury. Application of these principles to human clinical trials of hypothermia have been initiated in the setting of traumatic head injury, where very promising results have already been obtained.[2] By contrast, clinical trials of moderate hypothermia for acute ischemic stroke have not yet been reported. In this important publication, Schwab et al. establish the feasibility of brain and body temperature monitoring in acute ischemic stroke, note that brain temperature exceeds body-core temperature by 1–2°C, and establish that brain temperature modulation by systemic cooling is feasible. This important report should, hopefully, stimulate and pave the way for controlled therapeutic trials of hypothermia in acute stroke—a long overdue initiative.

M.D. Ginsberg, M.D.

References

1. Busto R, Dietrich WD, Globus MY-T, et al: Small differences in intraischemic brain temperature critically determine the extent of ischemic neuronal injury. *J Cereb Blood Flow Metab* 7:729–738, 1987.
2. Marion DW, Penrod LE, Kelsey SF, et al: Treatment of traumatic brain injury with moderate hypothermia. *N Engl J Med* 336:540–546, 1997.

Collaborative Systematic Review of the Randomised Trials of Organised Inpatient (Stroke Unit) Care After Stroke
Langhorne P, and the Stroke Unit Trialists' Collaboration (Royal Infirmary, Glasgow, Scotland)
BMJ 314:1151–1159, 1997   1–21

Introduction.—Evaluation of the benefits of organized inpatient (stroke unit) care after stroke has been difficult because of the complex nature of the intervention and its potential interaction with other aspects of care. A previous review of randomized trials indicated that stroke-unit care may reduce death and institutionalization after stroke. Randomized controlled trials were systematically reviewed.

Methods.—Studies were sought that allocated patients to an organized stroke unit or to conventional care. Excluded were studies that compared specific therapies within an organized stroke-care setting. Organization of service was divided into 3 predefined groups: dedicated stroke units, mixed assessment/rehabilitation units, and general medical wards. Outcomes were death, dependency, and need for institutional care at the end of follow-up. The principal investigators of the trials were asked to provide details of their trial design, duration of follow-up, and other relevant data.

Results.—Nineteen trials, including 3 with 2 treatment arms, were analyzed. Twelve trials randomly assigned 2,060 patients to a dedicated stroke unit or a general medical ward, 6 trials with 647 patients compared a mixed assessment/rehabilitation unit with a general medical ward, and 4 trials with 542 patients compared a dedicated stroke unit with a mixed assessment/rehabilitation unit. Stroke units were usually housed in a separate ward, employed coordinated multidisciplinary rehabilitation, and provided a specialized medical and nursing staff. With a median follow-up time of 1 year, stroke-unit care was associated with a reduction of death (odds ratio, 0.83), the combined outcomes of death and dependency (odds ratio, 0.69), and death or institutionalization (odds ratio, 0.75). Compared with conventional care, stroke-unit care reduced length of hospital stay by 8%. The benefits of stroke-unit care were independent of patient age and sex, stroke severity, and variations in stroke-unit organization.

Discussion.—Patients cared for in an organized stroke unit had higher survival rates and were less likely to be dependent and need institutional care than were patients cared for in general medical wards or mixed units. The benefits of stroke-unit care were not limited to any patient subgroups or to any specific model of stroke-unit care.

▶ This survey of 19 randomized trials comparing organized inpatient stroke care with conventional care establishes that stroke-unit care is associated, on average, with a 17% reduction in death, a 31% reduction in poor outcome (death or dependency), and a 25% reduction in the combined outcomes of death or institutionalization. Length of hospital stay was also reduced, compared with conventional care. In this era of encroaching managed care, these results should give one pause by raising the distinct possibility that expedient measures taken to reduce or minimize acute stroke care may, in fact, contribute to the chronic medical and financial burdens of this condition by increasing death and disability. This survey makes a strong case for the delivery of acute stroke care within organized inpatient units.

M.D. Ginsberg, M.D.

2 Headaches

Outcome of Early School-age Migraine
Metsähonkala L, Sillanpää M, Tuominen J (Turku Univ, Finland)
Cephalalgia 17:662–665, 1997   2–1

Background.—Studies have suggested that the outcomes of childhood migraine are good. However, there are few data on the relevant prognostic factors. The outcomes of migraine in school-age children were studied, along with the significant prognostic factors.

Methods.—Eighty-four children with migraine, who were followed up from ages 8–9 years to ages 11–12 years, were studied. The patients were identified from a population-based, unselected follow-up sample of a 1-year age cohort that had been followed up since birth. The prevalence of migraine among this cohort was about 3%, according to mail survey. At age 11–12 years of age, the patients were traced for in-person interviews. The outcomes of migraine from the early school years to puberty were assessed. Sex, headache characteristics, sociodemographic factors, and school attendance–related factors were evaluated for prognostic significance.

Results.—At follow-up, 95% of the children still had headaches and 63% still had migraine. Another 20% of children had migraine-type headaches, although they did not meet the International Headache Society criteria for a diagnosis of migraine. Eight percent of children had episodic tension-type headaches, whereas 4% had other types of headache. The mean number of migraine attacks per month at follow-up was 2.7 for boys vs. 1.8 for girls. The boys tended to use more drugs and to miss more school because of headache than girls, although the differences were nonsignificant. Frequent migraines appeared to be related to a problematic relationship between parents.

Conclusions.—Most school-age children with migraine are still having headaches by puberty, and the frequency of migraine attacks may increase in the interval. Factors related to poor prognosis—i.e., frequent attacks of migraine—include male sex and problems in parental relations.

▶ A number of early investigations have indicated that the long-term prognosis for migraine in children appears to be good. Long remissions are said to be common, although more than half have migraine in middle age.[1-4] This study, which uses International Headache Society criteria, paints a much different prognosis and one probably more in line with the clinical impressions of most clinicians. Migraine in children can be a grim problem and not one to be overlooked or treated lightly.

R.A. Davidoff, M.D.

References

1. Bille B: Migraine in school children. *Acta Paediatr Scand* 51:3S–151S, 1962.
2. Congdon PJ, Forsythe WI: Migraine in childhood: A study of 300 children. *Dev Med Child Neurol* 21:209–216, 1979.
3. Sillanpää M: Changes in the prevalence of migraine and other headaches during the first seven school years. *Headache* 23:15–19, 1983.
4. Tal Y, Dunn HG, Chrichton JU: Childhood migraine: A dangerous diagnosis? *Acta Paediatr Scand* 73:55–59, 1984.

Light-induced Discomfort and Pain in Migraine
Vanagaite J, Pareja JA, Støren O, et al (Univ Hosp, Trondheim, Norway; Hosp Ntra. Sra. de Sonsoles, Avila, Spain)
Cephalalgia 17:733–741, 1997   2–2

Background.—Few quantitative studies on photophobia in migraine have been published. In the current study, quantitatively measured dis-

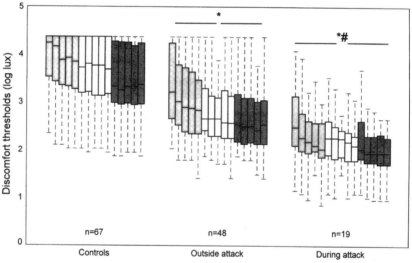

FIGURE 1.—Discomfort thresholds in controls and migraineurs (outside or during attack) on repeated stimulation, shown by box-and-whisker plots. Each box represents the median, 25th and 75th percentiles, and the whiskers the smallest and largest value that was not an outlier. Within each group, all 15 measurements are shown consecutively; right eye, measurements 1-5; left eye, measurements 6-10; both eyes, measurements 11-15. *Asterisk:* All thresholds in migraine patients were significantly different from corresponding thresholds in controls (p 0.0001). *Number sign:* All thresholds in patients during attack were significantly different from corresponding thresholds in migraineurs outside attack (*P* < 0.03) (Mann-Whitney test). (Reprinted from Light-induced discomfort and pain in migraine, by Vanagaite J, Pareja JA, Storen O, et al: from Cephalalgia 17:733–741, 1997 by permission of Scandinavian University Press.)

comfort and pain thresholds with monocular and binocular light stimuli in persons with and without migraine were compared.

Methods and Findings.—Sixty-seven patients with migraine, including 37 with aura and 30 without, and 67 healthy persons were studied. Patients were more photophobic during an attack than outside an attack. The patients were also more sensitive to light even between attacks than were healthy persons. Light sensitivity did not differ between migraine with and without aura. Unilateral pain affected light sensitivity on both sides. Seventy-four percent of patients reported light sensitivity outside an attack, and 100% during an attack. Sensitive patients had generally lower pain thresholds than nonsensitive patients, indicating some agreement between subjective and objective measures of photophobia (Fig 1).

Conclusions.—Photophobia appears to be intrinsic to migraine. Migraine pain increases photophobia, which seems to be unassociated with migraine characteristics such as nausea, migraine severity, pain character, and pain laterality.

▶ It is well known that intolerance of light is one of the most frequent symptoms associated with migrainous head pain. Between 65% and 90% of patients develop an amplified and usually unpleasant sensitivity to light during an attack. But as Vanagaite et al. show, migraineurs are also sensitive to light between attacks. This has therapeutic implications because previous studies have demonstrated that extended exposure to the strong or flickering light is a potent trigger for headaches in between 30% and 45% of migraine patients.[1, 2] Patients should pay attention to lighting at home and at work. Fluorescent lighting should be removed if it is a component in the generation of attacks. For some patients, tinted eye glasses are valuable both indoors and outdoors. Patients should be made aware of their options.

R.A. Davidoff, M.D.

References

1. Selby G and Lance JW: Observations on 500 cases of migraine and allied vascular headache. *J Neurol Neurosurg Psychiatry* 23:23–32, 1960.
2. Vijayan N, Gould S and Watson C: Exposure to sun and precipitation of migraine. *Headache* 20:42–43, 1980.

A Study of the Effects of Sumatriptan on Myocardial Perfusion in Healthy Female Migraineurs Using $^{13}NH_3$ Positron Emission Tomography

Lewis PJ, Barrington SF, Marsden PK, et al (Guy's and St Thomas' Hosps, London; Lewisham Hosp, London)
Neurology 48:1542–1550, 1997   2–3

Introduction.—Sumatriptan is a 5-HT$_{1D}$ agonist that is effective in relieving headaches in as many as 70% of patients with acute migraine when administered in a subcutaneous injection. Its ability to cause vasoconstriction in certain cerebral vessels may be what alleviates migraine attacks. Up to 5% of patients may experience chest symptoms, including tightness and heaviness. The effect of a single 6-mg subcutaneous dose of sumatriptan on myocardial perfusion (MP) was assessed using $^{13}NH_3$ PET in a double-blind, randomized, placebo-controlled, cross-over trial.

Methods.—Nineteen women with migraines, aged 35–65 years, who were at low risk for ischemic heart disease underwent 2 scanning sessions. During both scans, a baseline dynamic $^{13}NH_3$ PET scan was acquired followed by a $^{13}NH_3$ PET scan 10 minutes after subcutaneous injection of placebo or 6 mg of sumatriptan. Regional MP was evaluated in 5 myocardial regions using the Patlak system of image analysis.

Results.—The mean percent change from baseline in global MP was +9.5% and +6.6% after placebo and sumatriptan administration, respectively. None of the 5 myocardial regions had significant MP changes from baseline.

Conclusion.—A single 6-mg subcutaneous dose of sumatriptan does not create a significant change in regional or global myocardial perfusion in healthy women with migraine headaches.

▶ The ability of sumatriptan to abort migraine attacks is now well accepted, and all neurologists are knowledgeable regarding both its value and its side effects. The latter, particularly those such as tightness of the chest indicating potential cardiac problems, have given physicians some pause. Approximately 5% of individuals report vague chest discomfort, mainly a feeling of tightness or pressure in the chest. Other patients report chest discomfort radiating into the shoulders, arms, neck, or throat.

This carefully performed study shows that sumatriptan has no effect on myocardial perfusion in healthy women with migraine. The drug (and, presumably, the other "triptans" which have been released or will be released soon) appears to be safe if used only for individuals with severe, recurrent migraine that does not respond to less expensive medications, provided these do not have known cardiac problems and lack risk factors for coronary artery disease. Hence, the risk group would include postmenopausal women, men over 40 years of age, and those with hypertension, hypercholesterolemia, obesity, diabetes, history of smoking, or a strong family history of heart attacks.

R.A. Davidoff, M.D.

Double-blind, Placebo-controlled, Dose-finding Study of Rizatriptan (MK-462) in the Acute Treatment of Migraine

Gijsman H, Kramer MS, Sargent J, et al (Leiden Univ, The Netherlands; Merck Research Labs, West Point, Pa; Menninger Ctr for Clinical Pharmacology, Topeka, Kan; et al)

Cephalalgia 17:647–651, 1997   2–4

Background.—Rizatriptan, a potent $5HT_{1D}$ receptor agonist, has been shown to be tolerated in single doses of up to 60 mg in young, healthy volunteers. However, the initial dose-ranging study did not determine the minimal effective dose. The clinical efficacy and tolerability at doses of 10 mg and less were tested in the current study.

Methods.—Four hundred seventeen patients with moderate or severe migraine were enrolled in the multicenter, double-blind, placebo-controlled study. By random assignment, patients were given placebo or 2.5, 5, or 10 mg of rizatriptan. A second dose of the test drug was permitted at 2 hours if headache pain was still moderate or severe.

Findings.—There was an upward dose-response relationship among placebo, 2.5 mg, 5 mg, and 10 mg of rizatriptan in the primary efficacy measure of proportion of patients reporting pain relief. This relationship was apparent even at 30 minutes and was significant at 1.5 hours and thereafter. At 2 hours after the initial dose, pain relief was reported by 47.6% of patients given 10 mg of rizatriptan, by 45.4% given 5 mg, by 21.3% given 2.5 mg, and by 17.9% given placebo. Seventy percent of patients receiving 10 mg rizatriptan reported pain relief at 4 hours. AT 1.5 and 2 hours after dosing, patients receiving the 5 and 10 mg doses were significantly less functionally disabled than those receiving placebo. The 10 mg dose was consistently more effective than the 5 mg dose, although the differences were nonsignificant. The most common side effects were dizziness, somnolence, and asthenia/fatigue. No serious adverse events occurred.

Conclusions.—In patients with moderate or severe migraine, rizatriptan at doses of 5 and 10 mg are effective and generally well tolerated. The 2.5 mg dose was too low to be therapeutic.

▶ The efficacy of sumatriptan is well-established, and all neurologic clinicians are aware of its value and of its side effects. New "triptan" preparations are now available or are going to be released by the FDA shortly. Rizatriptan is one of the new products, and the results of the present study by Gijsman and colleagues show that it is well tolerated and effective. It remains to be shown, however, if the newer triptans (1) are more efficacious than sumatriptan; (2) work in patients whose headaches are not relieved by sumatriptan; (3) have fewer serious side effects; (4) are longer-lasting than sumatriptan; and (5) are less costly than sumatriptan. Comparative studies are eagerly awaited.

R.A Davidoff, M.D.

SUNCT Syndrome: A Clinical Review

Pareja JA, Sjaastad O (Trondheim Univ Hosps, Norway)
Headache 37:195–202, 1997   2–5

Introduction.—There is a group of patients with short-lasting, unilateral, neuralgiform headache attacks with conjunctival infection, tearing, and rhinorrhea (SUNCT syndrome). The long-term course of this syndrome is unpredictable; it may be symptomatic for awhile, followed by spontaneous remissions. Various mechanisms in both the trigeminal and extrageminal areas may precipitate attacks in some patients. Twenty-one cases have been reported so far, but the syndrome is likely more frequent than that. The clinical findings of these 21 patients with SUNCT syndrome are reviewed.

Patients.—The patients were 17 men and 4 women, with mean age at onset on symptoms approximately 51 years. Only 2 patients had a family history of migraine. The symptoms usually arose spontaneously, though there was a possible temporal relationship with another disorder in a few patients. The headaches occurred mainly in the orbital/periorbital area. Recurrences always developed on the same side, in an erratic pattern of attacks and remissions. The pain was rated as moderate to severe and characterized as burning, electrical, or stabbing. When headaches occurred, the patients also had prominent, ipsilateral, conjunctival injection with tearing and rhinorrhea or nasal obstruction. Many different precipitating events were reported, usually stronger than those needed to precipitate trigeminal neuralgia. Three patients had wholly spontaneous attacks, however.

Paroxysms usually lasted 10 to 60 seconds; at their longest, they ranged from 1 to 5 minutes. When attacks were occurring, their frequency was from less than once daily to more than 30 times per hour. Most patients had no observable abnormalities, though 2 had a documented vascular malformation in the ipsilateral cerebellopontine angle. Many different drugs and anesthetic blockade techniques were tried, including treatments for tic douloureux. Treatment was generally ineffective, however.

Discussion.—The clinical characteristics of SUNCT syndrome are reviewed. This syndrome should be considered in patients with unilateral, orbital/periorbital headache syndromes. The findings help to clarify the clinical picture of SUNCT syndrome; the differences from V1 tic are apparent.

▶ The SUNCT syndrome is one of the several short-lasting headaches that have recently been critically reviewed.[1] SUNCT is predominantly a male disorder, with most attacks lasting 15 seconds or more. In particular, it must be distinguished from trigeminal neuralgia involving V_1. The presence of prominent autonomic features of attacks of SUNCT and the lack of response to carbamazepine and mild autonomic symptoms during episodes of tic and response to carbamazepine should serve to make a differential diagnosis. The differential diagnosis has recently been reviewed by the authors of the present article.[2] Both disorders can be triggered by a variety of precipitating stimuli within the territory of the trigeminal nerve.

R.A. Davidoff, M.D.

References

1. Goadsby PJ, Lipton RB: A review of paroxysmal hemicranias, SUNCT syndrome and other short-lasting headaches with autonomic features, including new cases. *Brain* 120:193–209, 1997.
2. Sjaastad O, Pareja JA, Zukerman E, et al: Trigeminal neuralgia. Clinical manifestations of first division involvement. *Headache* 37:346–357, 1997.

Nontraumatic Subarachnoid Hemorrhage: Value of Repeat Angiography
du Mesnil de Rochemont RdM, Heindel W, Wesselmann C, et al (Univ of Cologne, Germany)
Radiology 202:798–800, 1997   2–6

Introduction.—The initial angiographic examination often fails to determine the source of bleeding in patients with nontraumatic subarachnoid hemorrhage (SAH). Because cerebral angiography carries the risk of complications, the use of repeat angiography to demonstrate the cause of bleeding has been questioned. A retrospective analysis of 391 angiographic examinations sought to define the benefits and risks of repeat studies in cases of nontraumatic SAH of unknown source.

Methods.—The study group included 159 women and 164 men with a mean age of 52 years. None had signs of skull or brain trauma. These patients underwent 323 initial examinations, 66 repeat studies, and 2 third examinations. In 34 of 66 patients having repeat studies, blood was located predominantly in the perimesence-phalic and pontine cisterns. Results of angiography were reviewed for the frequency with which the cause and location of a source of bleeding was detected at initial and repeat studies and for neurologic complications of the procedure.

Results.—Aneurysms were found in 195 patients (60.4%) at the initial angiographic examination and arteriovenous malformations in 11 (3.4%). Sixty-six of 117 patients with negative study results underwent repeat cerebral angiography. It was not determined why the remaining 55 patients had no further studies. None of the 117 patients had a second episode of bleeding. Repeat angiography showed 3 aneurysms, but all 3 could be detected retrospectively with the initial examination. Thus, the cause of bleeding remained unknown in 63 of 66 patients with repeat cerebral angiograms. The overall rate of angiography-related complications was 2.0%; 1 of the 8 affected patients (0.2%) had definitive neurologic deficits.

Conclusion.—Aneurysms and arteriovenous malformations are the most common sources of bleeding in patients with nontraumatic SAH. The source of bleeding is often not identified, however, and these patients generally have a good prognosis. Repeat angiography appears to be needed only for patients with a technically inadequate initial study, vasospasm, or further bleeding.

▶ The wisdom of following the tradition of performing repeat cerebral angiography for SAH when the initial angiogram is negative is severely questioned by the results of this investigation. Even in those few cases where the repeat angiogram identified the cause of the SAH, retrospective analysis of the initial angiogram showed that there was either a misinterpretation of the original study or that technical problems prevented proper visualization of the abnormality. Although all patients with nontraumatic SAH require an admission angiogram, if that 4-vessel angiogram is of high quality and shows no vasospasm or abnormalities, a repeat angiogram is not necessary. This approach is underscored by the real, albeit small, precentage of complications caused by cerebral angiography.

R.M. Quencer, M.D.

Syndrome of Orthostatic Headaches and Diffuse Pachymeningeal Gadolinium Enhancement

Mokri B, Piepgras DG, Miller GM (Mayo Clinic, Rochester, Minn)
Mayo Clin Proc 72:400–413, 1997   2–7

Background.—Intracranial hypotension is characterized clinically by postural headaches and sometimes nausea, vomiting, pain or tight feeling in the neck, dizziness, diplopia, photophobia, change in hearing, and blurred vision. Diffuse meningeal enhancement associated with intracranial hypotension is a recently reported phenomenon often associated with subdural collections of fluid, sagging of the brain, an increase in cerebrospinal fluid (CSF) protein, and a variable pleocytosis. The current study documents the clinical and imaging features, biopsy findings, etiologic factors, and outcomes in patients with intracranial hypotension, headaches, and diffuse pachymeningeal gadolinium enhancement on MRI.

Patients and Findings.—A total of 26 consecutive patients were studied. The patients were 15 men and 11 women, age 24–76 years. All had postural headaches, and some had additional symptoms. The cardinal MRI features were diffuse pachymeningeal gadolinium enhancement, 100%; subdural fluid collections, 69%; and evidence of brain descent, in 62% which resembled type I Chiari malformation in some patients. Only 46% had CSF opening pressures of 40 mm or less. Six patients had overdraining CSF shunts, and 11 had CSF leaks. Shunt revision or ligation and surgical correction of the leak resulted in clinical and MRI resolution in all treated patients. Four patients improved with epidural blood patch. Of 12 patients, 3 who were managed supportively continued to have symptoms. Histologic assessment revealed a thin subdural zone of fibroblasts and thin-walled vessels in an amorphous matrix.

Conclusions.—In many patients with the syndrome of low-pressure headaches and pachymeningeal gadolinium enhancement, the source of the CSF leak can be identified. Meningeal abnormalities probably can be attributed to reduced CSF volume and hydrostatic CSF pressure changes.

▶ All neurologists are familiar with the characteristics of the headache that sometimes follows a lumbar puncture. What is less common is the same syndrome occurring spontaneously in patients who have not had spinal taps and who do not have any obvious reason for a spinal fluid leak such as fracture at the base of the skull, otorrhea, or rhinorrhea. In this regard, the results of the study of Dr. Mokkri, et al are worthy of thought. The finding that may cause the clinician most concern is a diffuse enhancement of apparently thickened pachymeningeal membranes on MRI examination following injection of gadolinium. The differential diagnosis of such thickening includes various diseases of the meninges including meningitis, meningeal carcinomatosis, trauma, and previous subarachnoid hemorrhage. The point is made that myelography or computed tomographic myelography are appropriate tests for recognizing the source of the spinal fluid leak.

R.A. Davidoff, M.D.

Pseudomigraine With Temporary Neurological Symptoms and Lymphocytic Pleocytosis: A Report of 50 Cases

Gómez-Aranda F, Cañadillas F, Martí-Massó JF, et al (Univ Hosp Virgen del Rocío, Sevilla, Spain; Univ Hosp Reina Sofia, Córdoba, Spain; Hosp Nuestra Señora de Aránzazu, San Sebastián, Spain; et al)
Brain 120:1105–1113, 1997   2–8

Introduction.—During the 1980s, a number of published reports, each with 7 or fewer patients, described a transient syndrome with neurologic deficit accompanied or followed by migrainous headache and CSF pleocytosis of unknown origin. Most authors speculate that this syndrome, termed pseudomigraine with pleocytosis (PMP), is more common than usually recognized. A large series of patients with PMP was investigated for demographic, clinical, and laboratory findings.

Methods.—Data on patients with PMP were obtained from members of the Group for the Study of Headache within the Spanish Society of Neurology. Fifty patients met inclusion criteria: 1 or more episodes of transient neurologic deficit accompanied or followed by moderate-to-severe headache, CSF pleocytosis with lymphocytic predominance, negative etiologic studies, and spontaneous clinical resolution in less than 4 months.

Results.—The study group was 68% male and 32% female, with an age range of 14 to 39 years (mean, 28.1 years). None of the patients had a family history suggestive of PMP, but 13 had a personal history of migraine. Patients lived in different parts of Spain and became symptomatic during all seasons of the year. Ten patients had a recent history of viral-like illness when PMP was diagnosed. Most patients experienced multiple episodes (mean, 3.2). Headaches were throbbing in nature with a mean duration of 19 hours. Sensory symptoms were present in 78% of episodes, aphasic symptoms in 66%, and motor symptoms in 56%. All patients were free of symptoms between episodes. Protein was increased in the CSF of 96% of patients. All had CSF pleocytosis with a clear lymphocytic predominance and a mean of 199 lymphocytic cells/mm³. Both brain CT and MRI were always within normal limits, and extensive microbiological determinations were negative.

Discussion.—The etiology of PMP syndrome remains unknown, but the frequency of a viral-like illness preceding symptoms suggests that a viral infection could activate the immune system. Antibodies thus produced could induce an aseptic inflammation of the leptomeningeal vasculature. The syndrome should be considered in patients meeting the criteria for PMP defined in this study, especially when those affected are men in the third and fourth decades of life.

▶ Gómez-Aranda and colleagues make a strong case that lymphocytic pleocytosis occurring with migraine-like headaches and transient neurologic phenomena should not be regarded as a migraine. Differences between migraine and PMP included the observation that most of the patients with PMP were male; that the focal temporary neurologic phenomena of PMP were substantially longer than the aura of migraine, lasting on average 5 hours; and that paroxysmal attacks of PMP were self-limited with no recurrence observed after 2 months.

The authors suggest that the underlying pathophysiologic mechanism of PMP may be related to a "triggering of the immune system" by a preceding viral illness, as one quarter of their patients had a viral prodrome up to 3 weeks before the onset. Of course, other illnesses—such as viral illness, Mollaret's meningitis, Lyme disease, and neurosyphilis—need to be considered in the differential diagnosis. Regardless of the etiology, the illness is self-limited and without permanent sequelae.

J.R. Berger, M.D.

3 Neuromuscular Disease

MR Spectroscopy in Amyotrophic Lateral Sclerosis/Motor Neuron Disease
Pioro EP (Cleveland Clinic Found, Ohio)
J Neurol Sci 152:S49–S53, 1997
3–1

Objective.—In vivo assessments of neuronal and axonal abnormalities can be performed with proton magnetic resonance spectroscopy (^{1}H-MRS) and proton magnetic resonance spectroscopic imaging (^{1}H-MRSI). These studies have been used to evaluate patients with a wide range of CNS diseases, including amyotrophic lateral sclerosis/motor neuron disease (ALS/MND). Such studies could aid in confirming the diagnosis and understanding the pathogenesis of ALS/MND. The MR spectroscopic findings in ALS/MND were presented.

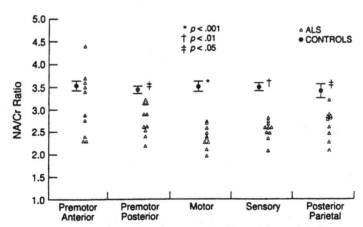

FIGURE 1.—Scatterplot of NA/Cr values in various cortical regions shows relatively constant means (approximately 3.5 ± SEM) in control individuals (n = 12) but significantly decreased ratios in the motor ($P < 0.001$), sensory ($P < 0.01$), posterior parietal ($P < 0.01$), and posterior premotor ($P < 0.05$) cortices of patients with amyotropic lateral sclerosis (*ALS*) (n = 10). In contrast, no significant difference in N-acetyl groups/creatine-phosphocreatine (*NA/Cr*) values is seen between patients and controls in the anterior premotor region. Data from Pioro et al. (1994). (Courtesy of Pioro EP: MR spectroscopy in amyotrophic lateral sclerosis/motor neuron disease. *J Neurol Sci* 152:S49–S53, 1997.)

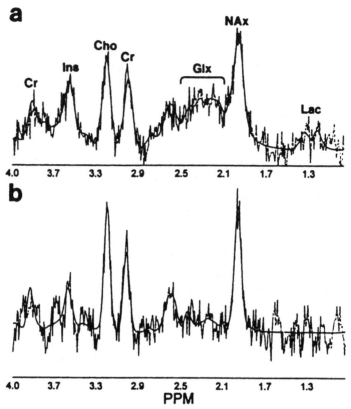

FIGURE 3.—LCModel analysis fit (*smooth line*) of proton MR spectroscopic imaging (¹H-MRSI) data (*irregular line*) obtained from the medulla of a patient with amyotrophic lateral sclerosis (AML) (**A**) and a control individual (**B**). The peaks identified include: creatine/phosphocreatine (*Cr*), *myo*-inositol (*Ins*), choline (*Cho*), *Glx* (glutamate + glutamine), *NAx* (*N*-acetylaspartate + *N*-acetylaspartylglutamate), and lactate (*Lac*). Note the higher Glx signal in the ALS patient (**B**) compared to the control individual (**A**). This Glx elevation is the result of increased glutamate and not glutamine. Resonant frequencies of the chemical species are expressed in parts per million (*PPM*). (Courtesy of Pioro EP: MR spectroscopy in amyotrophic lateral sclerosis/motor neuron disease. *J Neurol Sci* 152:S49–S53, 1997.)

Findings.—The brain metabolites choline (Cho), creatine/phosphocreatine (Cr), and N-acetyl (NA) groups are all depicted by both long and short echo time (TE) proton spectroscopy. Long TE spectroscopic studies of the sensorimotor cortex and brain stem of ALS patients show a significantly reduced NA/Cr ratio—an indicator of neural integrity—thus suggesting neuronal dysfunction or loss (Fig 1). The reduction in NA/Cr is proportional to the degree of clinical upper motor neuron deficit. Other metabolites relevant to ALS/MND, such as glutamate (Glu) and glutamine (Gln), are also depicted by short TE ¹H-MRS and ¹H-MRSI (Fig 3). Initial studies using short TE ¹H-MRSI to assess the medulla of patients with ALS/MND have found decreased NA/Cr values and elevated Glu+Gln/Cr ratios, the latter reaching higher levels in patients with a more rapid course of disease.

Discussion.—Noninvasive MR spectroscopic studies may provide useful insights into ALS/MND. Initial studies have demonstrated neuronal dysfunction and/or loss, most prominent in the sensorimotor cortex. Elevated Glu+Gln/Cr is present as well. This finding suggests the presence of abnormal glutamate metabolism in ALS/MND, whether occurring before or after the medullary neuronal and axonal degeneration.

▶ Magnetic resonance spectroscopy is one of the modern techniques for evaluating brain function and chemistry that has resulted from advances in neuroimaging. Magnetic resonance spectroscopy has its limitations with current machines because it can only investigate brain chemistry based on proton activities. Nevertheless, useful information can be derived. Here, Pioro reports decreased levels of a neuronal marker N-acetyl-aspartate (NAA), specifically in the sensorimotor cortex of patients with ALS. The low NAA levels seem to correlate particularly with upper motor neuron signs. There is an intriguing comment in the paper about a possible increase in glutamate and glutamine in ALS brains that needs further investigation.

W.G. Bradley, D.M., F.R.C.P.

Early and Late Losses of Motor Units After Poliomyelitis
McComas AJ, Quartly C, Griggs RC (McMaster Univ, Hamilton, Canada; Univ of Rochester, NY)
Brain 120:1415–1421, 1997   3–2

Background.—Patients who contracted poliomyelitis prior to the introduction of vaccinations develop a delayed illness progression, typified by further weakness. It has been hypothesized that this delayed progression is simply a more rapid onset of normal motor neuron aging, exacerbated by compensatory adjustments to the illness. Others believe that delayed progression is due to a continuing immunologic reaction to the previously infected motor neurons. To determine whether there is a delayed loss of functional motor neurons in these patients, muscle innervation was examined in those with a history of polio using motor-unit number estimation (MUNE).

Methods.—Motor-unit number estimation was used to evaluate muscle innervation in 76 patients with prior poliomyelitis. A motor nervous stimulus was gradually increased from a subthreshold value so that muscle response occurred in discreet steps, each reflecting the excitation of an additional motor unit. The motor-unit number estimation was determined by dividing the mean peak-to-peak amplitude of the increments into the peak-to-peak amplitude of the maximal respone of that muscle. Measurements of terminal motor latency and impulse-conduction-velocities were also performed. Sensory nerve conduction studies of the hands and feet were carried out.

Results.—Of the 76 patients, 68 were older than 70 years of age. Among these older patients, delayed musculoskeletal symptoms had appeared in

TABLE 3.—Comparison of MUNEs and M-Wave Amplitudes After a 2-Year Interval

	MUNE (%)	M-wave (%)
Initial values	106.7 ± 24.7	109.2 ± 19.0
After 2 years	93.3 ± 24.7	90.8 ± 19.0

A total of 95 muscles were studied. Values were expressed as percentages of means for each pair of observations. Reductions in MUNE and M-wave were both highly significant. (P < 0.001).
Abbreviation: MUNE, motor-unit number estimation.
(By permission of Oxford University Press. McComas AJ, Quartly C, Griggs RC: Early and Late Losses of Motor Units After Poliomyelitis *Brain* 120:1415–1421, 1997.)

64. The average latency interval between disease and the onset of delayed symptoms was approximately 38 years. There was an 87% incidence of denervated muscle in the previously affected limbs and a 65% incidence of denervated muscle in the previously unaffected limbs. There were significant differences in muscle denervation within the same limb. Surviving motor neurons in partially denervated muscles tended to be proportionally enlarged, similar to the enlargement observed in amyotrophic lateral sclerosis (ALS). This enlargement was not present in every muscle. Of the 188 muscles with electromographic features of chronic denervation examined, only 9 had fibrillations or positive sharp waves. After a 2-year interval, 95 muscles from 18 patients were re-examined. There was a 13.4% overall reduction in motor-unit number and an 18.4% reduction in M-wave amplitude. Both of these changes were highly significant (Table 3). The rate of motor-unit loss in the patients in this group was twice as high as that of healthy age-matched controls. The rate of motor unit loss varied between patients.

Conclusions.—Motor-unit number estimation was used to evaluate muscle innervation in 76 patients who had previously had poliomyelitis. Delayed denervation was detected in both clinically affected and unaffected muscles and appeared to be ongoing. This progression appeared to be more rapid than that occurring during normal aging. Axonal sprouting, similar to that seen in ALS, was detected in some cases.

▶ About 20% of patients who suffered poliomyelitis 25 or more years ago had a variety of complaints develop that are grouped together as the "postpolio syndrome." In the last few years, there has been a heated debate about whether such a syndrome exists and what the boundaries of that syndrome are. Postpolio muscular atrophy is the term applied to a condition in which there is slow but progressive deterioration of previously affected and reinnervated muscles. Studies from the Mayo group and Scandinavia have produced evidence suggesting that there is much variability from 1 patient to another, and from 1 muscle to another, during a 5-year follow-up, and that a progressive deterioration may in fact not occur. Many of us who have seen a good number of these patients are convinced that at least functionally, they do slowly deteriorate. Whether that is simply the effect of aging superimposed on neuromuscular function that is already at the limit is unclear. Data such as that produced by McComas and colleagues are of great importance to elucidate this question. These studies clearly indicate that in patients with the postpolio syndrome, there is a progressive loss of motor units and a decrease in the size of those motor units, which might be due either to terminal denervation or to loss of the largest motor units. This article will add fuel to the fire for those of us who believe that postpolio muscular atrophy is a true entity.

W.G. Bradley, D.M., F.R.C.P.

Epidemiological Study of Guillain-Barré Syndrome in South East England
Rees JH, Thompson RD, Smeeton NC, et al (UMDS Guy's Hosp, London)
J Neurol Neurosurg Psychiatry 64:74–77, 1998   3–3

Introduction.—Plasma exchange and administration of intravenous human immunoglobulin (IgG) shorten the duration of ventilation and inability to walk in patients with Guillain-Barré syndrome. The effects of these treatment approaches on long-term prognosis is unknown. The incidence, treatment, and outcome of Guillain-Barré syndrome in 79 patients in 1993–1994 in southeast England was compared with that of 100 patients from 1983–1984 in another part of southeast England.

Methods.—Patient outcome was compared for the 2 time periods. The effect of several variables (age, sex, previous diarrheal illness, treatment with IgG or plasma exchange, mechanical ventilation, transfer to or admission to a neurology center, and comorbidity) on 1-year outcome was assessed.

Results.—Of 79 patients, 35 were male and 44 were female (3 were children, 2 male and 1 female). The crude annual incidence of Guillain-Barré syndrome was 1.2/100,000 population; 1.5/100,000 when adjusted for undetected disease. Twenty of 79 patients (25%) needed mechanical ventilation for an average of 23 days. Treatment included IgG in 36 (46%) patients, plasma exchange in 5 (6%), both treatments in 11 (14%), steroids in 3 (4%), and no immunomodulatory treatment in 25 (32%). At 1-year follow-up, 6 (8%) patients had died (all were older than 60), 3 (4%) remained bedbound or ventilator dependent, 7 (9%) were unable to walk unaided, 14 (17%) were unable to run, and 49 (62%) had a complete or nearly complete recovery. There was a significant correlation between increasing age and poorer outcome.

Conclusion.—Even with the routine use of modern immunomodulatory treatments, patients with Guillain-Barré syndrome continue to have considerable morbidity and mortality.

▶ Early large studies of Guillain-Barré syndrome patients showed a death rate of 5% to 10%, with a permanent disability rate of about 5% to 10% on follow-up at ≥2 years after the acute attack. It has been the general impression (and hope) that with improved intensive care and the use of intravenous immunoglobulin or plasma exchange for treating Guillain-Barré syndrome, the mortality rate and prognosis would be improved. This regional survey from the Southeast of England, where medical care is generally of a high standard, indicates that the mortality and prognosis have not changed significantly over the years. The follow-up period of 1 year is shorter than is usually used in such studies, and a higher degree of recovery may be expected at a 2-year follow-up. Nevertheless, the 8% mortality must be noted.

W.G. Bradley, D.M., F.R.C.P.

Diagnostic Value of Sural Nerve Biopsy in Chronic Inflammatory Demyelinating Polyneuropathy
Molenaar DSM, Vermeulen M, de Haan R (Univ of Amsterdam)
J Neurol Neurosurg Psychiatry 64:84–89, 1998   3–4

Introduction.—Sural nerve biopsy is valuable in establishing the cause of peripheral neuropathies and should be performed only after careful clinical, laboratory, and neurophysiologic assessment. Its use in suspected chronic inflammatory demyelinating polyneuropathy (CIDP) has not been established. The additional diagnostic value of sural nerve biopsy was assessed in 64 patients in whom CIDP was suspected.

Methods.—Medical records were reviewed from 7 university hospitals in the Netherlands of patients who underwent sural nerve biopsy between 1989 and 1994. The additional diagnostic value of sural nerve biopsy was assessed with multivariate logistic regression. Data regarding 6 clinical features (remitting course, symmetric sensorimotor neuropathy in arms and legs, areflexia, raised CSF protein concentration, nerve conduction studies consistent with demyelination, and absence of comorbidity or relevant laboratory abnormalities) were entered into a logistical model. All

---

TABLE 2.—Clinical Features and Sural Nerve Biopsy in 23 Patients With CIDP and 41 Patients With Another Diagnosis: Sensitivity, Specificity, and Positive LR For the Diagnosis of CIDP

Clinical feature	Sensitivity	Specificity	Positive LR for CIDP
(1) Remitting course	0.39	0.88	3.21
(2) Symmetric sensorimotor neuropathy	0.70	0.78	3.17
(3) Areflexia	0.52	0.80	2.67
(4) Raised CSF protein concentration (>0.5 g/L)	0.87	0.44	1.55
Highly raised (>1 g/L)	0.57	0.88	4.63
(5) Neurophysiological studies consistent with CIDP	0.87	0.85	5.94
(6) Absence of comorbidity	0.65	0.63	1.78
(7) Sural nerve biopsy consistent with CIDP	0.61	0.78	2.77

Abbreviation: LR, likelihood ratio.
(Courtesy of Molenaar DSM, Vermeulen M, de Haan R: Diagnostic value of sural nerve biopsy in chronic inflammatory demyelinating polyneuropathy. *J Neurol Neurosurg Psychiatry* 64:84–89, 1998.)

significant features identified from this model and results of a sural nerve biopsy were forced into a second logistic model. The diagnostic performance of a neurologist proficient in diagnosis of peripheral nerve disorders was evaluated by receiver operating characteristics (ROC) curve analysis.

Results.—Outcome of the first logistic analysis indicated that CSF protein concentration >1 g/L and neurophysiologic analysis consistent with demyelination were strong predictors of CIDP. Upon forcing the significant features and the sural nerve biopsy data into the model, an independent predictive value of sural nerve biopsy could not be determined. Neurophysiologic studies consistent with demyelination, highly raised CSF protein concentrations, and absence of comorbidity were strong predictors for CIDP (Table 2). The neurologist was able to differentiate patients with and without CIDP. There was no significant improvement in his diagnostic performance when he was given results of sural nerve biopsy.

Conclusion.—There is no need to include sural nerve biopsy to confirm diagnosis of CIDP because it has no value in clinical practice.

▶ The diagnosis of CIDP is based on clinical and electrophysiologic findings at this stage. It would be very helpful if there was a pathologic accompaniment to allow nerve biopsy to be of diagnostic significance. This is an excellent study evaluating the sensitivity and specificity of the clinical features, neurophysiologic studies, and sural nerve biopsy in 64 patients. The sural nerve biopsy did not add to the reliability of the diagnosis in this series. Full details of the technical studies performed and the results in the sural nerve biopsies are not given, but teased fiber preparations were studied from all specimens, and morphometry and electron microscopy in over half.

I came to similar conclusions in a study of 10 sural nerve biopsies from patients with clinical and electrophysiologically diagnosed CIDP. Most had evidence of axonal degeneration, indicating some more proximal lesion, and only a small amount of segmental demyelination, and virtually no inflammatory infiltration was seen. It does not appear that sural nerve biopsy helps other than to exclude a vasculitis or some other etiology.

W.G. Bradley, D.M., F.R.C.P.

Association of IgM Type Anti-GM1 Antibodies and Muscle Strength in Chronic Acquired Demyelinating Polyneuropathy
Bech E, Andersen H, Ørntoft TF, et al (Aarhus Univ, Denmark)
Ann Neurol 43:72–78, 1998   3–5

Introduction.—The pathogenetic significance of anti-GM1 antibodies in chronic acquired demyelinating polyneuropathy (CADP) is not understood. The association between muscle performance and IgM anti-GM1 antibody titer levels in patients with CADP was assessed using an assay with internal calibrators combined with standardized isokinetic dynamometry.

TABLE 2.—Change of Muscle Strength and Anti-GM1 Levels During the Study Period

Case No.	Change of Isokinetic Muscle Strength (%)	Change of MRC Score (%)	Anti-GM1 Level at Start (AU)	Change of Anti-GM1 (%)
1	+29	ND	87	−24
2	−30	−20	55	+10
3	+24	+17	>200	−22
4	+89	+17	172	−39
5	−8	+2	25	+9
6	+600	+43	26	−48
7	+95	+50	56	−47 (two samples only)
8	+25	+16	130	−65

Abbreviation: MRC, Medical Research Council.
(Courtesy of Bech E, Andersen H, Ørntoft TF: Association of IgM anti-GM1 antibodies and muscle strength in chronic acquired demyelinating polyneuropathy. *Ann Neurol* 43:72–78, 1998, copyright ANA.)

Methods.—Eight patients with CADP underwent a standard diagnostic program including physical examination and biochemical, hematologic, and radiologic screening. Electrophysiologic testing was done, with special attention to the presence of peripheral motor conduction block, conduc-

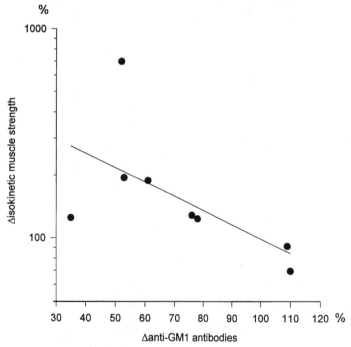

FIGURE 3.—The relationship between change of muscular strength evaluated by isokinetic dynamometry and the change of the levels of IgM anti-GM1 antibodies ($r = 0.78$, $P = 0.036$). (Courtesy of Bech E, Andersen H, Ørntoft TF: Association of IgM anti-GM1 antibodies and muscle strength in chronic acquired demyelinating polyneuropathy. *Ann Neurol* 43:72–78, 1998. Reprinted from Annals of Neurology by permission of Little, Brown, and Company, Inc., copyright ANA.)

tion velocities, F-wave latencies, and distal latencies. Anti-GM1 antibodies were monitored using a standardized enzyme-linked immunosorbent assay technique. Isokinetic muscle strength was assessed periodically during an observation period that ranged from 29 to 171 weeks (mean 24 weeks). *Results.*—Strength improved in 6 of 8 patients by a median of 54.5%. Anti-GM1 titers dropped in all 6 patients by 43%. Muscle performance dropped by 30% and 8%, respectively, in 2 patients, and anti-GM1 titers increased by 10% and 9%, respectively (Table 2). There was an inverse correlation between change in anti-GM1 and muscle performance (Fig 3). Clinical scoring of muscle performance using the Medical Research Council scale did not show an association with anti-GM1.

Conclusion.—The close relationship between muscle performance and titer level indicates that anti-GM1 has a pathogenic role in CADP or is closely related to the disease mechanism itself.

▶ This article describes 8 patients with chronic inflammatory demyelinating polyneuropathy, 3 of whom originally had multifocal motor neuropathy with conduction block. One of these later developed sensory symptoms and signs. Only 4 of these patients had increased anti-GM1 antibodies, and in none of them were their levels very high. The study is intended to review the relationship between anti-GM1 antibody titers and muscle strength in relation to treatment with intravenous immunoglobulin in 6 of the cases, plasma exchange in 1 of the cases, and spontaneous remission in 1 of the cases. Though an inverse relationship appeared between the anti-GM1 antibody titer and muscle strength, it still remains possible that the anti-GM1 antibodies are, in fact, an epiphenomenon and that some other antibody is producing the neurologic dysfunction. This is supported by the recent study of Hirota et al.,[1] indicating that only 1 out of 44 serum samples from patients with Guillain-Barré syndrome or multifocal motor neuropathy produced conduction block in right ventral root fibers in vitro, compared with 82% of fibers treated with anti-Ga1 C serum and 100% of fibers treated with tetrodotoxin. Rabid anti-GM1 sera produced conduction block in only 5% of cases.

W.G. Bradley, D.M., F.R.C.P.

Reference

1. Hirota N, Kaji R, Bostock M, et al: The physiological effect of anti-GM1, antibodies on saltatory conduction and transmembrane currents in single motor axons. *Brain* 120–2159–2169, 1997.

Peripheral Neuropathy Associated With Sicca Complex

Grant IA, Hunder GG, Homburger HA, et al (Mayo Clinic, Rochester, Minn)
Neurology 48:855–862, 1997   3–6

Introduction.—Patients with Sjögren's syndrome (SS) have peripheral neuropathy and sicca complex (xerophthalmia and xerostomia); extraglandular involvement such as arthritis and vasculitis is common. Sensory

TABLE 1.—Clinical and Serologic Features of Patients With Peripheral Neuropathy and Sicca Complex

Neuropathy type*	n	Sicca symptoms		Extraglandular features†		Serology					
		Present	Presenting feature	Present	≥2	SS-A	SS-B	ANA‡	RF§	Increased IgG	Increased ESR
Sensory											
Polyneuropathy	21	20	4	4	1	2/17	0/17	5/20	1/18	3/17	4/26
Ganglionopathy	12	10	0	1	0	2/12	1/12	2/11	0/11	3/9	2/10
Sensorimotor	9	9	1	4	2	1/8	0/8	3/9	1/8	4/9	1/9
Polyradiculoneuropathy	6	6	0	0	0	0/5	0/5	0/6	0/5	1/6	0/6
Trigeminal	4	3	1	1	0	0/3	0/3	0/4	0/2	1/3	1/3
Multiple mononeuropathy	3	3	1	3‖	2	0/4	0/4	1/4	1/4	0/4	2/4
Autonomic	1	1	0	0	0	0	0	0	np	0	0
Multiple cranial	1	1	0	0	0	0	0	0	0	0	0

*More than one type may be present in a given patient.
†Weight loss excluded.
‡Titer > 1:160.
§>79 units.
‖P < 0.05 compared with other neuropathy types.
Abbreviations: ANA, antinuclear antibody; *ESR*, erythrocyte sedimentation rate; *np*, not performed; *RF*, rheumatoid factor; *SS*, Sjögren's syndrome.
(Courtesy of Grant IA, Hunder GG, Homburger HA, et al: Peripheral neuropathy associated with sicca complex. *Neurology* 48:855–862, 1997. Reprinted from *Neurology* by permission of Little, Brown and Company, Inc.)

neuropathies are often associated with sicca complex in the absence of extraglandular features, however, and this combination may represent a distinctive syndrome. Disease characteristics in patients with sicca complex and peripheral neuropathy were studied retrospectively.

Methods.—Cases were identified through a computerized search of medical records of Mayo Clinic patients from 1989 to 1995. Two sets of diagnoses were of interest: sicca complex, keratoconjunctivitis sicca, or SS; and peripheral polyneuropathy, multiple mononeuropathy, or polyganglionopathy. Patients meeting established criteria for SS were categorized as having primary or secondary SS based on the presence or absence of another connective tissue disease.

Results.—Fifty-four patients, 42 women and 12 men with a mean age of 60 years, met study criteria for both sicca complex and peripheral neuropathy. Thirty-three patients met SS criteria; the primary form was present in 31. The diagnosis of SS was definite (4 criteria met) in 9 patients and probable (3 criteria met) in 24. Forty-seven (87%) patients were initially evaluated for peripheral neuropathy. Sensory neuropathies were predominant in all 54 patients and in the 33 who fulfilled SS criteria (Table 1). Sicca symptoms, present in 93%, were generally mild and were the presenting complaint in only 11% of patients. Saliva gland biopsies were performed in 33 patients and had positive results in 73%. Although vasculitic neuropathy was demonstrated in only 2 cases, 70% of nerve biopsies showed nonspecific epineural inflammation. There was little evidence of systemic disease, particularly in patients with sensory polyganglionopathy. The most specific serologic marker of SS, antibodies to extractable nuclear antigens, was present in 10.4% of patients.

Discussion.—This group of patients with coexisting neuropathy and sicca complex often met SS criteria. However, SS was seldom suspected by the referring physician, and most patients had a limited degree of systemic involvement. Neuropathies rather than sicca led the patient to seek medical care. Peripheral neuropathy and isolated sicca complex appear to form a distinctive syndrome in which sensory polyneuropathy and polyganglionopathy predominate. Tests of ocular or salivary involvement provide diagnostic information, but serology is very insensitive.

▶ This is a landmark study from the Mayo Clinic database describing 54 patients with associated sicca complex and peripheral neuropathy. The pleomorphism of the peripheral neuropathy is important, for no single type of neuropathy suggests sicca complex. Since xerophthalmia and xerostomia are often relatively mild, this disease association has to be thought of in almost every type of polyneuropathy in which no cause can be found. Antibody screening is not particularly helpful. A high index of suspicion and salivary or lacrimal gland biopsy is the only way to establish the diagnosis clearly. Although the study gives little in the way of information on treatment or response, immunosuppressant therapy in these cases is often beneficial.

W.G. Bradley, D.M., F.R.C.P.

Painful Proximal Diabetic Neuropathy: Inflammatory Nerve Lesions and Spontaneous Favorable Outcome

Said G, Elgrably F, Lacroix C, et al (Université Paris Sud; Service de Diabé-tologie–Hôtel Dieu de Paris)
Ann Neurol 41:762–770, 1997   3–7

Introduction.—Proximal diabetic neuropathy (PDN) of the lower limbs is a painful condition that usually improves spontaneously within months. Relapses on the other side are common, however, and disabling weakness and sensory loss may persist. Treatment with corticosteroids or with other immunomodulators is reported to bring dramatic relief in some cases. Improvement in 4 patients soon after undergoing a nerve biopsy was reported.

Methods.—The patients, 3 men and 1 woman, ranged in age from 47 to 82 years. All had non–insulin-dependent diabetes mellitus and were re-ferred for painful PDN of the lower limbs. Under local anesthesia, the patients underwent biopsy of the intermediate cutaneous nerve of the thigh. The quadriceps muscle was sampled during the same procedure, and specimens were prepared for analysis.

Results.—The nerve specimen from patient 1 showed a conspicuous inflammatory infiltrate around epineurial blood vessels (Fig 1). Mononu-clear cells predominated in the infiltrate, and a few fibers were undergoing axonal degeneration. Myelinated and unmyelinated fibers were markedly reduced. T lymphocytes made up 60% of the mononuclear infiltrate of specimens; B lymphocytes, 30%; and macrophages, 10%. In the nerve specimen from patient 3, the fascicles exhibited marked asymmetry, and only the largest fascicle (Fig 3) retained some fibers. Muscle biopsy speci-mens showed neurogenic atrophy in all 4 patients, with no inflammatory infiltration or abnormality of blood vessels. Pain disappeared within days after the nerve biopsy with no additional therapy. Two patients remain symptom-free at almost 1 year and more than 2 years after biopsy. The 2 other patients have residual proximal weakness.

Discussion.—All 4 patients with PDN experienced relief of pain after undergoing nerve biopsy to determine whether they had inflammatory nerve lesions that would justify treatment with corticosteroids or immu-nomodulators. The disappearance of pain may have been coincidental, or the procedure may have interrupted a sensory branch of a nerve producing pain.

▶ Painful lumbosacral plexopathies present a difficult differential diagnosis. This condition can occur in diabetes, with carcinomatous infiltration, with evidence of a vasculopathy and increased sedimentation rate,[1] and also without known cause. There have been suggestions that diabetic, inflam-matory, and idiopathic lumbosacral plexopathies can respond to immuno-suppressant therapy.[2] Diabetic lumbosacral plexopathy has been known for a long time to be eventually self-limiting in the majority of cases, with a moderately good eventual recovery within approximately 2 years. The ques-

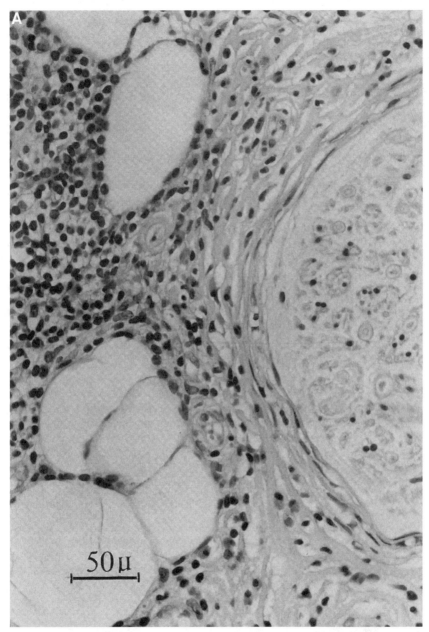

FIGURE 1.—Histologic appearance of the intermediate cutaneous nerve of the thigh of Patient 1 with non–insulin-dependent diabetes and proximal neuropathy of the lower limbs. **A,** cross section of the paraffin-embedded nerve specimen showing conspicuous inflammatory infiltration made of mononuclear cells, predominantly lymphocytes, in the epineurial area. (Hematoxylin-eosin.) (Courtesy of Said G, Elgrably F, Lacroix C, et al: Painful proximal diabetic neuropathy: Inflammatory nerve lesions and spontaneous favorable outcome. *Ann Neurol* 41:762–770, 1997. Reprinted from Annals of Neurology by permission of Little, Brown and Company, Inc., copyright ANA.)

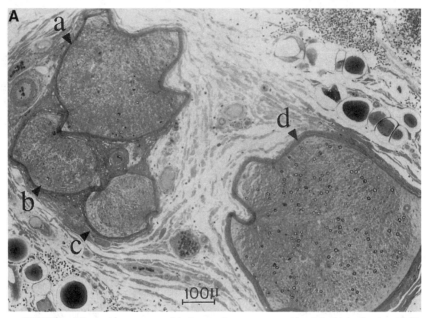

FIGURE 3.—Histologic appearance of the intermediate cutaneous nerve of the thigh of patient 3 with non–insulin-dependent diabetes and proximal neuropathy of the lower limbs. A, cross section of a nerve specimen showing asymmetrical loss of nerve fibers. Only the largest fascicle retained some fibers. (Courtesy of Said G, Elgrably F, Lacroix C, et al: Painful proximal diabetic neuropathy: Inflammatory nerve lesions and spontaneous favorable outcome. *Ann Neurol* 41:762–770, 1997. Reprinted from Annals of Neurology by permission of Little, Brown and Company, Inc., copyright ANA.)

tion raised by this study is whether prior reports of "therapeutic responsiveness" are real or represent simply spontaneous remission.

W.G. Bradley, D.M., F.R.C.P.

References

1. Bradley WG, Chad D, Verghese JP, et al: Painful lumbosacral plexopathy with elevated erythrocyte sedimentation rate: A treatable inflammatory syndrome. *Ann Neurol* 15:457–464, 1984.
2. Verma A, Bradley WG: High-dose intravenous immunoglobulin therapy in chronic progressive lumbosacral plexopathy. *Neurology* 44:248–250, 1994.

Charcot–Marie–Tooth Disease Type 1A With 17p11.2 Duplication: Clinical and Electrophysiological Phenotype Study and Factors Influencing Disease Severity in 119 Cases
Birouk N, Gouider R, Le Guern E, et al (Service d'Explorations Fonctionnelles, Paris; Hôpital de la Salpêtrière, Paris)
Brain 120:813–823, 1997   3–8

Background.—Differences in clinical, genetic, electrophysiologic, and histologic characteristics of Charcot-Marie-Tooth syndrome (CMT) led to a classification based on 7 types. Subsequent genetic studies resulted in a new classification of CMT, type 1A (CMT1A), which includes patients with 17p11.2 duplication or peripheral myelin protein 22 (PMP22) point-mutation. Such patients have the same genetic defect as those with CMT but exhibit a wide range of clinical disability. The clinical and electrophysiologic features of a large group of patients with CMT1A were presented.

Methods.—The 119 patients were examined by a single neurologist using a defined protocol. Data collected included age at onset, neurologic disability scores, functional disability score (FDS) based on the ability to walk and run, and findings of electrophysiologic and molecular studies. Patients were also examined for the presence of foot deformities, scoliosis, nerve hypertrophy, and associated signs.

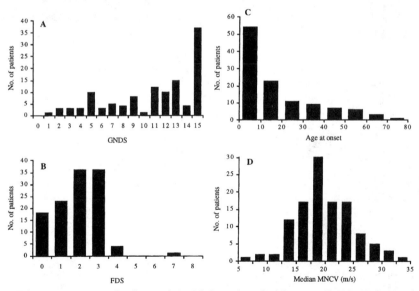

FIGURE 1.—Frequency distribution of (**A**) global neurologic disability score (*GNDS*), (**B**) functional disability scale (*FDS*), (**C**) age at onset, and (**D**) median motor nerve conduction velocity (*MNCV*) in 199 patients with 17p11.2 duplication. (Courtesy of Birouk N, Gouider R, Le Guern E, et al: Charcot-Marie-Tooth disease type 1A with 17p11.2 duplication: Clinical and electrophysiological phenotype study and factors influencing disease severity in 119 cases. *Brain* 120:813–823, 1997, by permission of Oxford University Press.)

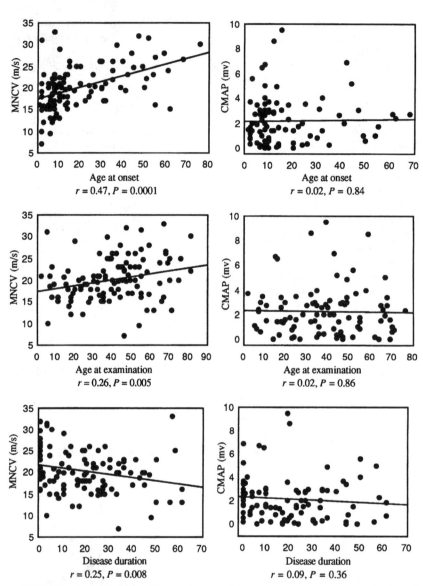

FIGURE 2.—Scatter diagrams with regression analysis between age at onset, age at examination and disease duration and between median nerve motor nerve conduction velocity (*MNCV*) (in m/sec) and median nerve, (*CMAP*) (in mV). Compound muscle action potential. (Courtesy of Birouk N, Gouider R, Le Guern E, et al: Charcot-Marie-Tooth disease type 1A with 17p11.2 duplication: Clinical and electrophysiological phenotype study and factors influencing disease severity in 119 cases. *Brain* 120:813–823, 1997, by permission of Oxford University Press.)

Results.—Fifty-five of 93 families with CMT1 tested positive for the 17p11.2 duplication and were classified as CMT1A. Of the 196 individuals with the 17p11.2 duplication, 119 had complete data. There were 65 female and 54 male patients ranging in age from 2 to 81 years. The mean age of the group at examination was 40.2 years; mean age at onset in symptomatic individuals was 19.4 years. Predominant clinical signs were muscle weakness and wasting in the lower limbs. Foot deformities and kyphoscoliosis were common. Even patients with no clinical sensory loss had abnormal sensory potentials and reduced motor nerve conduction velocity in all nerves. One third had the maximum score on the global neurologic disability score; FDS was stage 2 or 3 in 61% of patients, indicating that they had difficulty in walking or running but were still ambulatory. Motor nerve conduction velocity (MNCV) was less than or equal to 30 m/sec in all but 4 individuals who were at-risk relatives (Fig 1). Findings did not differ significantly between men and women or by parental transmission from the father or mother. Median nerve MNCV (Fig 2) was directly related to age at disease onset, and early onset together with greatly reduced median nerve MNCV were predictive of a more severe disease course.

Discussion.—In patients with CMT1A with 17p11.2 duplication, the disease was shown to be clinically progressive, whatever the age at onset. Although median nerve MNCV and compound muscle action potential did not change with time, neurologic deficits and functional disability increased. The phenotype is quite variable, even among siblings.

▶ From the time when the mutation responsible for an inherited disease is recognized, it becomes of great interest to examine genotype-phenotype correlations and to determine whether clinically atypical cases have the same mutation. The classification of CMT has been a fertile field for the splitters and lumpers. We now have the ability, at least in patients with chromosome 17p duplications, to ask these questions. It must be remembered, however, that there still may be subtle molecular genetic differences between different patients in terms of the specific size and location of the duplications. With that caveat, this is a very interesting study, with a number of lessons for our previous discussions about classification.

W.G. Bradley, D.M., F.R.C.P.

Hereditary Thermosensitive Neuropathy: An Autosomal Dominant Disorder of the Peripheral Nervous System
Magy L, Birouk N, Vallat JM, et al (Hôpital de la Salpêtrière, Paris; CHRU Dupuytren, Limoges, France)
Neurology 48:1684–1690, 1997   3–9

Introduction.—Eight patients with a hereditary neuropathy with an apparent thermosensitivity (HTN) of autosomal dominant inheritance were described. Fever caused by a variety of infectious diseases was found to be the triggering factor of the HTN, which is characterized by episodic attacks of muscle weakness.

Methods.—All family members underwent complete neurologic examinations and had detailed histories taken. Medical records were reviewed when available. The index patient and 14 relatives underwent electrophysiologic studies, and blood samples were collected from all participating individuals for molecular analysis. A biopsy specimen from the sural nerve of the index patient was obtained approximately 1 year after his last attack and examined microscopically.

Results.—The index patient, a 56-year-old man, experienced his first attack at age 41. The precipitating fever was caused by an upper urinary tract infection. Numbness was present in all 4 limbs, followed by severe quadriparesis and difficulty swallowing; complete areflexia was present. The patient recovered in 3 weeks, but experienced similar symptoms during subsequent episodes of fever. Electrophysiologic studies suggested a demyelinating polyneuropathy. The remaining 7 affected relatives, 3 men and 4 women, had similar fever-triggered attacks characterized by ascending muscle weakness, paresthesia, and areflexia. Four of the patients experienced up to 5 such reversible attacks. The mean patient age at onset was 13. One patient, a 7-year-old child, died during a severe episode with respiratory failure.

Discussion.—In this kinship with no consanguinity, clinically affected individuals were present in each generation. Because HTN is always transmitted by an affected individual, the disease is highly penetrant. Pathologic findings and electrophysiologic studies indicated the presence of a reversible demyelinating neuropathy. Thermal sensitivity of demyelinated nerves is well established, and thermosensitivity is an important feature of HTN. Loci causing other hereditary demyelinating neuropathies, such as Charcot-Marie-Tooth disease (CMT) type 1 and hereditary neuropathy with liability to pressure palsies (HNPP) were excluded by linkage analysis, demonstrating that HTN is not allelic to CMT type 1 or to HNPP.

▶ Patients with recurrent demyelinating neuropathies are generally suffering from chronic inflammatory demyelinating polyneuropathy, an autoimmune disease. Autoimmune processes can also lead to exacerbation in hereditary CMT. In this family the development of relapses of a demyelinating neuropathy from the development of a fever appears not to have been reported before. Detailed analysis of the family does not suggest that this is a banal observation, with exacerbation of a pre-existing demyelinating neuropathy with increased body temperature, a well-known phenomenon. It appears that fever does in some way produce active demyelination rather like the Guillain-Barré syndrome. Elucidation of the molecular mechanism for this disease will be very interesting.

W.G. Bradley, D.M., F.R.C.P.

Ocular Myasthenia Gravis: Response to Long Term Immunosuppressive Treatment
Sommer N, Sigg B, Melms A, et al (Eberhard-Karls-Univ Tübingen, Germany)
J Neurol Neurosurg Psychiatry 62:156–162, 1997   3–10

Background.—Myasthenia gravis is an autoimmune disease that sometimes manifests as a relatively mild ocular disease. The best method for treating ocular myasthenia gravis has not been determined. The results of the current therapies used to treat this condition were examined retrospectively.

Methods.—Of 178 patients with myasthenia gravis, 78 had ocular myasthenia gravis based on eye muscle weakness not resulting from other causes. In these 78 patients, myasthenia gravis had been diagnosed quite late, a mean (± SD) of 39.8 ± 93.5 months after symptoms developed. The mean disease duration was 8 years (range, 6 months to 58 years). The disease had been treated with immunosuppressants, corticosteroids, or thymectomy.

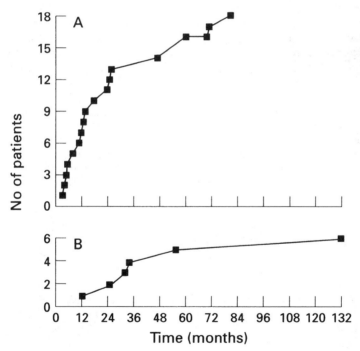

FIGURE 2.—Cumulative incidence of generalized symptoms in patients with initially purely ocular myasthenia gravis. **A** shows the patients without, **B** with immunosuppressive drug treatment. The median time to generalization was 16 months in **A** and 33 months in **B**. The risk of converting to generalized symptoms is greater during the first years, but is still present after many years. (Courtesy of Sommer N, Sigg B, Melms A, et al: Ocular myasthenia gravis: Response to long-term immunosuppressive treatment. *J Neurol Neurosurg Psychiatry* 62:156–162, 1997.)

Findings.—Generalized muscle weakness developed secondarily in 24 of 78 patients (31%) within 3–132 months after ocular symptoms became apparent. Treatments led to remission in 29 patients, improvement in 18, and no change in 7; no patient experienced a worsening of ocular symptoms. Pyridostigmine was given to 60 of 78 patients for an average of 45 months, and in 14 patients that was the sole treatment. Of those 14, 7 had considerable improvement, 6 had mild improvement, and 1 had no effect. Patients treated with the immunosuppressive drugs prednisolone (45 patients) or azathioprine or a combination (27 patients) were less likely to progress to generalized myasthenia gravis (only 12% did so, compared to 18 of 28 patients [64%] who did not receive immunosuppressants) (Fig 2). Thymectomy was performed in 12 patients an average of 50 months after symptom onset, and all but 1 were also treated with immunosuppressants. Of those 12, 6 achieved remission, 4 showed improved ocular muscle strength, and 2 subsequently had generalized disease.

Conclusions.—Overall, the prognosis for ocular myasthenia gravis is good. Treatment generally confines the disease to the eye muscles and achieves remission or improvement. In particular, early immunosuppressive treatment was associated with superior results. Thymectomy also provided a good outcome, but its results were not superior to those of medical management alone. On the basis of these results, in the majority of patients a combination of short-term pyridostigmine and prednisone is recommended. Long-term azathioprine may be required if prednisone therapy results in unacceptable side-effects.

▶ About a third of patients with ocular myasthenia gravis will have generalized symptoms, most within the first 5 years of the disease. Many of us believe that the use of immunosuppressants such as high-dose prednisone for purely ocular myasthenia is not indicated in view of the benignity of the disease and the severity of the side effects. However, if immunosuppressant therapy were to reduce the frequency of generalization, then this would add another factor in the equation. This article does appear to demonstrate a lower frequency of generalized myasthenia developing in patients receiving immunosuppressant therapy. It must be remembered that this is not a double-blind, controlled trial, which is still very much needed.

W.G. Bradley, D.M., F.R.C.P.

Clinical and Neurophysiological Features of Tick Paralysis
Grattan-Smith PJ, Morris JG, Johnston HM, et al (Univ of Sydney, Australia; Westmead Hosp, Sydney, Australia; Prince of Wales Children's Hosp, Sydney, Australia; et al)
Brain 120:1975–1987, 1997   3–11

Introduction.—Tick paralysis is an uncommon clinical problem. In Australia, most cases are caused by *Ixodes holocyclus*, which appears to be the most potent of the paralyzing ticks. The clinical and neurophysiologic features of 3 Australian boys and 3 girls, aged 2–12 years, with tick paralysis were described, along with a review of the literature.

Findings.—The findings suggested that tick paralysis is most common during the spring and summer and in children aged 1–5 years. The tick is usually found on the scalp; behind the ear is a common location. Initial prodromal symptoms are followed by an unsteady gait, then ascending, symmetric, flaccid paralysis. Cranial nerve involvement—notably, with both internal and external ophthalmoplegia—may occur early on. In the Australian children, the paralysis often got worse in the first day or two after the tick was removed; this is in contrast to paralysis caused by North American ticks. Children may require prolonged respiratory support. They recover eventually, although it may be several weeks before they can walk on their own. Treatment with tick antitoxin may be beneficial but carries a risk of acute allergic reactions and serum sickness. Neurophysiologic tests show low-amplitude compound muscle action potentials with normal motor conduction velocities, normal sensory studies, and a normal response to repetitive stimulation.

Discussion.—The clinical findings of tick paralysis were described, including the first description of the neurophysiologic effects. Although rare, this is a potentially fatal condition that should be suspected in all patients with signs of Guillain-Barré syndrome. The toxin of the Australian tick, *I. holocyclus*, is not completely understood but is similar in many ways to botulinum toxin.

▶ Tick paralysis is rare in humans despite the fact that many patients are infested with ticks in various parts of the world. In the United States it is said that recovery occurs within a few hours of removing the tick, but this was certainly not the experience in Australia, where this report comes from. A number of the patients continued to deteriorate and required ventilatory support for more than a week after removal of the tick. The toxin has been thought to be active at the neuromuscular junction, but in none of these patients was repetitive nerve stimulation abnormal. There was a reduction of compound muscle action potential, and in vitro studies have indicated an abnormality of the release of acetylcholine. The neuromuscular blockade was reversed by hypothermia. This article points out the need for hospitalization and careful observation of patients who have tick paralysis.

W.G. Bradley, D.M., F.R.C.P

A Novel Mitochondrial tRNA Phenylalanine Mutation Presenting With Acute Rhabdomyolysis

Chinnery PF, Johnson MA, Taylor RW, et al (Univ of New Castle upon Tyne, England)
Ann Neurol 41:408–410, 1997   3–12

Introduction.—Most cases of acute rhabdomyolysis or recurrent myoglobinuria with no apparent exogenous cause would have been classified as "idiopathic" until recently. A nuclear gene defect is now known to be the cause of many such cases. The first case of a mitochondrial tRNA gene point mutation presenting with acute rhabdomyolysis was reported.

> *Case Report.*—Man, 30, experienced muscle pain and weakness 3 hours after strenuous lifting. He had dark urine 6 hours later and stayed in bed the next day with general malaise. Although he was ambulant within 24 hours, his muscle strength did not return to normal for 2 weeks. Total serum creatine kinase level was grossly elevated 3 days after the episode (21,290 U/L); values returned to normal 2 weeks later. The patient had no family history of neuromuscular disease, and various clinical investigations yielded normal findings. Histochemical examination of a needle muscle biopsy specimen demonstrated classic subsarcolemmal accumulations of mitochondria. Cytochrome *c* oxidase activity was deficient in 68% of skeletal muscle fibers. The patient was found to have a respiratory chain defect associated with a novel heteroplasmic point mutation in the phenylalanine tRNA gene of the mitochondrial genome (mtDNA). Cytochrome *c* oxidase–negative fibers had significantly greater levels of mutant mtDNA than did cytochrome *c* oxidase–positive fibers (97% vs. 55%, respectively).

Discussion.—The diagnosis of acute rhabdomyolysis was confirmed by grossly elevated serum creatine kinase level after a period of weakness and muscle pain after strenuous exercise. The A-to-G transition at position 606 of the mitochondrial genome was believed to be the pathologic mutation responsible for the patient's syndrome. Histologic and biochemical investigations of skeletal muscle are needed in patients with apparently idiopathic myoglobinuria, and mitochondrial disease should be considered in the differential diagnosis of acute rhabdomyolysis.

▶ Rhabdomyolysis can occur as a result of toxic exposure, polymyositis, and in relation to disorders of energy metabolism such as carnitine palmitoyl transferase deficiency and disorders of glycolytic metabolism. A considerable number of patients with 1 or repeated attacks of rhabdomyolysis, however, do not have any of these conditions, and the underlying cause remains uncertain. This report of a patient with a mitochondrial DNA mutation causing acute rhabdomyolysis is very interesting, and prompts such detailed investigation in other patients with "idiopathic" rhabdomyolysis.

W.G. Bradley, D.M., F.R.C.P.

4 Pediatric Neurology

Measurement of Cerebral Blood Flow in Newborn Infants Using Near Infrared Spectroscopy With Indocyanine Green
Patel J, Marks K, Roberts I, et al (Hammersmith Hosp, London)
Pediatr Res 43:34–39, 1998   4–1

Introduction.—Cerebral blood flow (CBF) measurement in sick, newborn infants is useful in determining development of cerebral injury. Current methods expose infants to ionizing radiation or require a rapid change in arterial oxygen saturation (SaO_2), which is difficult to achieve in infants with severe respiratory insufficiency. An alternative method that may allow rapid and repeated measurements of CBF, by using near infrared spectroscopy (NIRS) with indocyanine green (ICG) dye as an intravascular tracer (CBF-ICG) is described.

Methods.—Six newborn infants with a median gestational age of 28 weeks (range, 26–38 weeks) and a median weight of 1.080 kg (0.885–3.730 kg) were assessed at postnatal age 10–60 hours. All infants required mechanical ventilation and supplemental oxygen. Indocyanine green dye 0.1 mg·kg was injected into an umbilical venous catheter. Blood ICG concentration was calculated using an optical umbilical artery catheter. Brain ICG concentration was measured by NIRS. The CBF-HbO_2 measurements were taken by rapidly increasing the inspired oxygen concentration; blood HbO_2 concentration was determined from SaO_2 measured by pulse oximetry. Brain HbO_2 concentration was evaluated by NIRS. A series of 3–5 CBF measurements were performed using each method before and after alternating the arterial carbon dioxide tension ($PaCO_2$). The methods were compared by using mean CBF values from several measurements of each method.

Results.—Ranges for measured variables were: 120–160[1] heart rate, 31–49 mm Hg mean arterial blood pressure, 85% to 98% mean SaO_2, 7.21–7.4 mean arterial pH, 7.2–12.2 kPa mean PaO_2, 4.0–6.8 kPa PaO_2, 4.1–9.9 mmol·L[1] blood glucose, and 14.2–16.6 g·dL[1] arterial hemoglobin. The $PaCO_2$ ranged from -0.2 to 0.5 kPa from the start to the end of each paired series of CBF measurements. Transcutaneous CO_2 tension varied from 0.3 and 0.5 kPa during the measured series. There was a significant correlation between the mean CBF-HbO_2 and the mean CBF-ICG (Fig 2). The mean difference between these 2 methods was -0.25 mL·100 g[1]·1[1].

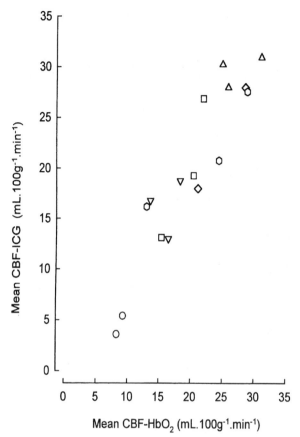

FIGURE 2.—Mean CBF-Hbo$_2$ vs. mean CBF-ICG. The mean CBF values from repeated measurements using each method at any give Paco$_2$ level are shown. The six infants are each denoted by a unique symbol. r = 0.93, P < 0.001; slope of the regression line intercept -2.76 mL·100 g^{-1}·min^{-1}. (Courtesy of Patel J, Marks K, Roberts I: Measurement of cerebral blood flow in newborn infants using near infrared spectroscopy with indocyanine green. *Pediatr Res* 43:34–39, 1998.)

Single CBF-ICG measurements were distributed with a standard deviation of 15%; for CBF-HbO$_2$, it was 24%.

Conclusion.—Intravenous ICG allowed rapid and repeated CBF measurements in 6 newborn infants with severe respiratory insufficiency at high risk of cerebral injury. This technique should help improve assessment of cerebral perfusion.

▶ Measuring cerebral blood flow in "real time" without perturbing the system and rapidly enough to account for acute changes in clinical state has not been possible until recently. Technical advances have made it possible to perform cerebral blood flow measurements at the bedside using NIRS. However, NIRS using hemoglobin as the tracer requires rapid changes in arterial oxygen saturation. This article points out that such changes may not be achievable in critically ill neonates. The authors present the use of injected indocyanine green as a reliable tracer for NIRS. This technique may be much more widely applicable than they indicate, since the induction of rapid changes in arterial oxygen saturation may be difficult to achieve in critically ill adults and older children with sever respiratory insufficiency.

N.F. Schor, M.D., Ph.D.

Etiology of Pediatric Ischemic Stroke
Ferrera PC, Curran CB, Swanson H (Albany Med Ctr, NY)
Am J Emerg Med 15:671–679, 1997   4–2

Introduction.—Ischemic strokes are rare in the pediatric population, but they occur with a slightly higher frequency than hemorrhagic strokes. Predisposing lesions in children are typically congenital, but may also be acquired. The most common initial manifestation of ischemic stroke in children usually is hemiplegia or hemiparesis. Children may also experience sensory impairment, aphasia, and hemianopsia. Fever and seizures are frequently seen in children with stroke. The cause, diagnostic testing, prognosis, and disposition of ischemic strokes are described.

Etiology.—The cause of ischemic strokes in children is frequently idiopathic. Children with stroke of unknown cause tend to have a high proportion of basal ganglia infarcts. Cortical infarcts occur most frequently in children with congenital heart disease, cerebral infections, and moyamoya disease (Table 1).

TABLE 1.—Brief List of Nontraumatic Causes of Ischemic Stroke

Common causes
    Congenital heart disease
    Acquired heart disease
    Infection (*Mycoplasma pneumoniae*, Coxsackie A9)
    Migraine
    Acquired immunodeficiency syndrome (AIDS)
    Systemic lupus erythematosus
    Sickle cell disease
    Protein C and S deficiencies
    Antiphospholipid antibody syndrome
    Malignancies
    Chemotherapy
Rare causes
    Moyamoya syndrome
    Fibromuscular dysplasia
    Polyarteritis nodosa
    Homocystinuria
    Ehlers-Danlos syndrome
    Marfan's syndrome
    MELAS* syndrome
    Spontaneous carotid artery dissection
    Neurofibromatosis

---

*Mitochondrial encephalopathy, lactic acidosis, and strokelike episodes.
(Courtesy of Ferrera PC, Curran CB, Swanson H: Etiology of pediatric ischemic stroke. *Am J Emerg Med* 15:671–679, 1997.)

Diagnostic Testing.—After thorough history taking and physical examination, the most important radiologic and laboratory examinations include cerebral CT, MRI, single-photon emission CT, xenon cerebral blood flow, and positron emission tomography, and complete blood cell count, erythrocyte sedimentation rate, and prothombin and partial thromboplastin times. Other laboratory studies may include tests for mitochondrial myopathy, encephalopathy, lactic acidosis, and strokelike episodes, homocystinuria, sickle cell disease, and proteins S and C deficiency. For suspected infectious or parainfectious processes, lumbar puncture may be required to examine the cerebral spinal fluid for elevated white blood cell count, high protein levels, or low glucose concentration. An ECG should be obtained to rule out cardiac structural abnormalities.

Prognosis and Disposition.—The literature is not in agreement about the prognosis of children with ischemic stroke, but many investigations have reported a high incidence of recurrent seizures. Mental retardation and epilepsy were commonly reported. Patients with hemorrhagic strokes are at greatest risk for immediate postinfarction mortality. Treatment depends on the underlying cause.

Conclusion.—Ischemic strokes in children have a variety of causes, and treatment should be based on the cause.

▶ Stroke is a relatively uncommon disorder in childhood. However, several underlying conditions place particular populations at high risk for childhood stroke. Furthermore, advances in medical technology have placed at the clinician's disposal a plethora of laboratory tests for the evaluation of the child with stroke. This review presents in a particularly organized and succinct way the etiologic and diagnostic considerations in the individual patient with childhood stroke. It then goes on to compare and contrast ischemic stroke in some specific disorders of childhood that are associated with increased stroke risk.

N.F. Schor, M.D., Ph.D.

Iron Deficiency: A Cause of Stroke in Infants and Children
Hartfield DS, Lowry NJ, Keene DL, et al (Univ of Saskatchewan, Saskatoon, Canada; Children's Hosp of Eastern Ontario, Ottawa, Canada)
Pediatr Neurol 16:50–53, 1997   4–3

Background.—Iron deficiency affects 20% to 25% of infants worldwide. Although it most commonly causes anemia, iron deficiency has also been implicated in neurologic sequelae such as irritability, lethargy, headache, developmental delay, and sometimes papilledema, pseudotumor cerebri, and cranial nerve abnormalities. One series of infants in whom iron deficiency caused stroke was reported.

Patients and Findings.—The patients were 5 girls and 1 boy, aged 6 to 18 months. All were iron deficient and had a mild viral infection of the upper respiratory or gastrointestinal tract before the occurrence of

TABLE 1.—Summary of Case Reports

Test	Patients					
	1	2	3	4	5	6
Diagnosis	Venous thrombus/venous infarction bilateral thalamus	SSS	Nonhemorrhagic infarct (basal ganglia/internal capsule)	Nonhemorrhagic infarct (middle cerebral artery)	SSS	Nonhemorrhagic infarct (middle cerebral artery)
Age	18 mo	12 mo	11 mo	18 mo	6 mo	18 mo
Sex	F	F	F	F	M	F
Past medical history	Nil	Nil	Nil	Nil	Developmental delay	Nil
Family history	Systemic lupus	Hyperlipidemia	Nil	Epilepsy	Nil	Epilepsy
Antecedent illness	Gastroenteritis	Gastroenteritis	URTI	Gastroenteritis	Gastroenteritis	Varicella
Hemoglobin (g/L)	67	77	126	114	45	98
Platelets (×10⁹/L)	972	380	693	373	657	653
MCV (normal*)	60	55	78	69	54	74
Iron (normal 10–29)		2	8		1	9
TIBC (normal 36–51)		43	57		61	68
Ferritin (normal 40–70)		<5			<4	
% Saturated transferrin		5	14		2	13
Metabolic screen		Negative	Negative	Normal	Negative	Negative
Echocardiogram			Small PFO	Normal	Normal	Normal
CT scan/MRI	Abnormal	Abnormal	Abnormal	Abnormal	Abnormal	Abnormal
Treatment	Iron	Heparin/warfarin	Iron/ASA	Iron	Iron/ASA	Iron/ASA
Outcome	Normal	Normal	Normal	Seizure disorder	Seizure disorder, developmental delay	Normal

*Normal mean corpuscular volume values: 3–12 months, 70; 1–5 years, 80–94.

Abbreviations: ASA, acetylsalicylic acid; *MCV*, mean corpuscular volume; *TIBC*, total iron-binding capacity; *PFO*, patent foramen ovale; *SSS*, superior sagital sinus thrombosis; *URTI*, upper respiratory tract infection.

(Reprinted by permission of the publisher from Hartfield DS, Lowry NJ, Keene DL, et al: Iron deficiency: A cause of stroke in infants and children. *Pediatr Neurol* 16:50–53, copyright 1997 by Elsevier Science Inc.)

ischemic stroke or venous thrombosis. Some of the infants had mild hydration, but this did not appear to be a significant component of their illness. All had been healthy before their events. Three patients had large venous thrombosis; 2 had infarcts in the distribution of a middle cerebral artery; and 1 had a completed stroke involving deep gray matter end arteries (Table 1). Four children recovered completely. In the remaining 2, seizure disorder developed. Outcomes appeared to be unaffected by the type of ischemic event.

Conclusions.—Iron deficiency was a consistent finding in these patients, for whom other known causes of childhood stroke were excluded. Thus, there is strong evidence that iron deficiency is associated with ischemic events in infants aged 6 to 18 months.

▶ Iron deficiency is an exceedingly common pediatric problem worldwide. Although "hard proof" is lacking in this regard, iron deficiency has been suspected of playing a role in the development of headaches and pseudotumor cerebri. This article presents a series of 6 children with iron deficiency and stroke. In most of these cases, other known risk factors for stroke (hyperlipidemia, metabolic abnormalities, cardiac anomalies, and a family history of early stroke) were examined and rejected. It is of particular interest that 3 of these children had venous thromboses, a major factor in pseudotumor cerebri as well. The authors present an excellent, concise review of the literature regarding the physiologic implications of anemia and their possible implications in cerebrovascular disease.

N.. Schor, M.D., Ph.D.

Characteristic Neuropathology of Leukomalacia in Extremely Low Birth Weight Infants

Deguchi K, Oguchi K, Takashima S (Natl Inst of Neuroscience, Tokyo; Kitasato Univ Sagamihara, Japan)
Pediatr Neurol 16:296–300, 1997   4–4

Background.—The pathogenesis of periventricular leukomalacia in extremely low birth weight infants remains to be characterized. These authors examined white-matter brain sections to see whether any common immunohistochemical markers could be identified in these infants.

Methods.—Examination of postmortem data identified 13 extremely low birth weight infants who had had periventricular leukomalacia without massive intracranial hemorrhages or anomalies. These 13 cases were matched with 9 controls who were similar in age (23–27 vs. 21–28 gestational weeks, respectively), time of death (2 days–5 months vs. 0–2 months), and birth weight (488–955 g vs. less than 1000 g). The presence of tumor necrosis factor-α (TNF-α), β-amyloid precursor protein (β-APP), and glial fibrillary acidic protein (GFAP) was assessed with immunoperoxidase techniques on coronal sections from the cerebral hemispheres.

Findings.—Leukomalacia was widespread, from deep to intermediate, in the white matter in all 13 cases. Most also showed spongy changes, cell necrosis, microglial activation, and proliferation of reactive astrocytes and foam cells, and 5 showed neovascularization. Cells positive for TNF-α were found in and around necrotic foci (but not in glial cells or neurons) in the cerebral cortex in 9 of 13 cases (69%) and in none of the controls. β-Amyloid precursor protein reactivity was found in axonal swellings in 11 of 13 cases (85%) and in none of the controls. Likewise, GFAP-positive cells around necrotic foci deep in the white matter, and spreading to the intermediate white matter, were evident in all 13 cases and in none of the controls.

Conclusion.—Brain tissue from extremely low birth weight infants with periventricular leukomalacia is characterized by axonal damage, astrocytosis, and microglial activation in the deep-to-intermediate white matter. These changes were widespread and may be caused by cerebral ischemia.

▶ Periventricular leukomalacia (PVL) is a known long-term sequela of extreme prematurity. Although this anatomical picture and its clinical manifestations have been ascribed to hypoxia, ischemia, and excitotoxic amino acid release, recent studies have attempted to determine the relative roles of necrosis and apoptosis in the cellular loss seen in this syndrome. This study may indirectly shed some light on this issue.

These authors examined the histopathology and immunologic evidence for the presence of GFAP, β-APP, and TNF-α in brains from extremely low birth weight infants with PVL. Their finding—specifically, that positivity for these agents did not occur in age-matched extremely low birth weight infants without PVL but was widespread in glia from such infants with PVL—suggests the hypothesis that cell loss occurs, at least in part, by apoptosis induced by cytokines such as TNF-α and other proteins such as β-APP, both of which have been shown to induce apoptosis in other systems. From the practical clinical standpoint, these results suggest immunohistochemical markers that may prove useful in defining the presence and severity of PVL in extremely low birth weight infants who succumb to their condition.

N.F. Schor, M.D., Ph.D.

Schizencephaly: Correlations of Clinical and Radiologic Features
Packard AM, Miller VS, Delgado MR, et al (Cornell Univ, New York; Univ of Texas, Dallas)
Neurology 48:1427–1434, 1997   4–5

Background.—Patients with the uncommon congenital disorder schizencephaly have a gray matter–lined cleft running from the pial surface to the ventricle. This can range from a thread of CSF to a wide communication between the subarachnoid space and ventricle. Patients frequently have bilateral clefts and associated CNS anomalies. Relatively few reports have addressed the range of neurodevelopmental outcomes associated

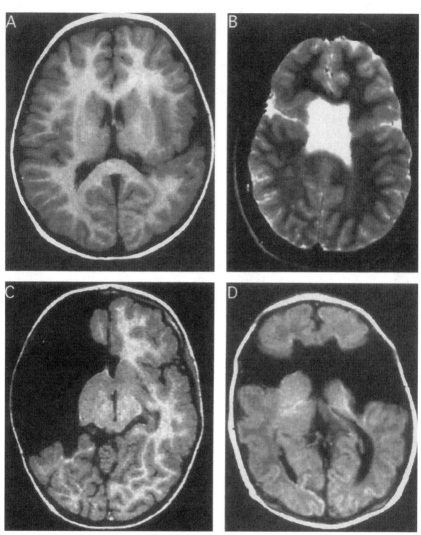

FIGURE 1.—MRI of the subtypes of schizencephaly. **A**, unilateral closed-lip schizencephaly (patient 8). **B**, bilateral closed-lip schizencephaly (patient 18). **C**, unilateral open-lip schizencephaly (patient 34). **D**, bilateral open-lip schizencephaly (patient 45). (Courtesy of Packard AM, Miller VS, Delgado MR, et al: Schizencephaly: Correlations of clinical and radiologic features. *Neurology* 48:1427–1434, 1997, copyright American Academy of Neurology, used with permission of Lippincott-Raven Publishers.)

with this condition. The neurodevelopmental and other findings of 47 children with schizencephaly are reported.

Methods.—All 47 children had a confirmed diagnosis of schizencephaly: 18 underwent cranial CT, 18 underwent cranial MRI, and 11 underwent both diagnostic studies. The study definition of schizencephaly was a gray matter–lined cortical cleft extending from the pial surface to the ventricle or a cleft closely associated with a focal ventricular abnormality. Patients with abutment of the 2 edges through the majority of the cleft were classified as having closed-lip lesions (Fig 1). The location, number, and nature of the clefts were assessed from the imaging studies, along with the presence of other CNS anomalies. Hospital charts and electroencephalographic records were reviewed as well. The patients' neurodevelopmental outcomes were classified as mild (normal language and motor skills or minimal motor deficits), moderate (moderate hemiparesis, learning disabilities, or language deficits, or severe (severe mental retardation, quadriparesis, severely impaired or absent language, or total dependency).

Findings.—Schizencephaly was unilateral in 62% of cases and bilateral in 38%. Sixty-two percent of clefts were open-lip lesions and 38% were closed-lip lesions. Ninety-one percent of patients had other CNS anomalies, including absence of the septum pellucidum in 45% of cases and absence of both the septum pellucidum and corpus callosum in 34%. Nine percent had findings consistent with septo-optic dysplasia (SOD). Excluding 12 patients with bilateral open-lip schizencephaly and extensive cerebral cortex loss, 57% of patients had an absent septum pellucidum, 14% had absence of both the septum pellucidum and corpus callosum, and 9% had SOD. At presentation, the major complaints were motor delay, hydrocephalus, and seizures. Hemiparesis or seizure was the most likely presenting complaint for children with closed-lip schizencephaly. For open-lip cases, the presentation was more variable. Eighty-seven percent of children had no symptoms during their first year of life. Seizures occurred in 58% of children and were unrelated to the subtype of schizencephaly. Seizures did start earlier for patients with open-lip schizencephaly. Seventy percent of patients with seizures had complex partial seizures. One-third of the children required a shunt because of progressive hydrocephalus.

Neurodevelopmental outcomes were classified as mild in 17% of patients, moderate in 32%, and severe in 51%. Outcomes were poorer for children with bilateral clefts and for patients with open-lip lesions. Outcomes were mildly abnormal for about half of children with unilateral, open-lip clefts, vs. 1 young infant with bilateral, closed-lip clefts. Neurodevelopmental outcomes were often predicted by the extent of cortical involvement. Outcomes were also better for children without other CNS anomalies. More than 90% of the children had some motor impairment. Sixty-eight percent had impaired language development, with 55% having severe impairment or total lack of speech. Seizures did not affect neurodevelopmental outcome.

Conclusions.—The clinical manifestations and neurodevelopmental outcomes of schizencephaly were studied. The clinical findings depended on the extent of the clefts and the presence of other CNS anomalies. Most children had motor deficits, which can be predicted from cranial imaging studies; language impairment was somewhat less. Neurologic impairment was severe for patients with schizencephaly involving 3 or more lobes.

▶ Disorders of migration constitute a significant percentage of the anomalies of brain development that result in long-term neurologic compromise. Of these, schizencephaly is among the best characterized and the easiest to distinguish radiologically. It results from a sequential failure of cortical cell bodies to migrate all the way out to the cortical surface, producing a gray matter–lined cleft extending from the pial surface to the cerebral ventricle. Despite this ready radiologic recognition, there have been relatively few studies that attempt to correlate in semi-quantitative fashion the radiologically defined degree and type of schizencephaly with functional and developmental outcome. This series of 47 children with schizencephaly represents an effort to do so and demonstrates that the degree of functional compromise is purely a function of the anatomic extent of the radiologically demonstrable defect. This is important and interesting because, in many developmental anomalies, the radiologic abnormality represents only the tip of the iceberg, while in schizencephaly it appears at least to correlate in degree with the long-term prognosis for these patients.

N.F. Schor, M.D., Ph.D.

Vigabatrin Versus ACTH as First-Line Treatment for Infantile Spasms: A Randomized, Prospective Study

Vigevano F, Cilio MR (Bambino Gesù Children's Hosp, Rome)
Epilepsia 38:1270–1274, 1997   4–6

Introduction.—Spasms, psychomotor development arrest, and hypsarrhythmic ECG pattern are commonly observed in infantile spasms (IS). The disease is considered symptomatic in the presence of known etiology or signs of brain damage preceding the spasm; when the etiology is unknown, the seizures are considered cryptogenic. The most effective treatment is adrenocorticotrophic hormone (ACTH) or oral corticosteroids. Earlier trials report that vigabatrin (VGB) is as efficacious as add-on therapy in resistant IS or as monotherapy. The efficacy and tolerability of VGB and ACTH were compared as first-line therapy in IS.

Methods.—Age range of 22 males and 20 females with newly diagnosed and previously untreated IS was 2–9 months at onset. Patients were randomized to receive VGB 100–150 mg/kg/day or Depot ACTH 10 IU/day in this response-mediated crossover trial. The alternative drug was administered if spasms did not disappear after 20 days of therapy or if there was intolerance. The ACTH dose was constant; VGB dosage was increased to as high as 150 mg/kg/day.

Results.—Spasms ceased in 11 (48%) patients randomized to VGB and 14 (74%) randomized to ACTH. Patients responding to VGB did so within 1–14 days. Seven of 11 patients responded within 3 days. The rate of drowsiness, hypotonia, and irritability was 13% in patients treated with VGB, compared with 37% in patients treated with ACTH. Treatment with VGB was more effective than ACTH for cerebral malformations or tuberous sclerosis. Patients with perinatal hypoxic/ischemic injury were best treated with ACTH. Efficacy of both drugs was similar in the treatment of cryptogenic IS. Interictal EEG abnormalities disappeared sooner in patients randomized to ACTH than to VGB. In a second phase of the trial, the alternative drug was administered to patients who were resistant. Spasms halted in 2 of 5 patients treated with VGB and in 11 of 12 patients treated with ACTH. At 3 month follow-up, relapse of spasms occurred in 6 patients treated with ACTH and 1 treated with VGB. Half the patients who received VGB experienced a therapeutic response.

Conclusion.—This is the first prospective trial comparing VGB and ACTH as first-line treatment of IS. The dose of Depot ACTH was low, but its side effects made it essential to limit treatment time. These data support the belief that VGB offers an effective and maybe safer therapy for management of IS than VGB.

▶ The treatment of infantile spasms has long been problematic. The use of ACTH is frought with side effects, and families must learn both the injection technique and the monitoring needs of infants so treated. Other anticonvulsants have been used in symptomatic infantile spasms, but current dogma holds that ACTH is the optimal treatment for cryptogenic and the most effective treatment for symptomatic infantile spasms. This article presents evidence that oral vigabatrin therapy may be a viable alternative to ACTH. It indicates that there are subgroups of infantile spasm patients that might be most likely to benefit from vigabatrin therapy. Furthermore, although vigabatrin did not have as high a success rate as ACTH in cryptogenic patients, response when it occurred was rapid enough to allow one to make an informed decision to switch to ACTH in selected patients. The response to vigabatrin appeared to be longer lasting than that achieved with ACTH.

N.F. Schor, M.D., Ph.D.

West Syndrome: Cerebrospinal Fluid Nerve Growth Factor and Effect of ACTH
Riikonen RS, Söderström S, Vanhala R, et al (Univ of Helsinki; Univ of Kuopio, Finland; Univ of Uppsala, Sweden)
Pediatr Neurol 17:224–229, 1997   4–7

Introduction.—West Syndrome is an age-limited encephalopathy of infants distinguished by infantile spasms, hypsarrhythmia, and progression to mental retardation. The pathogenesis is unknown, but defects and delay in brain maturation are suspected. Infantile spasms are either symptomatic or cryptogenic. Several growth factors and their receptors are present in the nervous system. A neurotrophic factor is a protein that is important in the regulation of neuronal survival and differentiation. One neurotrophic factor, β-nerve growth factor (NGF) is present in the CNS. Patients with infantile spasms were assessed to determine if there are subgroups that differ in CSF concentrations of NGF and if the therapeutic treatment of spasms with adrenocorticotropic hormone (ACTH) changes the levels of NGF.

CSF NGF, pg/ml   CSF NGF, pg/ml

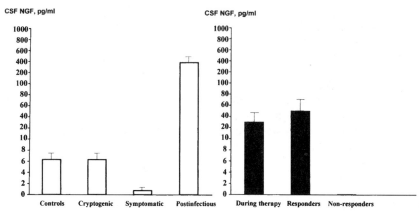

FIGURE 1.—Cerebrospinal fluid (*CSF*) nerve growth factor (*NGF*) concentrations (mean ± SEM) in patients with West syndrome. **Left,** before ACTH therapy: patients with cryptogenic spasms ($n = 6$), patients with symptomatic noninfectious spasms ($n = 27$), and patients with symptomatic postinfectious spasms ($n = 5$). **Right,** during ACTH therapy: all patients ($n = 17$), responders ($n = 10$), and nonresponders ($n = 6$). Significant differences are revealed between patients with cryptogenic spasms and patients with symptomatic postinfectious spasms ($P = 0.001$) and between responders and nonresponders ($P = 0.024$). (Reprinted by permission of the publisher from Riikonen RS, Söderström S, Vanhala R: West syndrome cerebrospinal fluid nerve growth factor and effect of ACTH. *Pediatr Neurol* 17:224–229, copyright 1997 by Elsevier Science Inc.)

Methods.—Using human NGF as a standard for a 2-site enzyme-linked immunosorbent assay method, levels of NGF were determined in the CSF of 38 children with infantile spasms and 22 controls. The CSF samples were obtained before beginning ACTH therapy in 32 patients and during maximum therapy in 11 patients.

Results.—The mean NGF level was 6.3 pg/mL, 0.77 pg/mL, and 378.56 pg/mL, respectively, in children with infantile spasms of cryptogenic causes, noninfectious symptomatic causes, and postencephalitic spasms. Treatment with ACTH produced a greater increase in CSF NGF concentrations in patients with a good response, compared with those with poor response (Fig 1).

Conclusion.—Absent or low concentrations of NGF in the CNS in patients with symptomatic infantile spasms might indicate massive neuronal death that would show up as atrophy on CT scans. This is the first investigation to demonstrate regulation of NGF in humans. ACTH modulated NGF gene activity, which has already been observed in animal experiments for glucocorticoids.

▶ A growing body of evidence is implicating aberrations in growth factor and proto-oncogene activity in a host of human diseases. Many of these disorders primarily affect the adult nervous system. The present article raises the possibility that the mechanism of action of ACTH in abrogation of seizures in patients with symptomatic infantile spasms involves a restoration of abnormally low NGF production in the brain. Although the authors point out that the decrease in NGF levels in the CSF is probably secondary to cell loss and not etiologic in the neurologic dysfunction seen in these children, they demonstrate that clinical anticonvulsive response is correlated with an ACTH-induced increase in CSF levels of NGF. Conversely, children with symptomatic infantile spasms whose NGF levels do not increase in response to ACTH treatment do not experience good seizure control as a group. That this is not the whole story in West syndrome is demonstrated by the findings that patients with cryptogenic infantile spasms have "normal" CSF NGF levels and that those with postinfectious infantile spasms have high NGF levels. These comparisons must be interpreted with caution, given the neurologic dysfunction of most of the children included in the control group. Nonetheless, the suggestion that ACTH alters CSF concentrations of a molecule of clear developmental and neuroprotective import in a disorder with developmental and neurodegenerative precipitants and consequences deserves carefully designed follow-up.

N.F. Schor, M.D., Ph.D.

Myoclonus and Epilepsy in Childhood
Dulac O, for the Commission on Pediatric Epilepsy of the International League Against Epilepsy (Hôpital Saint Vincent de Paul, Paris)
Epilepsia 38:1251–1254, 1997   4–8

Background.—The Commission on Pediatric Epilepsy of the International League Against Epilepsy (ILAE) and the participants of an ILAE-sponsored workshop in 1996 have agreed on certain terminology and descriptions.

Terms and Descriptions.—There are 4 main types of myoclonus: cortical myoclonus (CM), thalamocortical myoclonus, reticular reflex myoclonus (RRM), and negative myoclonus (NM). Myoclonus is termed *epileptic* when it occurs along with cortical epileptiform discharges. In some patients, the latter may be shown only by back-averaging. Positive myoclonus may occur with epilepsy in various conditions. In progressive encephalopathies, myoclonus is of the cortical type. In nonprogressive generalized epilepsy, myoclonus primarily involves idiopathic generalized epilepsy and is of the thalamocortical type. In congenital nonprogressive encephalopathy of various causes, including malformations or chromosome aberrations, myoclonus consists of long-lasting episodes of myoclonus with continuous generalized spikes and slow wave activity on EEG, combined with neurologic deterioration, in infancy or childhood. In neonatal myoclonic encephalopathy, bursts of massive myoclonus are combined with an EEG suppression-burst pattern. Patients with benign myoclonic epilepsy of infancy (BMEI) and myoclonic astatic epilepsy (MAE) have myoclonus status characterized by erratic myoclonus, primarily involving face and extremities, together with obtundation and diffuse slow waves and spikes. Epileptic NM is a heterogeneous condition that can originate from various areas of the brain, including the premotor cortex and motor cortex. This condition may be associated with the slow wave of a spike-wave complex or the negative transient of the polyspike of a polyspike-wave complex. It may be generalized or focal.

Treatment.—There are several major antimyoclonic agents. Piracetam is mainly active in the cortical myoclonus. Valproate and ethosuximide are mainly active in generalized myoclonus of idiopathic generalized epilepsy. Benzodiazepines have a wide spectrum of activity. Carbamazepine, phenytoin, and vigabatrin are not effective against myoclonus and may actually worsen it.

▶ It is often said that myoclonus can have its origin anywhere in the central nervous system. This brief report from the ILAE presents the consensus view arrived at a meeting held in France in May 1996. It deals primarily with epileptic myoclonus, and arrives at a clinical nosology that is useful from diagnostic, prognostic, and treatment standpoints. It is important to keep in mind, however, that myoclonus may not be epileptic in nature, and may, in fact, have its origins in the spinal cord rather than the brain.

N.F. Schor, M.D., Ph.D.

5   Movement Disorders

Mutation in the α-Synuclein Gene Identified in Families With Parkinson's Disease
Polymeropoulos MH, Lavedan C, Leroy E, et al (NIH, Bethesda, Md; Univ of Medicine and Dentistry of New Jersey, Piscataway; Seconda Universita degli Studi di Napoli, Naples, Italy; et al)
Science 276:2045–2047, 1997   5–1

Background.—In some cases, heritable factors may predispose a person to Parkinson's disease. Cosegregation of gene markers on chromosome 4q21–q23 with the Parkinson's disease phenotype has previously been shown in a large Italian kindred. These gene markers map to the same region as α-synuclein, a presynaptic nerve terminal protein believed to influence neural plasticity. The molecular association of α-synuclein with the Parkinson's disease phenotype was investigated in the same Italian kindred and in a group of unrelated Greek families.

Methods.—Genotype analysis in the Italian kindred revealed that the α-synuclein gene completely segregated with the Parkinson's disease phenotype, with 1 mutation in α-synuclein at position 209 from G to A. Comparison with a selection of 314 chromosomes from other people indicated that none of them carried this G209A mutation. Once cosegregation was thus confirmed in the Italian kindred, Greek patients with the Parkinson's disease phenotype were identified and examined for this G209A mutation.

Findings.—The G209A mutation was found in 3 of the Greek kindreds. As in the original Italian kindred, this mutation cosegregated with the Parkinson's disease phenotype. The α-synuclein mutation was found in all 4 families with the Parkinson's disease phenotype, but not in any of 314 control chromosomes studied.

Conclusions.—A mutation in the α-synuclein gene may account for the development of Parkinson's disease in families with a highly penetrant, autosomal dominant inheritance. Although this mutation may account for only a few percent of cases of Parkinson's disease, its further study may give insights into the pathogenesis of this disease.

▶ Most Parkinson's disease is sporadic, and familial cases generally do not follow classic mendelian patterns of inheritance. Only in 4 families that exhibit an autosomal dominant pattern of inheritance has the genetic mutation been identified. The mutation involves a substitution of alanine for threonine in a region of the α-synuclein protein whose secondary structure predicts an α-helical formation bounded by β sheets. This mutation may predispose the protein to autoaggregate into β sheets. The authors note that the disease caused by this mutation is reminiscent of diseases such as Gerstmann-Sträussler and Creutzfeldt-Jakob diseases, in which missense mutations in the prion protein are implicated in amyloid production. In both of these disorders, the physical chemical properties of mutant cellular proteins appear to be important in initiating and propagating neuronal lesions that lead to the disease. Although this mutation was not found in patients with sporadic disease, it is hoped that studies in the synuclein protein family may provide insights into the etiology and pathogenesis of idiopathic Parkinson's disease.

J. Sanchez-Ramos, M.D., Ph.D.

High-frequency Stimulation of the Globus Pallidus for the Treatment of Parkinson's Disease
Pahwa R, Wilkinson S, Smith D, et al (Univ of Kansas, Kansas City)
Neurology 49:249–253, 1997   5–2

Background.—Long-term levodopa treatment for Parkinson's disease (PD) is complicated by the development of motor fluctuations and dyskinesias. In patients with PD, posteroventral pallidotomy may improve tremors, bradykinesia, rigidity, and dyskinesias. Long-term stimulation of the globus pallidus was performed to duplicate the positive outcomes of pallidotomy while decreasing the risk of permanent neurologic deficit in patients with advanced PD.

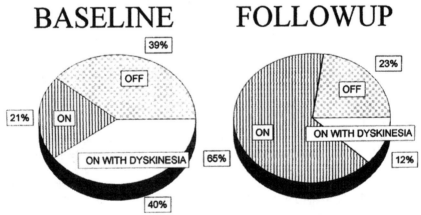

FIGURE.—Data from patient diaries at baseline and follow-up. (Reprinted from Pahwa R, Wilkinson S, Smith D, et al: High-frequency stimulation of the globus pallidus for the treatment of Parkinson's disease. *Neurology* 49:249–253, 1997, copyright American Academy of Neurology, used with permission of Lippincott-Raven Publishers.)

Methods.—Five patients with disabling PD were included in the study. The lead for long-term stimulation of the globus pallidus was implanted stereotactically with the aid of microelectrode recordings in the globus pallidus pars interna, and an electric pulse generator was implanted in the subclavicular region. Three patients had bilateral implants.

Findings.—Three months after the last follow-up, 4 patients considered themselves to be markedly improved, and 1 considered himself to be moderately improved. The amount of time in the "on" state rose from 21% before stimulation to 65% 3 months later (Figure). All subscales of the Unified Parkinson's Disease Rating Scale improved significantly. The adverse effects of stimulation were minimal. An asymptomatic intracranial bleeding event, transient hemiparesis during surgery, and the need for surgical repositioning of the lead occurred in 1 patient each.

Conclusions.—Long-term pallidal stimulation is safe and effective in patients with PD complicated by motor fluctuations and dyskinesias. Most objective and subjective scales showed significant improvement in scores after pallidal stimulation.

▶ At first glance, this experimental treatment seems preferable to a permanent pallidal lesion for alleviation of severe levodopa-induced dyskinesias. This short-term study clearly demonstrates efficacy, only minor surgical complications. However, the long-term risks and benefits of a permanently implanted electrode need to be investigated.

J. Sanchez-Ramos, M.D., Ph.D.

Changes in Cerebral Activity Pattern Due to Subthalamic Nucleus or Internal Pallidum Stimulation in Parkinson's Disease
Limousin P, Greene J, Pollak P, et al (Inst of Neurology, London; Joseph Fourier Univ, Grenoble, France)
Ann Neurol 42:283–291, 1997   5–3

Background.—Previous studies using positron emission tomography (PET) have demonstrated reduced activation of supplementary motor areas (SMAs), the anterior cingulate cortex, and the dorsolateral prefrontal cortex during free-choice joystick movements in patients with Parkinson's disease. Patients treated with high-frequency electrical stimulation of the internal pallidum (GPi) or subthalamic nucleus (STN) show clinical improvement. This technique provides a reversible effect that can be altered by changing the electrical stimulation patterns. The effects of STN and GPi stimulation on cortical activation patterns during subject-selected movements were examined.

Methods.—Participants were 12 patients with Parkinson's disease being treated by high-frequency electrical stimulators: 6 of the STN and 6 of the GPi. The patients were studied by $H_2^{15}O$ PET to assess possible changes in regional cerebral blood flow (rCBF) accompanying changes in movement performance. The PET studies were performed with the patient at rest and

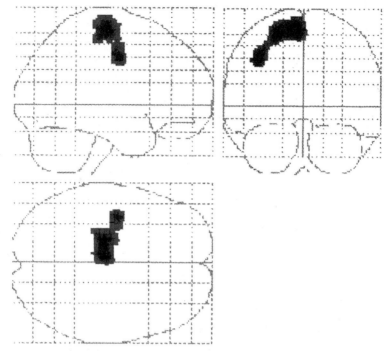

FIGURE 1.—Relative deactivations due to main effect of effective subthalamic nucleus stimulation ([M−S+] + [M+S−] vs. [M−S+] + [M+S+]). *Abbreviations: M−*, rest; M+, movement; S+, effective stimulation; S−, ineffective stimulation. (Courtesy of Limousin P, Greene J, Pollak P, et al: Changes in cerebral activity pattern due to subthalamic nucleus or internal pallidum stimulation in Parkinson's disease. *Ann Neurol* 42:283–291, Copyright ANA, 1997, by permission of Little, Brown and Company.)

during free-choice joystick movements, performed during periods of effective and ineffective electrical stimulation.

Results.—Effective stimulation of the STN was associated with significantly increased rCBF in the supplementary motor area, cingulate cortex, and dorsolateral prefrontal cortex, compared with ineffective stimulation. In contrast, effective GPi stimulation was not accompanied by rCBF changes in any of these areas. Most of the difference in movement-related activity between the 2 stimulation sites was localized to the dorsolateral prefrontal cortex (Fig 1).

Conclusions.—The effects of high-frequency electrical stimulation in Parkinson's disease demonstrate the importance of nonprimary motor areas in controlling movement in patients with this condition. Input from the STN plays an important role in controlling these motor areas. The specific action of STN stimulation on the dorsolateral prefrontal cortex may explain the clinical differences between stimulation of the STN vs. the GPi.

▶ Both STN and GPi have been targets for surgical approaches (focal lesioning and deep brain electrical stimulation) in the treatment of Parkinson's disease. High-frequency electrical stimulation of STN activates several areas of cortex that are not activated by stimulation of GPi. In particular, STN stimulation induced a pattern of regional blood flow to supplementary motor cortical areas, especially the dorsal lateral prefrontal cortex, similar to that seen during free-choice joystick movements in normal individuals. Despite the difference in pattern of cortical activation, the clinical benefits measured (movement time, Parkinson's disease rating scales) were equivalent whether GPi or STN was stimulated.

Several issues were not addressed that merit future investigation. Because the STN is a smaller target than GPi, are the risks of STN stimulation greater than GPi stimulation? With respect to risks and benefits, how does deep brain stimulation of STN or GPi compare with surgical lesions of the same structures?

J. Sanchez-Ramos, M.D., Ph.D.

Posteroventral Medial Pallidotomy in Advanced Parkinson's Disease
Lang AE, Lozano AM, Montgomery E, et al (Toronto Hosp; Univ of Arizona, Tucson)
N Engl J Med 337:1036–1042, 1997   5–4

Objective.—There is renewed interest in the use of neurosurgical procedures for the treatment of Parkinson's disease, especially posteroventral medial pallidotomy. Reports have described dramatic improvement in patients with advanced Parkinson's disease undergoing this procedure; however, the studies have been limited by their small size and short-term follow-up. Forty patients with Parkinson's disease who underwent posteroventral medial pallidotomy during a 2½-year period were followed up.

Methods.—Serial evaluations were performed with the patients on and off their optimal medical regimen. All patients were evaluated before surgery, and 39 were evaluated at 6 months, 27 at 1 year, and 11 at 2 years after surgery. Overall score on the Unified Parkinson's Disease Rating Scale was the main efficacy outcome.

Results.—The 6-month evaluation revealed a 28% improvement in off-period score for overall motor function, with the contralateral limbs showing the greatest improvement. Off-period score for activities of daily living increased by 29%. On-period score for contralateral dyskinesias improved by 82%, whereas on-period score for ipsilateral dyskinesias improved by 44%. The 2-year follow-up studies showed lasting improvement in dyskinesias and total scores for off-period parkinsonism, contralateral bradykinesia, and rigidity. However, the improvement in ipsilateral dyskinesias disappeared after 1 year, while the gains in postural stability and gait were lost after only 3–6 months. Patients who needed assistance with activities of daily living before surgery had about a 50% chance of becoming independent afterward. The patients tolerated the surgery well and showed no significant changes in medication use.

Conclusions.—For patients with advanced-stage Parkinson's disease, pallidotomy can significantly reduce dyskinesias and off-period disability. A variety of benefits were documented, many of which persist during 2 years' follow-up. However, other improvements, including the reductions in ipsilateral dyskinesias and axial symptoms, disappear in the year after surgery. Pallidotomy produces no improvement in on-period symptoms that do not respond to dopaminergic therapy.

▶ This article carefully reviews the benefits and risks of pallidotomy in 40 patients, with 11 of them followed up to 2 years. A much longer follow-up report on many more patients would be extremely helpful for the practitioner who must decide when, and for whom, this procedure should be performed.

J. Sanchez-Ramos, M.D., Ph.D.

Pallidotomy in Parkinson's Disease Increases Supplementary Motor Area and Prefrontal Activation During Performance of Volitional Movements: An H₂¹⁵O PET Study

Samuel M, Ceballos-Baumann AO, Turjanski N, et al (Hammersmith Hosp, London; Inst of Neurology, London; Neurologische Klinik der Technischen Universität, München, Germany; et al)
Brain 120:1301–1313, 1997   5–5

Purpose.—There is renewed interest in the performance of posteroventral medial pallidotomy for the treatment of Parkinson's disease. Patients with this condition show selective impairment of supplementary motor area and right dorsal prefrontal cortex activation during volitional limb movements. Patients undergoing pallidotomy show improved motor performance while off medication; as such, they might also show increased supplementary motor area and dorsal prefrontal cortex activation. This hypothesis was tested using $H_2^{15}O$ positron emission tomography (PET).

Methods.—Six patients with Parkinson's disease undergoing unilateral right posteroventral pallidotomy were studied. The patients had a median total motor Unified Parkinson's Disease Rating Scale (UPDRS) score of 52.5 in the "off" condition. Before and 3–4 months after pallidotomy, each patient underwent $H_2^{15}O$ PET. The scans provided measurements of regional cerebral blood flow with the patients at rest and while performing regularly paced joystick movements with the left hand. Statistical parametric mapping was performed to compare the levels of activation during prepallidotomy and postpallidotomy scans.

Results.—The patients' median total motor UPDRS score in the "off" state decreased by 35% after pallidotomy. On joystick testing, their mean response times in response to pacing tones improved by 14%. These movements were associated with relatively increased activation of the supplementary motor area and right dorsal prefrontal cortex and decreased activation of the right pallidum.

Conclusions.—In patients with Parkinson's disease, pallidotomy appears to reduce pallidal inhibition of the thalamocortical circuits. At the same time, it at least partially reverses impairment of the supplementary motor area and activation of the dorsal prefrontal cortex. Thus the functional benefits of pallidotomy appear to result from increased activity of the cortical areas involved in motor planning and receiving projections from the basal ganglia.

▶ Similar to the preceding study (Abstract 5–3) on deep brain stimulation, pallidotomy improves movement time and other signs of Parkinson's disease. This benefit is associated with activation of the prefrontal cortex and supplementary motor area. Both of these studies demonstrate the functional connections between basal ganglia and specific cortical areas and their importance for normal execution of free-choice paced movements.

J. Sanchez-Ramos, M.D., Ph.D.

Huntington's Disease
Craufurd D (St Mary's Hosp, Manchester, England)
Prenat Diagn 16:1237–1245, 1996   5–6

Introduction.—Huntington's disease (HD), an inherited degenerative disorder of the central nervous system, follows a progressive course from motor abnormalities at diagnosis to a hypokinetic state in the later stages. Although onset of HD is usually between the ages of 30 and 50 years, testing can now identify those with a dominantly inherited mutation in a gene on chromosome 4p. Issues involved in predictive testing and prenatal testing for HD were addressed.

Genetics.—Huntington's disease is inherited as an autosomal dominant trait with complete penetrance. Although HD cannot be cured or its onset delayed, modern molecular genetic techniques have improved the outlook for affected families. The mutation responsible for HD is a $(CAG)_n$ trinucleotide repeat sequence close to the 5' end of the gene. Whereas most unaffected individuals have alleles with 11–31 copies of the (CAG) repeat, those affected usually have greater than 38 repeats. As with other disorders caused the unstable $(CAG)_n$ mutation, transmission of the gene by the father results in an earlier age at disease onset or increasing clinical severity in successive generations.

Predictive Testing.—A direct test measuring the number of repeats at the HD locus now allows carrier status to be predicted with greater speed and accuracy. All descendants of someone with a favorable test result are not at risk; an unfavorable result may lead to psychological problems and discrimination by insurance companies or potential employers. When requested, testing should be performed only in the context of a suitable protocol for counselling and support.

Prenatal Testing.—Carriers can undergo prenatal testing, either by linkage or direct mutation testing, to help them decide whether to have children. Results are obtained in the first trimester by chorionic villus biopsy. Prenatal exclusion testing, which allows at-risk pregnancies to be terminated without revealing the genetic status of the at-risk parent, offers an alternative for prospective parents who do not wish to be tested themselves but cannot risk passing HD to another generation. Various ethical problems are presented, however, such as when an at-risk couple chooses not to terminate the pregnancy after test results are unfavorable. An international survey identified fewer than 250 prenatal tests performed from 1986 through 1994, yet several thousand predictive tests took place during this period.

Discussion.—The development of new approaches to treatment of HD fosters optimism, but the current testing choices have created new responsibilities and ethical problems. Genetic counsellors must help individuals make informed decisions based on their particular situations.

▶ In this era of molecular diagnosis, issues of prenatal and adult predictive diagnosis are going to have more impact on the delivery of neurologic care, with all of its ethical and social implications. Nowhere is this case more cogently made than in the instance of HD, a disorder from which most patients become symptomatic only after their childbearing years, and for which there is currently much stigma and no palliation or cure. This article delineates and discusses the ethical and social dilemmas raised by genetic diagnostics and suggests possible solutions to these problems. It is of direct and immediate relevance, not only for HD, but for an enormous host of diseases for which we now and in the future can make molecular diagnoses.

N.F. Schor, M.D., Ph.D.

Long-term Effects of Tetrabenazine in Hyperkinetic Movement Disorders
Jankovic J, Beach J (Baylor College of Medicine, Houston)
Neurology 48:358–362, 1997   5–7

Background.—Tetrabenazine (TBZ), initially introduced as an antipsychotic agent, is currently used most often outside the United States to treat hyperkinetic movement disorders. The outcome of long-term TBZ therapy was investigated in a large group of patients with various hyperkinetic movement disorders.

Methods.—Five hundred twenty-six patients with severe hyperkinetic movement disorders treated with TBZ in the past 15 years were studied. Follow-up data were complete for 400. The mean duration of TBZ therapy was 28.9 months.

Findings.—Marked improvement was documented in 89.2% of the patients with tardive stereotypy, 83.3% of those with myoclonus, 82.8% of those with Huntington's disease, and 80.5% with tardive dystonia. Seventy-nine percent of patients with other movement disorders also showed marked improvement, as did 62.9% of patients with idiopathic dystonia and 57.4% of those with Tourette's syndrome. The most common adverse effects were drowsiness, occurring in 36.5%; parkinsonism, in 28.5%; depression, in 15%; insomnia, in 11%; nervousness or anxiety, in 10.3%; and akathisia, in 9.5%. Dosage reductions controlled these adverse effects.

Conclusions.—Tetrabenazine is effective and safe in the treatment of various hyperkinetic movement disorders. Unlike typical neuroleptics, TBZ apparently does not cause tardive dyskinesia.

▶ This review of the long-term benefits and adverse effects of TBZ, despite methodological shortcomings, demonstrates its remarkable utility and favorable therapeutic index for a range of hyperkinetic movement disorders. In particular, TBZ is very effective treatment for tardive dyskinesias. Unfortunately, TBZ is not yet available in U.S. pharmacies, which means that many patients must seek the medication in European pharmacies where it has been available for many years.

J. Sanchez-Ramos, M.D., Ph.D.

Hyperekplexia: Abnormal Startle Response Due to Glycine Receptor Mutations
Andrew M, Owen MJ (Univ of Wales, Cardiff)
Br J Psychiatry 170:106–108, 1997   5–8

Objective.—Patients with a grossly exaggerated response to unexpected stimuli are said to have hyperekplexia, or "startle disease." Responses include generalized hypertonia and stiffness, causing the patient to fall, frequently resulting in injury but usually not unconsciousness. Neonatal hyperekplexia, or "stiff baby syndrome," increases the risk of death from apnea and aspiration pneumonia, along with hypokinesia. Current knowledge of hyperekplexia is reviewed, including the genetic aspects.

Diagnosis.—The diagnosis of hyperekplexia is not difficult to make, if one is aware of the syndrome. The diagnosis is usually made by the history of an episode following a loud noise or other stimulus, with corroboration from an observer. Hyperekplexia is distinguished from startle epilepsy by the findings of preserved consciousness and the absence of electroencephalographic evidence of epilepsy. The patients may have a broad-based, unsteady, "insecure" gait, resulting from uncertainty and fear of falling. The patient may have scars from previous falls. Hyperekplexia is often misdiagnosed as epilepsy, hysteria, or malingering.

Management.—Treatment with clonazepam can dramatically reduce the startle response, though not eliminate it completely. When this treatment is unsuccessful, it is often because the dosage is too low. Valproate may also be useful. Even with a response to drug treatment, the patient may have difficult-to-manage secondary handicaps, including anxiety disorders, depression, alcohol abuse, drug side effects, and isolation and distress for the patient and family. Successful drug treatment may uncover complex residual social and psychologic problems.

Neonatal Hyperekplexia.—Newborn infants with hyperekplexia have a brief pathologic startle reflex followed by a sustained tonic spasm. Sudden infant death and recurring apnea have been reported. This diagnosis should be considered in infants with apnea, aspiration pneumonia, episodic muscular rigidity, hyperexcitability, or near-miss sudden infant death syndrome. Early clonazepam therapy may be life-saving.

Genetics.—In many families, hyperekplexia is inherited in autosomal dominant fashion with nearly complete penetrance. Previous reports have described associated mutations in the α_1 subunit of the glycine receptor (GLRA I). Both recessive and dominant mutations have been documented. Studies in mouse mutants suggest that cases without these mutations may have mutations in the β subunit of the glycine receptor.

Discussion.—Hyperekplexia is an abnormal startle reflex resulting from mutations of a neurotransmitter gene. Both dominant and recessive inheritance can result from different mutations in the same gene. This may be relevant to other neuropsychiatric disorders arising from mutations in ligand-gated ion channels. Genetic counseling and diagnostic evaluation of neonatal hypertonia may be aided by mutation analysis of GLRA I.

▶ An exaggerated startle response to unexpected noises or other stimuli such as unexpected touch, associated with stiffening of the body and falling down with arms held firmly by the side of the body, without loss of consciousness, should suggest the syndrome of hyperekplexia. This condition has often been misdiagnosed as hysteria, malingering, or epilepsy. This article provides a brief but excellent summary of the clinical aspects, differential diagnosis, and treatment of hyperekplexia. The review includes recent molecular advances that tie together multiple levels of understanding, ranging from molecular genetics of the glycine receptor to physiology of ligand-gated ion channels and varied clinical expression of the disorder.

J. Sanchez-Ramos, M.D., Ph.D.

6 Neuroradiology

Proton (¹H) MR Spectroscopy for Routine Diagnostic Evaluation of Brain Lesions
Burtscher IM, Ståhlberg F, Holtås S (Univ Hosp, Lund, Sweden)
Acta Radiol 38:953–960, 1997   6–1

Background.—Recent improvements in equipment and evaluation tools have enabled high-quality magnetic resonance spectroscopy (MRS) to be obtained on standard 1.5 T units in a clinically useful time frame. The use of MRS in the daily routine of a modern standard unit was described in the current study.

Methods.—Fifty-two patients with brain lesions underwent proton MRS, with spin-echo (SE) and stimulated echo acquisition mode (STEAM) sequences used for chemical-shift imaging and single-volume spectroscopy. The quality of the spectra was graded from 1 to 3, with 1 being best. The main factors affecting the quality of the spectra were also determined.

Findings.—Eighty-five percent of the measures were graded as 1, 12% as 2, and 3% as 3. Poor spectral quality resulted mainly from malpositioning of the volumes of interest (VOI), hemorrhage, and/or postoperative changes within the VOI. Confidence in the MR diagnosis was increased by MRS findings in 18 of the 40 patients with a final diagnosis. In 3 patients, MRS contributed significantly to the preoperative diagnosis. The spectra were not specific in 10 patients and difficult to determine in 9 because of decreased quality.

Conclusions.—In clinical routine, brain MRS can provide a high percentage of interpretable spectra. In this series, findings on MRS often increased confidence in the MR diagnosis of brain lesions.

► Could it be that MR spectroscopy will become an integral part of MR imaging of the brain? This article from Sweden indicates that in one-third of cases, MRS performed as part of an MR examination gives important additional information concerning an abnormality seen on routine MR. In the United States, MRS, in the vast majority of centers, is used only to answer a specific question such as whether a ring-enhancing lesion is more likely a tumor or an abscess, or whether a certain mass might represent a hamartoma or a neoplasm. To employ MRS routinely will require more investigations such as this one, validating the efficacy of routine MRS. What will be required is an investigation of a large number of patients with information on how MRS influenced patient care, the evaluation of other MRS methods such as long TE sequences, detailed descriptions of the spectral peaks, and the value of spectroscopic imaging vs. single voxel spectroscopy.

R.M. Quencer, M.D

Clinical Utility of Diffusion-weighted Magnetic Resonance Imaging in the Assessment of Ischemic Stroke

Lutsep HL, Albers GW, DeCrespigny A, et al (Stanford Univ, Calif)
Ann Neurol 41:574–580, 1997   6–2

Introduction.—Management decisions in cases of acute stroke must consider both the location and the age of the acute ischemic lesion. Diffusion-weighted imaging (DWI), a method that detects small changes in water diffusion that occur in ischemic brain, has shown promise in early lesion localization and may assist in determining lesion age. Patients with cerebral ischemia were studied with phase-navigated spin-echo DWI and T2-weighted MRI (T2W MRI).

Methods.—During a 1-year period, 109 DWI scans were obtained in patients with symptoms of brain ischemia; 103 patients had clinical diagnoses of cerebral ischemia. Maps of apparent diffusion coefficients (ADCs) synthesized from DW images have shown that ADCs are below normal levels in the first 4 days after ischemia and elevated after 10 days. Both ADC values and T2 ratios of image intensity were measured from the ischemic region and from the corresponding contralateral brain region. Patients' clinical histories were reviewed to determine the contribution of DWI to clinical diagnosis or management.

Results.—Scans were obtained within 24 hours of symptoms onset in one third of patients and within 2 days in one half of patients. The mean time between symptom onset and scanning was 10.4 days. Diffusion-weighted imaging detected 6 lesions not seen on 2T-weighted imaging and discriminated 2 new infarcts from old lesions. The DWI technique was found to be most useful when performed within 48 hours of the event. In 26 patients, the precise time of stroke onset could be determined. The evolution of ADC values and T2 ratios was evaluated in these cases. The ADC values were low during the first week after stroke onset, then became elevated; T2 ratios were near normal in the acute period but increased thereafter.

Conclusion.—Compared with T2W MRI alone, DWI yielded additional clinically relevant findings in 8% of patients. When imaging revealed an acute lesion and was obtained within 72 hours of symptom onset, DWI contributed additional information in 21% of cases. Assessment of ADC values, together with measurements of T2-weighted imaging signal intensity, may determine the time of stroke onset more accurately.

▶ Recent publications and presentations at national neuroscience meetings have demonstrated the increased sensitivity of DWI for the detection of cerebral lesions not otherwise seen on conventional T1- and T2-weighted spin echo imaging. Where this technique has its greatest clinical potential is in the evaluation of acute stroke, i.e., within the first 6 hours after symptom onset. It is the detection of an alteration of the normal diffusion of water (hypointense signal on DW images) to an abnormal diffusion (hyperintense signal) that allows one to presume the presence of ischemia, even with normal-appearing T2-weighted images. With this finding, one may consider thrombolytic therapy during this early stage of a developing stroke.

R.M. Quencer, M.D.

An Accurate, Cost-effective Approach for Diagnosing Retrocochlear Lesions Utilizing the T2-weighted, Fast-Spin Echo Magnetic Resonance Imaging Scan
Linker SP, Ruckenstein MJ, Acker J, et al (Univ of Tennessee, Memphis; Baptist Mem Hosp, Memphis, Tenn)
Laryngoscope 107:1525–1529, 1997   6–3

Purpose.—There is debate over the best diagnostic approach to patients with possible retrocochlear causes of auditory dysfunction. The screening test of choice is evoked potential audiometry; however, there is evidence that auditory brain stem response (ABR) may miss small tumors in the internal auditory canal and cerebellopontine angle. Enhanced MRI scans can detect these lesions with a high level of accuracy, but are time-consuming and prohibitively expensive. T2-weighted, fast-spin echo MRI was prospectively evaluated as a potential screening study for the diagnosis of retrocochlear lesions.

Methods.—Participants included 155 patients referred for evaluation of possible retrocochlear lesions. All underwent T2-weight, fast-spin echo MRI. All scans were performed and read by a radiologic group experienced in this technique.

Results.—The limited MRI scans provided excellent visualization of the inner ear, seventh and eighth cranial nerves, internal auditory canal, cerebellopontine angle, and brain stem (Fig 1). The scans took 15–20 minutes to perform. Of 155 scans performed, 5 were read as positive for the presence of tumors. Full enhanced MRI scans or surgery confirmed the presence of a mass in 4 of the 5 cases. Full MRI scans were performed in 4 patients with negative limited scans, confirming the absence of retrocochlear lesions. The global cost of the limited MRI scans was $475.

Conclusions.—T2-weighted, fast-spin echo MRI may be a very useful screening test for retrocochlear lesions. The limited scans are quickly performed, inexpensive, and provide excellent visualization of the relevant structures. When the limited scan is positive, a full MRI scan may not be

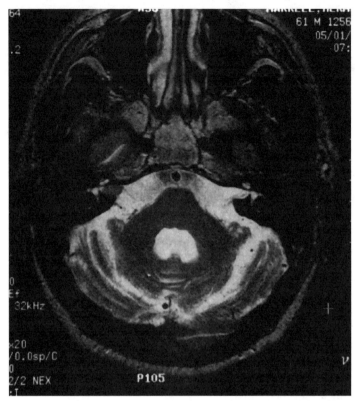

FIGURE 1.—T2-weighted, fast spin echo MRI scan from this series showing a left-sided vestibular schwannoma. Note the filling of the right internal auditory canal (IAC) with CSF, allowing for the excellent visualization of the seventh and eighth cranial nerve complex, typical of a normal scan. (Courtesy of Linker SP, Ruckenstein MJ, Acker J, et al: An accurate, cost-effective approach for diagnosing retrocochlear lesions utilizing the T2-weighted, fast-spin echo magnetic resonance imaging scan. *Laryngoscope* 107:1525–1529, 1997. Copyright Triological Society.)

necessary. Replacing ABR with limited MRI scans appears to be a cost-effective approach to the evaluation of suspected retrocochlear lesions.

▶ Acoustic neuromas make up 5% to 10% of all intracranial tumors and have a clinical incidence of 1 in 100,000. Enhanced MRI scans with eighth nerve cuts is the most sensitive and specific test to identify this tumor. This type of scan cannot be used as a screening test for this tumor because of the cost. The test is clearly indicated in patients with unexplained, unilateral or significantly asymmetric (greater than 15 dB at 2 or more frequencies) sensorineural hearing loss (SNHL) or tinnitus. In patients with more symmetric SNHL, bilateral tinnitus, or noise exposure, the auditory evoked response (AER) has been used as a screening test. The AER frequently misses small tumors, and the sensitivity and specificity may be as low as 63% and 64%, respectively. by decreasing the criteria for increased wave I-III interval, sensitivity goes up but at the expense of specificity.

This article nicely discusses the cost analysis of tests for acoustic neuromas including limited MRI scans. Limited MRI scans were done on 155 patients, and full MRI scans were done on most patients with a suspicious cerebellopontine angle lesion. Sensitivity and specificity of limited MRI cannot be determined from this study, but is reported to be 100% and 99%, respectively, in another study.[1] On a cost basis, it makes sense to use limited MRI scans instead of AERs as a screening test.

R.J. Tusa, M.D., Ph.D.

Reference

1. Shelton C, Harnsberger HR, Allen R, et al: Fast spin echo magnetic resonance imaging: Clinical application in screening for acoustic neuroma. *Otolaryngol Head Neck Surg* 114:71–76, 1996.

The Value of Proton MR Spectroscopy in Pediatric Metabolic Brain Disease

Zimmerman RA, Wang ZJ (Children's Hosp, Philadelphia)
AJNR 18:1872–1879, 1997   6–4

Introduction.—Magnetic resonance (MR) spectroscopy noninvasively depicts the biochemistry of brain tissue. It has been used in the evaluation of pediatric metabolic diseases for only about a decade. Described are the challenges of using this technology and its clinical application in children with metabolic brain diseases.

Challenges.—Even with improvements in the magnetic field gradient coils and shorter time frames, there are other problems with the procedure. The young patient of interest may be medically unstable and is not likely to be cooperative without sedation. These patients usually need medical support plus time out of the ICU. Tests are frequently not reimbursable in the United States, and the prolonged use of the MR imager takes potential time away from paying patients. The ability of proton MR spectroscopy to accumulate statistically sufficient information about rare disorders is challenging. The metabolic pathways and substrates generated within the living, intact, and in vivo human brain are not completely understood (Table 1). This is compounded when trying to understand a complex metabolic brain disease.

Clinical Applications.—Pediatric metabolic disorders affecting the brain can be classified simply as peroxisomal, lysosomal, mitochondrial, aminoacidopathic, and primary white matter disorders. Proton MR spectroscopy has been used to evaluate the major metabolites observed within the brain in several series of patients within the classification system. It has proved useful in evaluating the state of disease and response to therapy in patients with a variety of pediatric metabolic brain diseases.

Conclusion.—Proton MR spectroscopy contributes specific information not available with MR imaging. It gives data regarding state of disease and response to treatment for patients with a wide range of pediatric metabolic

TABLE 1.—Major Metabolites Observed in the Brain

Metabolite	Role	Clinical Significance
N-acetylaspartate (NAA)	Present in neuronal cell and synthesized in mitochondria. Physiological role is poorly understood. It is also an osmolite.	NAA is a neuronal marker. Neuronal damage and cell death cause decrease in NAA. Overall, NAA is the most sensitive metabolite to central nervous system disorders. Sometimes a small decrease in NAA is reversible, and may not indicate permanent cell damage. NAA is increased in Canavan disease.
Total creatine and phosphocreatine (Cr)	Involved in energy metabolism of cells.	Level of Cr is relatively stable in metabolic diseases; however, Cr may decrease, and it is not a reliable internal reference.
Choline-containing compound (Cho)	Membrane component and an osmolite.	Cho is sensitive to myelin disorders and is often decreased; however, it may be increased when cell membrane turnover is increased, usually in the early or acute stage of a demyelinating disease. Cho is increased in malignant brain tumors.
Myo-inositol	Present only in glial cells. It is a hormone messenger and osmolite.	Myo-inositol is a glial marker. It is sensitive to osmolarity and reflects the serum sodium level. Myo-inositol is increased in hypernatremia and decreased in hyponatremia. Its level may change in white matter diseases.
Glutamate and glutamine	Glutamate is an excitatory neurotransmitter, glutamine is involved in the recycle of glutamate	Glutamine is increased in hepatic encephalopathy. Total glutamate and glutamine are increased in human immunodeficiency virus and other viral infections.
Glucose	Fuel for brain cells	Glucose level is low under normal conditions. Elevation of glucose may be observed in diabetics.
γ-aminobutyrate (GABA)	Inhibitory neurotransmitter	Higher GABA as a result of medication helps to suppress seizures.
Taurine	Osmolite and bile acid	Taurine appears to be important in neonates.
Lactate	Product of anaerobic glucose metabolism.	Lactate elevation is found in hypoxia, stroke, and mitochondria diseases. Lactate elevation may be found in other disorders, too, but the reasons for this are not fully understood.

(Courtesy of Zimmerman RA, Wang ZJ: The value of proton MR spectroscopy in pediatric metabolic brain disease. *AJNR* 18:1872–1879, 1997, copyright American Society of Neuroradiology.)

brain diseases. With improved technology and more knowledge and experience, this noninvasive procedure will likely have an increasingly important role in the evaluation of metabolic diseases.

▶ A substantial subset of patients with childhood neurologic disease owe their physiologic dysfunction to known metabolic abnormalities. An additional group of such patients has clear physiologic dysfunction without identifiable anatomic abnormalities, and may well also harbor as yet unknown metabolic aberrations. The impracticality of obtaining brain tissue from patients with suspected metabolic disorders isolated to brain has limited the in vivo detection of such abnormalities. However, technological advances in MR spectroscopy have now made it possible to noninvasively quantitate many functionally important molecules in the brain. This article summarizes the present and potential applications, limitations, and practical (e.g., economic) issues of MR spectroscopy for pediatric neurometabolic disease.

N.F. Schor, M.D., Ph.D.

Magnetization Transfer Study of HIV Encephalitis and Progressive Multifocal Leukoencephalopathy
Dousett V, and the Groupe d'Epidémiologie Clinique su SIDA en Aquitaine (Hopital Pellegris-Tripode, CHU de Bordeaux, France; Université de Bordeaux II, France)
AJNR 18:895–901, 1997   6–5

Introduction.—Magnetization transfer (MT) in MR imaging is a technique that is particularly sensitive to tissue destruction. A study of HIV-positive patients was conducted to determine whether MT could differentiate a pure demyelinating process, progressive multifocal leukoencephalopathy (PML), from a far less destructive disease, HIV encephalitis.

Methods.—Study participants were 11 healthy controls and 2 groups of patients who were HIV-positive: 10 patients with clinical and radiologic findings of PML and 13 patients with HIV encephalitis (Fig 1). Brain imaging was performed with a 1.5-T MR unit and a transmit-receive head coil. An off-resonance pulse was applied before each excitation, achieving MT by saturating the macromolecular matrix in the steady state. Magnetization transfer ratios (MTRs) were calculated in the lesions of PML and HIV encephalitis and in the normal-appearing white matter in patients and controls. For both types of lesions, 2 MTR values were calculated and averaged at sites of hyperintense white matter signal.

Results.—The mean MTR value of hyperintensities in the deep white matter of patients with HIV encephalitis was 40%; the lowest value was 36%. This differed significantly from the mean MTR value for PML lesions, which was 22%; the lowest value in this group was 14%. Normal-appearing white matter from healthy controls had a mean MTR value of

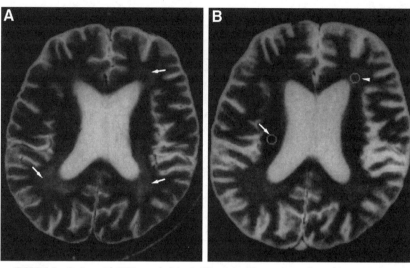

FIGURE 1.—Patient with HIV encephalitis. **A,** T2-weighted image shows deep white matter hyperintensity in the periventricular areas *(arrows)*. **B,** magnetization transfer image with cursors indicating region of interest in 1 lesion site *(arrowhead)* and normal-appearing white matter in another site *(arrow)*. (Courtesy of Dousset V, and the Groupe d'Epidémiologie Clinique du SIDA en Aquitaine: Magnetization transfer study of HIV encephalitis and progressive multifocal leukoencephalopathy. *AJNR* 18:895–901, 1997. Copyright by the American Society of Neuroradiology.)

47%. The MTR of normal-appearing white matter was significantly higher in controls than in patients with PML or HIV encephalitis.

Discussion.—It is important to differentiate between PML and HIV encephalitis because the latter can be treated and has a much better prognosis. In this series, PML was the cause of death in all 10 affected patients, whereas 4 of 13 patients with HIV encephalitis died of cachexia or nonneurologic infections. The pathogenesis of PML is JC papovavirus, an opportunistic agent, and the disease is characterized by demyelination. The pathogenesis of HIV encephalitis is uncertain, but myelin destruction is not usual. When the diagnosis is doubtful, MTR values may distinguish between PML and HIV encephalitis.

▶ Various MRI findings that attempt to distinguish the white matter lesions of progressive multifocal leukoencephalopathy (PML) from those of HIV encephalitis have been published. Among these findings are the more centrally located white matter abnormalities in PML, the more frequent parietal–occipital location of PML, and the hypointensity of white matter on T1-weighted images in PML. Because there may, however, be an overlap between PML and HIV encephalitis when these imaging criteria are used, a more quantitative method for distinguishing between these 2 is welcomed. Specifically, the destruction of white matter seen in PML results in a significantly decreased magnetization (MT) ratio when compared with HIV encephalitis. The use of MT ratios is encouraged when distinction between the 2 is believed to be clinically important.

R.M. Quencer, M.D.

Single-photon Emission CT Findings in Acute Japanese Encephalitis
Kimura K, Dosaka A, Hashimoto Y, et al (Kumamoto City Hosp, Japan; Kumamoto Univ, Japan)
AJNR 18:465–469, 1997   6–6

Background.—Japanese encephalitis (JE), characterized neurologically by extrapyramidal signs such as tremors, dystonia, and rigidity in the acute stage, is often severe, and there is rapid progression to a state of coma. It usually appears in the summer and early fall. Epidemics of JE have occurred throughout Asia. The value of single-photon emission CT (SPECT) in the diagnosis of this disease was determined.

Methods.—Ten patients with viral encephalitis were examined. The mean age was 69 years. Four patients had JE, and 6 had herpes simplex encephalitis or encephalitis of unknown origin. All patients underwent ^{99m}Tc-hexamethylpropyleneamine oxime (HMPAO) SPECT within 15 days of the onset of symptoms, and 2 patients with JE underwent SPECT in a later stage of the disease. Magnetic resonance imaging was performed in all patients after SPECT.

Findings.—All patients with acute-stage JE had a marked increase in HMPAO uptake that matched the hyperintense region seen on MR images in the thalami and putamina bilaterally. Follow-up SPECT studies in 2 patients with JE showed a reduction of HMPAO deposition in the high uptake regions. None of the patients with other types of JE had an increased accumulation of HMPAO in the thalami or putamina.

Conclusions.—Single-photon emission CT is useful for differentiating JE from herpes simplex encephalitis and encephalitis from other causes. This imaging modality may be a useful diagnostic tool in the early stages of JE.

▶ The hyperemic state and the resulting increased perfusion in the thalami and putamina in cases of acute viral encephalitis is the basis for the increased HMPAO accumulation in Japanese encephalitis. This type of activity is similar to the findings seen in the temporal lobes and limbic system in patients with herpes encephalitis but appears to differ from those with non-herpetic encephalitis. The value of a SPECT-HMPAO study is illustrated in Fig 1 of the original article where, by the T2-weighted MR image alone, the underlying cause of the thalamic hyperintensities is not obvious. The SPECT study is useful because the dramatic activity in the thalami and putamina is typical of Japanese encephalitis.

R.M. Quencer, M.D.

A Pain in the Ear: The Radiology of Otalgia

Weissman JL (Univ of Pittsburgh, Pa)

AJNR 18:1641–1651, 1997   6–7

Introduction.—The radiologic approach to patients with otalgia is dependent upon findings on physical examination. Primary otalgia is caused by ear disease; secondary otalgia (referred ear pain) is referred to the ear from structures remote from the ear. Diseases of the mouth and face are the most common sources of referred otalgia. The trigeminal nerve is the usual pathway for referred otalgia. Primary and secondary sources of otalgia were discussed.

Sensory Innervation.—Four cranial nerves (V, VII, IX, and X), the upper cervical plexus, and cervical sympathetic fibers are responsible for sensation from the ear and adjacent structures. These pathways are involved in primary and referred otalgia (pain caused by distant structures that receive sensory innervation from the same cranial nerves as the ear).

Sources of Primary and Secondary Otalgia.—Diseases of the auricle, external auditory canal, and tympanic membrane are sources of primary otalgia. The trigeminal nerve, facial nerve, and glossopharyngeal nerve are pathways that mediate referred otalgia. Referred otalgia may be caused by diseases of the nasopharynx and retropharynx, paranasal sinuses and nasal cavity, oropharynx and oral cavity, temporomandibular joint, parotid gland, hypopharynx and larynx, thyroid gland, esophagus, and trachea; as well as neuralgias, myofascial pain syndromes, pain of spinal nerve origin, and carotidynia and eagle syndrome.

Conclusion.—Patients with otalgia can be diagnostically challenging to clinicians and radiologists. Normal CT or MRI findings can indicate that pain is referred to the ear from remote sources.

▶ Of all the causes of facial pain, ear pain (otalgia) can be the most problematic. Not only is otalgia a frequent complaint, frequently nothing is found on neurologic examination. Otolaryngologists usually pick up the cause of primary otalgia (processes involving the internal auditory canal and middle ear), whereas, neurologists need to be familiar with the causes of referred otalgia (processes involving structures innervated by cranial nerves V, VII, IX and X, which also innervate the ear).

The most common cause of referred otalgia is temporal mandibular joint (TMJ) disease. Classically, this occurs in the morning or while the patient chews. The best way to detect TMJ is to place each forefinger in the external auditory canals and rest each thumb about ¾ inch anterior to the ear. This isolates the TMJ between the thumb and forefinger. Then have the patient open and close the jaw. If the patient reports tenderness in that area, TMJ should be suspected. Subluxation and crepitance of the joint are less useful signs, as they are very common in patients without clinical TMJ and they are not always present in those with early TMJ. Treatment should include night splint, reduced chewing, and avoidance of wide jaw opening.

Other causes of referred pain that should be familiar to neurologists include Gradenigo's syndrome (otalgia and abducens weakness from spread of otitis media to the petrous apex), Ramsay Hunt syndrome, and glosso-pharyngeal neuralgia. When the examination does not yield results, petrous bone CT or MRI scans of the head may be helpful.

R.J. Tusa, M.D., Ph.D.

Cervical Spondylotic Amyotrophy: Magnetic Resonance Imaging Demonstration of Intrinsic Cord Pathology
Kameyama T, Ando T, Yanagi T, et al (Nagoya Univ, Japan)
Spine 23:448–452, 1998   6–8

Introduction.—Cervical spondylotic amyotrophy is characterized by severe muscular atrophy in the upper extremities in patients with cervical spondylosis. Sensory deficits may be absent or insignificant. It has not been determined whether the pathophysiology of this syndrome involves selective damage to the ventral roots or to anterior horns. Reports on 3 patients with segmental muscular atrophy in whom MRI confirmed intrinsic cord disease as the cause of the syndrome are given.

Methods.—Age range of 3 men with segmental muscular atrophy of the proximal upper extremities was 52–72 years. Patients underwent MRI to determine the pathophysiology of cervical spondylotic amyotrophy.

Results.—Sagittal T2-weighted MRIs confirmed the cause of the syndrome as intrinsic cord disease in all 3 patients. Multiple linear high-signal intensity areas were observed within the compressed spinal cord. These lesions extended to more than one segment on sagittal images and small symmetric intramedullary high-intensity areas on axial images in all 3 patients (Fig 1). These lesions were thought to be irreversible cystic lesions, not potentially reversible edema. In autopsy findings of cervical compression myelopathy, these cysts have been observed to extend from the central gray matter to the anterior horns. Thus, surgery would not have been effective in any of these 3 patients.

Conclusion.—Multisegmental damage to the anterior horns is one pathologic feature of cervical spondylotic amyotrophy. This may be caused by dynamic cord compression through circulatory insufficiency. An understanding of the pathophysiology associated with cervical spondylotic amyotrophy is crucial for determining appropriate therapeutic strategies.

▶ The location of signal abnormalities within the spinal cord on axial spin echo T2-weighted images give clues as to the underlying disease causing the presenting clinical condition. Separation of laterally placed abnormalities (white matter) vs. centrally placed abnormalities (gray matter or watershed regions) is often a clue pointing to ischemic disease, demyelinating disease, or primary degenerative disease. Striking central/paracentral lesions in a patient with significant discogenic spondylosis point to a mechanism whereby hypoperfusion of the gray matter results because of the strategic

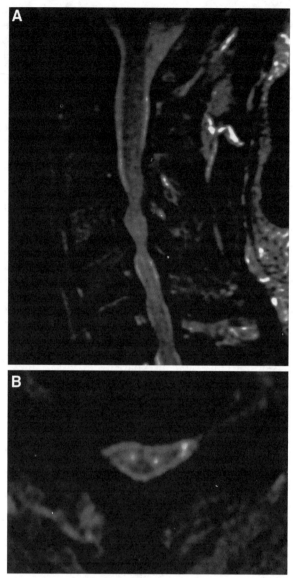

FIGURE 1.—In Case 1, sagittal T2-weighted magnetic resonance image (spin echo: repetition time [msec] 1,500, echo time [msec] 90) shows the spinal cord compressed by disk protrusions from C3–C4 to C6–C7, with greatest severity at C4–C5. Linear region of high-signal intensity is observed within spinal cord, extending from C4–C5 to C5–C6 (**A**). Axial T2*-weighted magnetic resonance image (field echo: repetition time [msec] 700, echo time [msec] 18, flip angle 15 degrees) at C5–C6 demonstrates small symmetric areas of high-signal intensity within the spinal cord, which appear to be located in the anterior horns bilaterally (**B**). (Courtesy of Kameyama T, Ando T, Yanagi T: Cervical spondylotic amyotrophy; Magnetic resonance imaging demonstration of intrinsic cord pathology. *Spine* 23:448–452, 1998.)

location of the anterior perforating arteries. The major differential diagnoses based solely on the location of the symmetric signal abnormalities within the cord would be ischemia/infarction, a primary degenerative process of the cord involving the anterior horn cells (amyotrophic lateral sclerosis, spinal muscular atrophy), and the result of a neurotropic viral infection.

R.M. Quencer, M.D.

7 Sleep Disorders

Contributions of the Pedunculopontine Region to Normal and Altered REM Sleep
Rye DB (Emory Univ, Atlanta, Ga)
Sleep 20:757–788, 1997   7–1

Background.—The pedunculopontine (PPN) region of the upper brainstem is a critical modulator of activated behavioral states, such as wakefulness and rapid eye movement (REM) sleep. The expression of REM sleep–related physiology relies on a subpopulation of PPN neurons that release acetylcholine (ACh), which acts on muscarinic receptors. Serotonin's potent hyperpolarization of cholinergic PPN neurons is important in models of REM sleep control. The article reviewed recent work from various neuroscience disciplines and constructed a framework for defining the role of the PPN and laterodorsal tegmental (LDT) region in normal and abnormal behaviors in which state control is a major feature.

Discussion.—Increasing experimental evidence and clinical experience suggest that the responsiveness of the PPN region and thus REM sleep modulation involves closely adjacent glutamatergic neurons and alternate afferent neurotransmitters. The most conspicuous and most likely to be relevant clinically are the dopamine-sensitive GABAergic pathways exiting the main output nuclei of the basal ganglia and adjacent forebrain nuclei. These GABAergic pathways are ideal for differentially modulating the physiologic hallmarks of REM sleep, as each originates from a functionally unique forebrain circuit and terminates in a unique pattern on brain stem neurons with unique membrane features. Changes in the quality, timing, and quantity of REM sleep that characterize narcolepsy, REM sleep behavior disorder, and neurodegenerative and affective disorders appear to reflect changes in the responsiveness of cells in the PPN region governed by these afferents, an increase or decline in PPN cell number, or muscarinic ACh receptors mediating increased responsiveness to ACh derived from the PPN.

▶ This is an excellent review of recent knowledge of the neuroanatomy and neurophysiology of the generation and regulation of REM sleep. A wealth of information is presented in an exceptionally well-organized fashion. The reader should find the information elucidative of the current state of knowledge in this area. The author also offers some possible mechanisms for relationships between REM sleep regulation and clinical disorders associated with alterations of REM sleep. Better understanding of these relationships should help to serve as a useful bridge between newer knowledge of neurophysiologic processes in the pedunculopontine region and the expanding knowledge of clinical sleep disorders.

B. Nolan, M.D.

Pontine Lesions in Idiopathic Narcolepsy
Plazzi G, Montagna P, Provini F, et al (Univ of Bologna, Italy; Johns Hopkins Univ, Baltimore, Md; Case Western Reserve Univ, Cleveland, Ohio)
Neurology 46:1250–1254, 1996   7–2

Introduction.—Brain tumors, brain stem lesions, and hypothalamic syndromes have all been reported in patients with narcolepsy, and there may be a genetic predisposition (linked to the HLA-DR2 haplotype) that enhances the effect of these causal lesions. Three patients were described who had longstanding disabling narcolepsy and were HLA-DR2 positive but showed no other neurologic manifestations.

Case Report 2.—Man, 66, had experienced excessive daytime somnolence and sleep attacks from the age of 16 years. Migraine attacks preceded by a visual aura started to occur several times a year at age 20. The condition progressed as the patient grew older, and at age 40 he experienced cataplectic falls when laughing and while playing tennis. Treatment with dextroamphetamine, then viloxazine, brought about moderate improvement in alertness and cataplexy. At the time of evaluation, results of his general medical and neurologic examinations were normal. A 48-hour dynamic

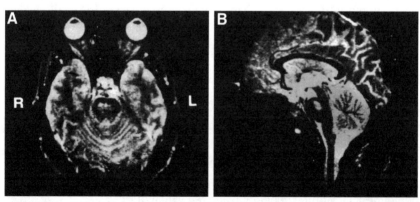

FIGURE 2.—Patient 2. **A,** axial (spin echo: 1,800/100; 7-mm slice thickness) and **B,** sagittal (spin echo: 1,800/100; 5-mm slice thickness) T2-weighted MR images show bilateral hyperintense lesions without mass effect in the central portion of the rostral pons. (Reprinted from Neurology, courtesy of Plazzi G, Montagna P, Provini F, et al: Pontine lesions in idiopathic narcolepsy. *Neurology* 46:1250–1254, 1996, by permission of Little, Brown and Company, Inc.)

polygraphic recording revealed 4 episodes of sleep during the daytime. These episodes were characterized by shortened rapid eye movement (REM) latency and 5 cataplectic attacks. Tissue typing was positive for HLA-DR2. On MRI, (Fig 2), bilateral hyperintense lesions were seen in the central portion of the rostral pons. The patient has had some functional improvement with viloxazine (200 mg/day) therapy.

Discussion.—Although all 3 of the patients reported here were considered to have "idiopathic" narcolepsy, MRI revealed lesions in the pons. All had the classic signs of narcolepsy, which appeared in adolescence and responded only partially to therapy. The only other neurologic signs or symptoms appeared in patient 2, who had migraine with aura. Pontine structural alterations in these patients were considered causally related to the narcolepsy. The location of these lesions correspond to the pontine reticular regions, the site of structures that regulate REM sleep.

▶ It seems unlikely that the striking pontine abnormalities described in these 3 older patients with narcolepsy are coincidental. Because the disorder typically becomes clinically apparent in the second or third decade of life, abnormalities seen in these patients in the sixth and seventh decades may possibly be caused by progression of the underlying disorder, as the authors suggest. Another possible explanation is that the changes seen may somehow be related to treatment, or nontreatment as the case may be. Although the patients were apparently highly symptomatic, the details regarding treatment are limited. As the treatment for narcolepsy still leaves a great deal to be desired, improved future understanding of the development of pontine abnormalities in the course of the disorder would be most welcome.

B. Nolan, M.D.

Idiopathic Hypersomnia: A Series of 42 Patients
Bassetti C, Aldrich MS (Univ of Michigan, Ann Arbor)
Brain 120:1423–1435, 1997   7–3

Background.—Idiopathic hypersomnia is characterized by nonimperative sleepiness, long unrefreshing naps, prolonged night sleep, and difficulty reaching full wakefulness with sleep drunkenness. Although narcolepsy initially was considered a separate syndrome from idiopathic hypersomnia, more recent evidence suggests some overlap. The relationship between these 2 syndromes was determined by reviewing clinical data from a large population with sleep disorders.

Study Design.—A database of more than 4,000 patients who had been examined from 1986 to 1995 at the Sleep Disorders Center of the University of Michigan was reviewed. During this period, 258 patients had narcolepsy diagnosed and 63 received a diagnosis of idiopathic hypersomnia. Patients with upper airway resistance syndrome or with insufficient

TABLE 2.—Clinical, Polygraphic, and Genetic Findings in Idiopathic Hypersomnia and Narcolepsy

Parameter	Idiopathic hypersomnia	Mono-symptomatic narcolepsy*	Narcolepsy with cataplexy*
Subjects (n)	42	28	39
Mean age at diagnosis (years)	35	34	46
Female : male	27 : 15	13 : 15	25 : 14
Caucasian : African-American : Asian	39 : 3 : 0	20 : 7 : 1	27 : 11 : 1
Automatic behavior	61%†	25–35%‡	31–38%‡
Sleep paralysis§	40%	27–36%‡	49–58%‡
Hypnagogic hallucinations§	43%	14–30%‡	74–75%‡·‖
Hours of sleep per weekday	8.4 ± 1.9	7.7 ± 0.4	7.8 ± 0.3
Time to get going in the morning (min)	42	48	36
Sleep efficiency	93 ± 5%	93 ± 5%	86 ± 12%‖
Total sleep time (min)	464 ± 50	468 ± 47	432 ± 75
Number of awakenings (>1 min)	20 ± 11	9 ± 7¶	17 ± 10
Slow wave sleep (% of total sleep)	8 ± 5	8 ± 4	5 ± 4
REM sleep (% of total sleep)	18 ± 7	19 ± 4	16 ± 6
Mean sleep latency on MSLT	4.3 ± 2.1†	2.8 ± 1.1	2.2 ± 1.2
Periods of sleep onset with REM/ chances on polysomnogram + MSLT	12/303 (4%)†	93/188 (49%)	106/210 (50%)
DR2 (number of positives/total tested)	6/18 (33%)†	4/7 (57%)	9/11 (82%)
DQ1 (number of positives/total tested)	13/18 (72%)	7/7 (100%)	9/10 (90%)

*Data from Aldrich (1996). Monosymptomatic narcolepsy was defined as narcolepsy by International Classification of Sleep Disorders criteria (1990) with > 2 periods of sleep onset with REM or MSLT but with no definite cataplexy.
†P < 0.05 vs. monosymptomatic narcolepsy and narcolepsy with cataplexy.
‡Range of percentage obtained from questionnaire or clinical assessment.
§Occasionally, often or always.
‖P < 0.05 vs. idiopathic hypersomnia and monosymptomatic narcolepsy.
¶P < 0.05 vs. idiopathic hypersomnia and narcolepsy with cataplexy.
*Abbreviations: MSLT, Multiple Sleep Latency Tests; REM, rapid eye movement.
(Courtesy of Bassetti C, Aldrich MS: Idiopathic hypersomnia: A series of 42 patients. *Brain* 120:1423–1435, 1997, by permission of Oxford University Press.)

clinical data for diagnosis were excluded from the study group. The study group consisted of 42 patients with diagnosed idiopathic hypersomnia who met the following criteria: excessive daytime sleepiness for more than 1 year, absence of cataplexy, average sleep latency on Multiple Sleep Latency Tests (MSLT) of less than 10 minutes, no more than 1 sleep-onset rapid eye movement (REM) period on MSLT, apnea + hypopnea index of less than 10, periodic limb-movement index of less than 20, no improvement after increased nighttime sleep, and no other apparent cause of sleepiness. A retrospective clinical assessment and sleep studies review was performed for all study participants. A prospective clinical assessment was performed with 28 participants.

Findings.—Of the 42 participants with idiopathic hypersomnia, only 29% had the classic symptoms of nonimperative sleepiness, long unrefreshing naps, prolonged nighttime sleep, and difficulty awakening. Sleep recordings were generally normal (Table 2). Another 32% had symptoms similar to narcolepsy with irresistible sleepiness, short and refreshing naps, normal awakening, no cataplexy, no REM abnormalities, and good response to stimulants. The remaining 39% of patients with idiopathic hypersomnia had intermediate characteristics. There was no increase in human leukocyte antigens detected in narcolepsy patients. There was a good response to stimulants in three fourths of these patients, and one fourth had spontaneous improvement. Possible etiologies including viral illness, head trauma, and primary mood disorder were detected in 10 of the study participants.

Conclusions.—Idiopathic hypersomnia is a rare sleep syndrome that remains a diagnosis of exclusion. Only a minority of cases fulfilled all classic criteria. Idiopathic hypersomnia usually began in adolescence or young adulthood with hypersomnia, normal-to-prolonged nighttime sleep, and awakening difficulties. Sleep recordings were usually normal. Spontaneous remissions were common, and both stimulants and antidepressants could be beneficial. Current classifications of hypersomnias probably require revision.

▶ This retrospective review of a large series of patients with careful clinical evaluation highlights the relative rarity of idiopathic hypersomnia. In the authors' experience, idiopathic hypersomnia appears to be less than one fourth as common as narcolepsy. However, more than twice the number of idiopathic hypersomnia patients were excluded because of insufficient data and diagnosed as "excessive-daytime-sleepiness-not-otherwise-specified." Clinical and laboratory evaluation can sort out most of the more common causes of hypersomnia including sleep-induced respiratory abnormalities, narcolepsy, and proposed variants. Considering the frequent limitations of obtaining a clinical history and also the limitations of current diagnostic tests, it is perhaps somewhat surprising that there are so few "idiopathic" cases. The authors' elucidation of the common features of idiopathic hypersomnia and their experience with response to stimulant or, at times, antidepressant medication are worthy of note.

B. Nolan, M.D.

Regional Cerebral Blood Flow Throughout the Sleep-Wake Cycle: An H$_2$^{15}O PET Study
Braun AR, Balkin TJ, Wesensten NJ, et al (NIH, Bethesda, Md; Walter Reed Army Inst of Research, Washington, DC)
Brain 120:1173–1197, 1997   7–4

Introduction.—The best technical approach currently available for examination of sleep is that of H$_2$^{15}O–positron emission tomography (PET), which makes it possible to visualize functional brain activity during discrete sleep stages and to study multiple sleep stages in the same individual during a single night. Normal male volunteers took part in a study designed to assess dynamic changes in brain function throughout the sleep-wake cycle by measuring cerebral blood flow (CBF) with H$_2$^{15}O-PET.

Methods.—The volunteers had a mean age of 24.5 years; 33 were right handed. None had any known medical, neurologic, or psychiatric conditions that might affect brain function. All underwent sleep deprivation or sleep restriction procedures before the PET studies. After these procedures, participants were positioned in the PET scanner and polysomnographically monitored for the duration of the study. Cerebral blood flow was measured before sleep onset, during deep slow-wave sleep (SWS), during rapid eye movement (REM) sleep, and upon waking after recovery sleep.

Results.—Compared with the period of presleep wakefulness, deep sleep (SWS) was characterized by a global reduction in partial pressure of carbon dioxide (pCO_2–corrected CBF of 26.0%. Among centrencephalic structures, the most significant reductions in analysis of covariance–corrected regional CBF (rCBF) during SWS were found in the posterior putamen. Significant decreases were detected throughout the midbrain and throughout the basal forebrain, and reduced CBF was apparent throughout the thalamus. Heterogeneous changes in rCBF were seen in the neocortex. Compared with SWS, postsleep wakefulness was characterized by a global increase in pCO_2-corrected CBF of 11.4%. A global increase of +16.8% occurred in the transition from SWS to REM sleep. Compared with SWS, REM sleep showed activation of paralimbic and limbic areas. Activity in the frontoparietal association cortices remained depressed in REM sleep, and there was selective activation of certain postrolandic sensory cortices.

Discussion.—The course of the human sleep-wake cycle is characterized by fundamental, state-dependent changes in the functional organization of the brain. Centrencephalic structures are important in the genesis of each sleep or wakefulness state. Comparisons of wakefulness and SWS and REM sleep indicate that shifts in the level of activity of the striatum are the most significant detected changes. Deactivation of the heteromodal association areas, the single feature common to both REM and nonREM sleep states, may be a defining characteristic of sleep.

▶ It has been known for some time that there are dramatic differences in the functional activity of the nervous system related to the different states of wakefulness, nonREM, and REM sleep. The sophisticated work presented in this article provides us with greater localization of the differences in CBF between wakefulness flow patterns and regional differences in selected sleep states. The reported differences in CBF in basal ganglia in sleep are interesting and provide evidence for a greater involvement of these structures than is generally appreciated. The careful correlation of CBF measures to simultaneous measures of awake and sleep states makes the information presented particularly compelling.

B. Nolan, M.D.

REM Sleep Behavior Disorders in Multiple System Atrophy

Plazzi G, Corsini R, Provini F, et al (Univ of Bologna, Italy)
Neurology 48:1094–1097, 1997   7–5

Background.—Multiple system atrophy (MSA), characterized by any combination of autonomic failure with parkinsonism, with absent or poor response to levodopa, and with cerebellar and pyramidal signs, usually does not include the features of REM sleep behavior disorders (RBD). However, several patients with MSA reporting intense motor or verbal paroxysmal episodes during sleep have been described recently in the literature. The frequency of RBD in patients with MSA, its clinical relevance, and whether RBD is associated with demographic or clinical features were investigated.

Methods and Findings.—Thirty-nine consecutive patients with MSA were included in the study. Sixty-nine percent reported nocturnal motor paroxysmal episodes associated with dreams, suggesting the clinical diagnosis of RBD. In 44% of these patients, RBD preceded the clinical onset of MSA by more than 1 year. In 26%, RBD onset was concomitant with the appearance of motor or autonomic symptoms, and in 30%, it occurred at least 2 years afterward. Ninety percent of the patients with MSA had RBD according to polysomnographic recordings. Other findings on polysomnography were nonclinical obstructive sleep apnea in 6 patients, laryngeal stridor in 8, and periodic limb movements during sleep in 10.

Conclusions.—In patients with MSA, RBD is the most common clinical sleep manifestation and polysomnographic finding. Such sleep disorder often precedes the appearance of other MSA symptoms by years. Extended polysomnographic montages are recommended in the sleep studies of patients with MSA.

▶ REM sleep behavior disorder is a troubling and potentially injurious condition. Patients and families can usually give descriptions of behaviors that are often dramatic, and sometimes aggressive and injurious, which suggest the presence of the disorder. Because interventions may alleviate the symptoms and prevent possible injury to patients as well as bedpartners, clinicians should be alert for the occurrence of RBD. This report highlights the authors' finding of frequent association of RBD and MSA. Inquiring about and recognizing such distressing symptoms should help the astute clinician to suspect the potential association of RBD with MSA or other neurologic disorder.

B. Nolan, M.D.

Sleep-disordered Breathing and Neuropsychological Deficits: A Population-based Study

Kim HC, Young T, Matthews CG, et al (Univ of Wisconsin—Madison)
Am J Respir Crit Care Med 156:1813–1819, 1997   7–6

Introduction.—Unrecognized sleep-disordered breathing (SDB) is highly prevalent in the population, although the associated morbidity and mortality are uncertain. Patients with clinical SDB are found to have pathologic sleepiness and problems with memory, concentration, and task performance. Evidence of such neuropsychological deficits was sought in general population subjects with SDB.

Methods.—Data were used from the Wisconsin Sleep Cohort Study, a prospective, population-based study designed to clarify the natural history of SDB. Overnight polysomnography was performed in 841 employed men and women aged 30–60 years. The data were used to calculate each individual's apnea-hypopnea index (AHI), defined as the frequency of apneas and hypopneas per hour of sleep. Before undergoing sleep testing, each individual was evaluated on a battery of neuropsychological tests, including such functional areas as motor skills, attention, concentration, information processing, and memory. Self-reported sleepiness was evaluated as well.

Results.—The AHI was less than 5 in 642 individuals and 5 or greater in 199. On principal factor analysis of the neuropsychological test results, 2 common factors were identified: a psychomotor efficiency factor and a memory factor accounting for 54% of the variance. On multiple regression analysis, the psychomotor efficiency factor was significantly and negatively associated with logarithmically transformed AHI (LogAHI). This relationship was independent of age, sex, or education and was unexplained by subject-reported sleepiness. LogAHI was unrelated to the memory factor (Table 7).

Conclusions.—A significant association exists between undiagnosed SDB and neuropsychological deficit, particularly in the domain of psychomotor efficiency. These cases of SDB may interfere with coordination of fine visuomotor control and information via sustained attention and concentration. The relationship is linear, suggesting that even individuals with

TABLE 7.—Mean Neuropsychological Factor Scores* by Sleep-disordered Breathing Categories

Variable	n	Psychomotor Efficiency		Memory	
		Mean* ± SEM	p Value	Mean ± SEM	p Value
Apnea-Hypopnea Index (AHI)					
< 5	642	0.038 ± 0.036	0.035	0.021 ± 0.039	0.279
≥ 5	199	−0.123 ± 0.066		−0.067 ± 0.070	

*Least square mean adjusted to the mean age, and gender and educational status distributions of our sample.
(Courtesy of Kim HC, Young T, Matthews CG, et al: Sleep-disordered breathing and neuropsychological deficits: A population-based study. *Am J Respir Crit Care Med* 156:1813–1819, 1997. Official Journal of the American Thoracic Society, copyright American Lung Association.)

mild SDB have some neuropsychological impairment. The effects of an AHI of 15 on psychomotor efficiency can be equated to those of 5 additional years of age or to one half of the effects of hypnosedative use.

▶ The authors report their experience with a large and well-studied cohort. The study is well designed and comprehensive. Of particular interest is the demonstrable adverse effect of relatively mild abnormalities of AHI. The data offer support for the treatment of mild SDB when impaired daytime performance is an issue. This study used self-report measures for daytime sleepiness. Nevertheless, the results appear to support the growing body of data that appear to implicate nocturnal hypoxemia rather than daytime somnolence as the culprit in impaired performance. Future longitudinal study of this cohort should not only add to the current cross-sectional data, but also further improve our knowledge of SDB and better assess the value of treatment interventions.

B. Nolan, M.D.

8 Neuro-oncology

Motor Neuron Syndromes in Cancer Patients
Forsyth PA, Dalmau J, Graus F, et al (Mem Sloan-Kettering Cancer Ctr, New York; Univ of Calgary, Canada; Univ of Alberta, Edmonton, Canada; et al)
Ann Neurol 41:722–730, 1997   8–1

Introduction.—Motor neuron disease (MND) may be a paraneoplastic syndrome in certain cases. Findings in 14 patients studied suggest that MND may be a paraneoplastic syndrome when a specific paraneoplastic marker (such as the anti-Hu antibody) or unusual symptoms are present.

Methods.—The 14 patients had a pure or predominant MND syndrome and cancer. Ten patients were examined, and the medical records and samples of serum and CSF were reviewed in the other 4. Autopsy material was available in paraffin blocks from 2 patients. Patients were classified into 3 groups according to the presence of anti-neuronal antibodies, type of neurologic syndrome, and histology of the cancer.

Results.—Three patients (group 1) had anti-Hu antibodies, had rapidly progressive MND, and showed less prominent symptoms of involvement of other areas of the nervous system. The mean age of group 1 patients was 66 years; 2 had small-cell lung cancer (SCLC) and 1 had prostate cancer. Neurologic symptoms appeared 4–10 months before diagnosis of SCLC and 1.5 months after diagnosis of prostate cancer. The finding of anti-Hu antibodies in 1 patient with SCLC led to diagnosis of the cancer, despite negative results of a chest CT scan and normal bronchoscopy findings. Group 2 patients were 5 women (mean age, 62 years) with breast cancer. Their signs of upper motor neuron (UMN) disease initially resembled primary lateral sclerosis and appeared from 62 months before to 79 months after diagnosis of breast cancer. These patients had no metastases or spinal cord compression. The 6 patients in group 3 had UMN disease resembling amyotrophic lateral sclerosis, with symptoms appearing between 47 months before and 48 months after their cancer diagnosis. Neurologic symptoms were unchanged in 4 patients after treatment of the tumor, worsened in 1, and subjectively improved in 1.

Discussion.—In group 1, MND associated with the anti-Hu antibody was considered unequivocally paraneoplastic. Four of the 5 women in group 2 had symptoms of UMN disease occur within 3 months of cancer diagnosis or tumor recurrence, thus strongly suggesting the paraneoplastic nature of the MND. Certain patients with MND should be evaluated for an underlying cancer. Treatment of cancer in patients with MND may improve or stabilize their neurologic symptoms.

▶ The possible association of MND disease or amyotrophic lateral sclerosis with neoplasia has been hotly debated ever since Lord Brain first suggested that the 2 conditions might be associated. In general, the protagonists have believed that an underlying neoplasm, such as a plasma-cell dyscrasia, a lymphoma, or a carcinoma can cause the motor-neuron degeneration. The contrary view is that these are both relatively common disorders of the elderly, and that an association may be coincidental. It might be expected that epidemiologic studies could answer this question, but if a more intensive search for an underlying neoplasm is made in the population with amyotrophic lateral sclerosis than in a "control normal" population, as is inevitable, then epidemiologic studies are invalid. The best proof of the paraneoplastic origin of a motor-neuron degeneration would be that removal of the cancer led to arrest or cure of the MND. There are extremely few such cases described in the literature. Another way of fulfilling "Koch's postulates" would be to demonstrate the presence of antibodies that bind to and kill motor neurons. The presence of anti-Hu antibodies in group 1 of this study might fulfill this criterion. The third way of showing that the paraneoplastic cause of a MND syndrome is very likely to show that the syndrome is very different from cases without neoplasm. The authors suggest that this is the case with regard to their group 2 patients, although there are many similar patients without evidence of an underlying cancer seen in clinics for amyotrophic lateral sclerosis. This is an important article that should be read carefully by those interested in this topic.

W.G. Bradley, D.M., F.R.C.P.

Small-Cell Lung Cancer, Paraneoplastic Cerebellar Degeneration and the Lambert-Eaton Myasthenic Syndrome
Mason WP, Graus F, Lang B, et al (Mem Sloan-Kettering Cancer Ctr; Cornell Univ, New York; Univ of Barcelona; et al)
Brain 120:1279–1300, 1997   8–2

Background.—Paraneoplastic cerebellar degeneration (PCD) is characterized by the onset of subacute cerebellar dysfunction associated with cancer, most commonly of the lung, ovary, or breast. Antibodies to neuronal antigens expressed by the tumor, onconeural antibodies, are often detected in association with this condition. In patients with small-cell lung cancer, PCD can occur both in the presence and the absence of Hu antineuronal antibodies (HuAb). Degeneration may also be associated with Lambert-Eaton myasthenic syndrome (LEMS). The sera of 57 PCD were examined to study the clinical implications of antineuronal antibodies.

Study Design.—Sera were collected from 57 patients with small-cell lung cancer and PCD and from a control group of 109 patients with small-cell lung cancer, but without PCD symptoms. Serum samples were assayed for HuAb, as well as P/Q- and N-type voltage-gated calcium channel antibodies. Antibody titers were classified as high, low, or negative. Low and negative samples were grouped together for the purpose of analysis.

Findings.—Of the 57 patients in the PCD group, 25 had high titer, 4 had low titer, and 28 were HuAb negative. None of the 109 control patients had high HuAb titers. The patients with high titer were more likely to be female, to have multifocal neurologic disease, and to be severely disabled compared to HuAb− PCD patients. Nine of the patients with PCD developed LEMS. Of the 7 patients with LEMS who were tested for antibodies to P/Q-type voltage-gated calcium channel antibodies, all were positive, as were 20% of the PCD patients who were HuAb−. Only 2% of control patients had these antibodies. Neither cancer therapy nor immunomodulation altered the course of PCD, but LEMS symptoms improved. Neurologic disease was the cause of death in 65% of HuAb+ PCD patients and 10% of HuAb− PCD patients. The patients with PCD did not survive as long as age-, tumor-stage, and treatment-matched patients without PCD. The pathologic findings of 5 HuAb+ PCD patients at autopsy included diffuse encephalomyelitis with severe loss of Purkinje cells in 4 patients and involvement of posterior nerve roots or dorsal root ganglia in 3 patients. Autopsy studies of 3 HuAb− PCD patients revealed severe loss of Purkinje cells without inflammatory infiltrates.

Conclusions.—A group of 57 patients with small-cell lung cancer and paraneoplastic cerebellar degeneration were evaluated and compared to a group of patients with cancer, but without PCD. In PCD patients, HuAb antibodies were not necessarily present at high titer. Approximately 15% of the PCD patients developed Lambert-Eaton myasthenic syndrome, irrespective of HuAb status. All LEMS patients were P/Q-type voltage-gated calcium channel antibody positive, as were 20% of HuAb+ PCD patients without clinical symptoms of LEMS. Patients who were HuAb+ PCD were more likely to be female, to have multifocal neurologic disease and to be severely impaired than HuAb− PCD patients. Paraneoplastic cerebellar degeneration was associated with a more rapid onset of death. Inflammatory infiltrates were more common in the brains of HuAb+ PCD patients than in HuAb− PCD patients. In patients without known cancer, detection of HuAb should increase the index of suspicion for small-cell lung cancer. In patients with this type of cancer, the development of a cerebellar syndrome should raise the suspicion of PCD. Neither treatment of the tumor nor the PCD appears to modify the cerebellar disorder in most patients, although it may modulate the symptoms of LEMS, if present. Patients with LEMS have antibodies against voltage-gated calcium channel proteins, as do many PCD HuAb− patients. This suggests that antibodies to voltage-gated calcium channel proteins may also play a role in PCD.

▶ Antibodies are not everything! Individuals with no symptoms may have high titers of antibodies that in other individuals are responsible for severe disease. This has been known for many years. The discovery that Lambert-

Eaton syndrome and paraneoplastic antibody-mediated cerebellar degeneration could be 2 of a number of different neurologic manifestations of small-cell lung cancer was an important breakthrough. We are now trying to discover the details of this relationship. Of undoubted importance are anti-Hu antibodies in cerebellar degeneration, and antibodies against the P/Q and N-type voltage-gated calcium channels in the Lambert-Eaton syndrome. It would be wonderful if there were a simple direct relationship, but this is clearly not the case. Factors inducing variability include that the antibodies can be directed against different epitopes of the antigen, and that may induce differing degrees of complement activation and lymphocytic infiltration. This extensive paper highlights that there are clinical differences between patients who are antibody-negative and antibody-positive, which will be of use in clinical practice. The most intriguing and unresolved matter is "how it all works."

W.G. Bradley, D.M., F.R.C.P.

Cerebral Complications of Murine Monoclonal CD3 Antibody (OKT3): CT and MR Findings
Parizel PM, Snoeck H-W, van den Hauwe L, et al (Univ of Antwerp, Belgium)
AJNR 18:1935–1938, 1997   8–3

Introduction.—An increasing number of systemic and neurologic adverse reactions and complications have been reported in patients treated with OKT3, a mouse monoclonal antibody directed against human T-lymphocytes. The primary use of the drug is to treat acute corticosteroid-resistant allograft rejection. This study describes a patient who developed an acute neurologic syndrome after IV administration of OKT3.

Case Report.—A boy, 13 years, had reflux nephropathy and dysplastic kidneys. When end-stage renal failure developed, he received 2 kidneys from a 2-year-old donor. Six weeks later the boy experienced acute allograft rejection and was treated for 3 days with methylprednisolone (1 g/day). Clinical response was inadequate, however, and OKT3 was initiated in a dosage of 3 mg/day. Seven days later the patient experienced 2 episodes of generalized seizure, increased lethargy, a decrease in mental function, and progression to coma.

Imaging with CT and MR revealed confluent cerebral lesions at the corticomedullary junction. With contrast administration the lesions were found to have produced blood-brain barrier dysfunction. The patient received a diagnosis of OKT3-induced encephalopathy with cerebral edema and capillary leak syndrome. With supportive therapy, the boy's neurologic status improved rapidly. Subsequent CT scans demonstrated progressive disappearance of brain edema.

Discussion.—In some previous cases, patients treated with OKT3 experienced an acute clinical syndrome known as cytokine-release syndrome (CRS). Patients typically showed clinical symptoms of CRS within 30 to 60 minutes after the start of treatment. In this case, the late onset of neurologic symptoms, 7 days after the start of OKT3 treatment, was unusual. Neuroimaging findings appear to be related to the increased vascular permeability induced by the drug. Clinicians and neuroradiologists should be aware of CNS complications associated with OKT3.

▶ The spectrum of neurological disorders affecting transplant patients is quite broad. The specific etiology of an underlying encephalopathy or focal neurological disorder often remains elusive. Among the diagnostic considerations are opportunistic infections secondary to immunosuppression, metabolic encephalopathy, cerebrovascular disease, and the side effects of pharmacotherapy. Dr. Parizel and colleagues describe a patient who presented with seizures and altered mental status accompanied by dramatic abnormalities on CT scan and MRI that occurred in association with the use of OKT3 to prevent renal transplant rejection. The possibility that a therapeutic immunomodulator may be the cause of neurological disease always needs to be considered in this population.

J.R. Berger, M.D.

9 Epilepsy

A Potassium Channel Mutation in Neonatal Human Epilepsy
Biervert C, Schroeder BC, Kubisch C, et al (Univ of Bonn, Germany; Univ of Hamburg, Germany; Univ of Melbourne, Australia)
Science 279:403–406, 1998   9–1

Introduction.—Most forms of idiopathic epilepsy have a genetic component, but only a few have specific syndromes that are single-gene disorders. Benign familial neonatal convulsions (BFNC) is an autosomal dominant, idiopathic epilepsy of infancy. It is characterized by unprovoked partial or generalized clonic convulsions and occasional apneic spells occurring during wakefulness and sleep. Seizures usually start about day 3 of life and commonly disappear after several weeks or months. About 10% to 15% of patients have febrile or afebrile seizures in later childhood. The gene loci for BFNC has been mapped to chromosomes 20q13.3 and 8q24. Most familial disorders are linked to chromosome 20. Reported are gene defects in patients with BFNC.

Findings.—Cosmid DNA from a previously described contig in the chromosomal region 20q13.3 was used to isolate a 3.4-kb partial cDNA clone from a human fetal brain cDNA library and extend it by 4 kb toward the 5' end by rapid amplification of cDNA ends. A search of the GenBank database indicated that the 5' open reading frame is about 50% identical to KvLQT1 and that a 1160-base pair (bp) stretch is identical to a partial cDNA isolated earlier. The KVLQT1 potassium channel gene is now renamed KCNQ1. The present homolog KCNQ2 is now named. The KCNQ homolog (KCNQ3) on human chromosome 8q24 has also been identified close to the second locus (4) for BFNC. Ion channels regulating neuronal excitability have been suggested as possible epilepsy genes. The KCNQ2 genomic structure (13) and screen (14) was partially determined in a large Australian white pedigree that was linked earlier to chromosome 20q13 (15) for mutations in KCNQ2. A 5-bp insertion was detected at the triplet encoding amino acid 534 in a segment highly conserved between KCNQ2 and KvLQT1. This resulting frameshift could result in a premature stop, which would truncate more than 300 amino acids. This insertion cosegregated with BFNC, but not febrile convulsions, in the pedigree and was not detected in a control panel of 231 independent white blood donors. The functional effects of this mutation were assessed for its causative role in BFNC. When *Xenopus laevis* oocytes were injected with

KCNQ2, complementary RNA (cRNA) demonstrated a current (16) that slowly activated at voltages more positive than -60 mV and was fully activated at 0 mV. The open channel was just barely inwardly rectifying. Ion substitution experiments showed that the current was potassium-selective and had a K > Rb > Cs > Na permeability sequence. These currents are similar to those of KvLQT1 in their permeability sequence, voltage dependence, and kinetics.

Conclusion.—Potassium channels are integral in the repolarizing action potentials. Mutations in the KCNA1 potassium channel produce episodic ataxia, a nonepileptic disorder with paroxysmal cerebellar symptoms and seizures in some patients. Since BFNC is related to the loss of function of a potassium channel, the pathologic neuronal hyperexcitability in this syndrome is probably caused by impaired repolarization. Support for this concept of idiopathic epilepsies as ion channel disorders comes from earlier observation of a nicotinic acetylcholine receptor subunit defect in a form of human partial epilepsy and of calcium channel defects in some inherited forms of epilepsy in mice. No other gene defects have been detected in human idiopathic epilepsies.

▶ The past few years have seen the discovery of gene loci involved in the pathogenesis of many neurologic disorders. Very few of these, indeed, relate to the pathogenesis of epilepsy. By defining an aberrant gene in a family with benign familial neonatal convulsions, determining the homology of the gene product to known genes, and testing the function of the product of the aberrant gene expressed in an ex vivo system, these authors demonstrate the power of molecular biologic techniques for the understanding of disorders of the nervous system.

N.F. Schor, M.D., Ph.D.

Outcome Following Surgery in Patients With Bitemporal Interictal Epileptiform Patterns
Holmes MD, Dodrill CB, Ojemann GA, et al (Univ of Washington, Seattle)
Neurology 48:1037–1040, 1997   9–2

Introduction.—Most physicians prefer that all, or almost all, recorded seizures originate from one temporal lobe or the other before performing surgery in patients with drug-resistant temporal lobe epilepsy. There is disagreement regarding whether complete lateralization of seizures to one side is required for good outcome after surgery. Reported are surgical outcomes in a series of patients with medically intractable epilepsy and bitemporal epileptiform patterns who underwent invasive monitoring and surgical therapy. Factors associated with seizure-free outcome were identified.

Methods.—Forty-four patients with intractable seizures were surgically treated between December 1990 and April 1995. Average age of 27 women and 17 men was 31 years, and average duration of seizures was 20 years. Seizures were due to history of febrile seizures (8 patients), head trauma accompanied by loss of consciousness (7), meningitis or encephalitis, (6), status epilepticus (3), perinatal difficulties (1), and no known risk factor for epilepsy (19). All patients had independent, bilateral, basal-temporal, interictal epileptiform patterns on standard EEGs.

Results.—At a minimum follow-up of 1 year, 22 patients (50%) were seizure-free, 14 (32%) had at least a 75% decrease in seizures, and 8 (14%) had less than a 75% decease in seizures. Three factors were independently associated with good outcome: concordance of MRI findings, history of febrile seizures, and 100% lateralization of intracranially recorded ictal onset to the side of surgery. Seizure-free outcome was more likely in the presence of more than one of these factors. When 2 factors were present, 83% (15/18) patients were seizure-free, and when 1 factor was present, 35% (7/20) were seizure-free. Six patients with none of these factors were not seizure-free.

Conclusion.—It is possible to reasonably predict which patients with bitemporal epileptiform abnormalities will have a good surgical outcome, based on 3 independent factors.

▶ Temporal lobectomy performed in patients with a single, well-localized epileptic focus results in complete remission from the seizures in 80% to 90%. One criteria that had been considered in selecting patients was the absence of bilateral independent foci on routine EEGs. This article found that localized MRI findings and consistent lateralization of ictal seizure activity were better predictors of outcome. Thus we can, and should, consider patients for surgery with bilateral EEG abnormalities.

E.R. Ramsay, M.D.

Neuropsychological, Intellectual, and Behavioral Findings in Patients With Centrotemporal Spikes With and Without Seizures
Weglage J, Demsky A, Pietsch M, et al (Univ of Münster, Germany)
Dev Med Child Neurol 39:646–651, 1997   9–3

Introduction.—Benign epilepsy with centrotemporal spikes (BECTS), or rolandic epilepsy, is a common epilepsy syndrome in childhood. Nearly 15% to 25% of children with seizures have BECTS. These are usually simple partial seizures characterized by nocturnal (rarely, daytime) events that awaken the patient and clonic activity of one side of the face and upper and lower extremities. Most patients with a rolandic focus never have overt seizures. Seizures occur in the 2 to 14-year age range, with peak incidence at age 6 to 8 years. It is somewhat more common in boys than in girls. Patients with rolandic foci, with and without seizures, were compared with healthy controls to determine any differences in neuropsychologic, intellectual, and behavioral findings.

Methods.—Forty 6- to 12-year-old children with untreated rolandic epilepsy by electrographic criteria only and 40 healthy controls matched for age, sex, and socioeconomic status underwent standard EEG recordings with unipolar and bipolar registration. All patients with BECTS had centrotemporal spikes on EEG examination. Neuropsychologic, intellectual, and behavioral outcomes were compared in patients and controls.

Results.—Compared with controls, patients with BECTS had significant impairment in IQ, visual perception, spatial orientation, short-term memory, psychiatric status, and some subtests in fine motor performance tasks of the dominant right hand: follow lines, aiming, tapping, long pins, and pursuit rotor. Clinical neurologic status was not impaired. These children had behavioral problems, according to their mothers.

Conclusion.—Patients with left, as opposed to right, centrotemporal spikes had similar test results because there is a frequent shift in lateralization of the focus with rolandic epilepsy. The cause of behavioral maladjustment remains unknown. Children with chronic disease are at higher risk for emotional and behavioral problems. It is possible that EEG abnormalities influence behavioral status. This needs to be clarified with further investigation to determine if problems could be avoided with drug-induced normalization of EEGs. A rolandic focus with or without seizures may not be so benign as once believed.

▶ The syndrome of so-called benign rolandic epilepsy is frequently encountered in clinical pediatric and pediatric neurology practice. The current dogma is that this disorder usually has no long-term implications for the child, and the need for anticonvulsants, if it is there at all, is often outgrown. This study raises the possibility that there are, in fact, neurobehavioral consequences of benign rolandic epilepsy. As is often the case with studies of this genre, some caveats apply to the interpretation of these data. The differences found, though statistically significant, are rather small, and may hold somewhat less functional or clinical significance. In addition, as the authors point out, primary differences cannot be distinguished in this study from differences that result from the way in which the family, child, and others involved with them reacted to the diagnosis or the treatment. Nonetheless, this study raises a very provocative question in a high incidence disorder of childhood.

N.F. Schor, M.D., Ph.D.

Epilepsy and Attention Deficit Hyperactivity Disorder: Is Methylphenidate Safe and Effective?
Gross-Tsur V, Manor O, van der Meere J, et al (Hadassah-Hebrew Univ, Jerusalem; Univ of Gröningen, The Netherlands)
J Pediatr 130:670–674, 1997   9–4

Background.—Both epilepsy and attention deficit hyperactivity disorder (ADHD) are relatively common childhood disorders, affecting 1% and 3% to 5% of children, respectively. It is believed, however, that at least 20% of children with epilepsy may also have ADHD, making appropriate clinical management of the dual disorders an important concern. The use of psychostimulants, such as methylphenidate (MP), in the treatment of ADHD accompanied by epilepsy has been controversial because of the imputed ability of the drugs to lower seizure threshold. MP has been used successfully in a small number of children with the dual diagnosis; however, a larger, systematic study of the potential value of the drug in such cases remains to be conducted. The safety and efficacy of MP in the clinical management of children with both ADHD and a seizure disorder were examined in this prospective study.

Methods.—Thirty children, aged 6.4 to 16.4 years, with ADHD and epilepsy participated in this 4-month study. Each child received only his or her normal antiepileptic drug (AED) during the first 8 weeks, and received both the AED and MP, at 0.3 mg/kg once daily before school, during the final 8 weeks of the study. The children were evaluated clinically and cognitively prior to and following the 2-month methylphenidate intervention. In addition, blood AED concentrations and results of electroencephalographic and continuous-performance task tests were determined within 1.75 hours of methylphenidate or placebo administration.

Results.—Twenty five of the 30 children experienced no seizures in the absence of MP. None of these 25 children experienced seizures when MP was added to the therapeutic regimen. Of the 5 children who did have seizures prior to MP use, seizure activity increased in 3, was unchanged in 1, and was absent in 1 when MP was in use. Electroencephalographic abnormalities were identified in 23 children prior to MP use, with changes occurring in 7 children, including 4 with previously-normal electroencephalograms, after MP use had begun. Continuous-performance task test performance improved during MP use, while blood AED concentrations were unaffected. Reported side effects of MP were largely transient, excluding a long-term loss of appetite, and did not require discontinuing use of the drug.

Conclusions.—MP use benefited 70% of children with ADHD and epilepsy. Seizures were not precipitated in any seizure-free children by exposure to MP, and the EEG changes apparently associated with MP are consistent with induced variation rather than exacerbation. MP appears to be safe and effective for use in children with ADHD and epilepsy. The use of MP in children with continued seizure activity requires caution; however, the relative benefits of the drug may support its use even in such patients.

▶ Epilepsy and ADHD are among the most common problems addressed by child neurologists. Somewhere between 20% and 30% of children with epilepsy have clinically-defined ADHD. ADHD is known to be exacerbated and, some would contend, produced during treatment with anticonvulsants. Furthermore, it is often said that pharmacologic treatment of ADHD decreases the seizure threshold of patients with epilepsy. This crossover-design study suggests that MP is safe and effective in patients with ADHD who are being adequately treated with anticonvulsants for seizure disorders.

This is a finding that affects a significant percentage of the patients seen in the typical child neurology practice.

N.F. Schor, M.D., Ph.D.

A Prospective, Randomized Study Comparing Intramuscular Midazolam With Intravenous Diazepam for the Treatment of Seizures in Children

Chamberlain JM, Altieri MA, Futterman C, et al (Georgetown Univs, Washington, DC; Fairfax Hosp, Falls Church, Va; Univ of Maryland, Baltimore)
Pediatr Emerg Care 13:92–94, 1997   9–5

Introduction.—Patients with status epilepticus need emergency ventilatory and oxygenation support until seizures can be controlled pharmacologically. One recommended treatment is IV diazepam followed by IV phenytoin. However, gaining IV access may be difficult in some patients and in some situations, including the pediatric office setting. The benzodiazepine drug midazolam has anticonvulsant activity at least as good as that of diazepam and offers complete absorption with IM administration. A randomized trial of IM midazolam vs. IV diazepam for the treatment of ongoing seizures is reported.

Methods.—The controlled clinical trial included 24 children with motor seizures that lasted at least 10 minutes. This was chosen as the time frame in which most physicians would initiate anticonvulsant therapy. All children were seen in a pediatric emergency department. Patients who had an established IV line or had received anticonvulsant drugs for the current seizure episode were excluded. They were randomized to receive either IM midazolam, 0.2 mg/kg to a maximum of 7 mg, or IV diazepam, 0.3 mg/kg, to a maximum of 10 mg. The treatment was considered successful if the seizure stopped within 5 minutes, successful but delayed if it took 5 to 10 minutes to stop the seizures, and unsuccessful if the seizure was still occurring 10 minutes after administration. At this point, further treatment with IV diazepam or phenytoin was started. The study compared the

TABLE 2.—Comparisons Between Study Groups in Duration of Seizures
Prior to and in Response to Treatment*

	Midazolam	Diazepam	P
Duration prior to arrival	41.2 ± 49.6	28.3 ± 32.0	NS†
Time after arrival to administer medication	3.3 ± 2.0	7.8 ± 3.2	0.001
Time to cessation after medication	4.5 ± 3.0	3.4 ± 2.0	0.32
Time to cessation after arrival	7.8 ± 4.1	11.2 ± 3.6	0.047

*One treatment failure in each group has been excluded. All times are in minutes (mean ± SD).
†The Mann-Whitney U test was used. For all other comparisons, the Student's t test was used.
(Courtesy of Chamberlain JM, Altieri MA, Futterman C, et al: A prospective, randomized study comparing intramuscular midazolam with intravenous diazepam for the treatment of seizures in children. *Pediatr Emerg Care* 13:92–94, 1997.)

efficacy of the 2 treatments, as well as the time to seizure cessation, including the time required to start the IV line.

Results.—Both treatments effectively stopped seizures. Only 2 patients, 1 in each group, failed to respond to initial benzodiazepine treatment. Seizure control was more likely to be delayed in the midazolam group. However, midazolam treatment was started in a mean of 3 minutes of arrival in the emergency department, compared with 8 minutes in the diazepam group. Total time to cessation of seizures was 8 and 11 minutes, respectively (Table 2). In all patients but 1, seizures stopped within 15 minutes of arrival. Recurrent seizures developed in 4 patients in each group, including 1 case of recurrence within 15 minutes. There was no evidence of respiratory depression, and no complications.

Conclusions.—For children with ongoing motor seizures, IM midazolam is just as effective as IV diazepam. Because IM midazolam can be given more quickly, the total time to seizure cessation is shortened. Although the study was small, the differences are clinically important and unlikely to have arisen by chance. Intramuscular midazolam may be a useful treatment for ongoing seizures when immediate IV access is not available, such as in the office or prehospital setting.

▶ Status epilepticus is among the most common neurologic diagnoses in the emergency room. Much debate has centered on the choice of IV anticonvulsants for the initial treatment of this true emergency situation. While IV treatment of the child and the expertise and equipment it requires are staples of the emergency room, this is not the case for all private pediatricians' offices or adult hospitals. The finding of these authors that IM midazolam was as effective, as safe, and as long-lasting, and quicker to administer than IV diazepam represents the identification of a welcome alternative to IV medication for status epilepticus that presents in settings or in patients when intravenous access is not possible or practical.

N.F. Schor, M.D., Ph.D.

10 Neuro-Otology

Migraine-related Vestibulopathy
Cass SP, Furman JM, Ankerstjerne JKP, et al (Univ of Pittsburgh, Pa)
Ann Otol Rhinol Laryngol 106:182–189, 1997   10–1

Background.—The vestibular symptoms of migraine are varied and not specific. These authors reviewed the common symptoms of, diagnoses of, and treatments for migraine-related vestibulopathy.

Methods.—The charts of 100 patients, 7 to 83 years of age, with migraine-related vestibulopathy were reviewed retrospectively. The diagnosis had been made based on the following factors: a personal or family history of migraine headaches, a history of motion sickness or visually evoked vertigo, and vestibular symptoms that were not characteristic of other vestibular syndromes. Vestibular laboratory testing was performed and patients were assessed by computerized moving platform posturography.

Findings.—Migraine with aura ($N = 50$) or without aura ($N = 46$) were the most common classifications, with aura without headache present in only 4 patients. Slightly over three fourths of patients had a family history of migraine and the same percentage reported discomfort with space or motion. Disequilibrium, lightheadedness, and unsteadiness were common (Table 2). Almost three fourths of patients had normal posturography, but rotation chair testing revealed that nearly half had an abnormal directional

TABLE 2.—Character of Symptoms in Migraine-related Vestibulopathy

		No. of Patients
Movement-associated dysequilibrium, lightheadedness, and unsteadiness		79
Seconds to minutes	14	
Hours	41	
Days to weeks	25	
Always	34	
True vertigo		21
Seconds	10	
Minutes	38	
Hours	52	

(Courtesy of Cass SP, Furman JM, Ankerstjerne JKP, et al: Migraine-related vestibulopathy. *Ann Otol Rhinol Laryngol* 106:182–189, 1997.)

preponderance. About three fourths had abnormal results on vestibular function testing, yet all but 1 patient had normal MRI or CT scans.

Conclusion.—The headache was treated by prescribing antimigraine medications and avoiding dietary triggers of migraine. Vestibular symptoms were treated by motion sickness medications, vestibular rehabilitation, and behavioral or medical therapy to relieve any associated anxiety or panic disorders.

▶ Visual disturbance is the most common and accepted migraine aura. Dizziness is also a common complaint among patients with migraine, but isolated dizziness has not received widespread acceptance as a migraine aura, partly because dizziness is a very common symptom that is caused by a variety of problems. Benign paroxysmal vertigo of childhood is the only symptom of dizziness that has its own organization, the International Headache Society (IHS) for Migraine. The article by Cass et al. reports the experience from a "dizzy clinic" that includes both neurologists and otolaryngologists. Although the authors did not specifically state that they followed the IHS classification for migraine, the criteria they used are in line with this classification.

One of the more interesting parts of the paper is Table 2, which characterizes the symptoms of their population. The majority of patients experienced head-movement–induced disequilibrium and lightheadedness for hours during the "migraine aura." Although the authors attribute this to a vestibular problem, vertigo is really the only symptom that can clearly be attributed to vestibular dysfunction. Only 20% of their patients had true vertigo. Unfortunately, the authors did not discuss the percentage of cases in which dizziness was associated with a "migraine" headache. Therefore, these cases still remain a "migraine diagnosis" of exclusion.

Although the authors report a number of abnormal vestibular test results in these patients, testing does not help with the diagnosis and is usually not necessary in the workup in patients with spells of dizziness. The single test that is probably useful is an audiogram in patients with spells of dizziness and hearing loss; this is to rule out Meniere's disease, an entity that can cause spells of vertigo lasting for the same length of time as migraine. In summary, this is a good descriptive paper regarding migraine-induced dizziness. Vestibular tests are not specific and, generally, not helpful in the diagnosis.

R.J. Tusa, M.D., Ph.D.

Migraine-associated Vertigo
Savundra PA, Carroll JD, Davies RA, et al (Natl Hosp for Neurology & Neurosurgery, London)
Cephalalgia 17:505–510, 1997   10–2

Introduction.—The association between migraine and vertigo is not well defined, in part because of the lack of standardized definitions of both

TABLE 2.—Site of Vestibular Disturbance in Subjects With Vertigo

Group	Central	Peripheral	Combined	None
Migraineur ($n=99$)	6	37	9	47
Non-migraineur ($n=125$)	1	117	0	7
95% confidence interval	*	*	*	*

*Significant difference.
(Reprinted by permission of Scandinavian University Press, from Savundra PA, Carroll JD, Davies RA, et al: Migraine-associated vertigo. *Cephalalgia* 17:505–510, 1997, by permission of Scandinavian University Press.)

disorders. A retrospective analysis of 363 patients who had sought treatment for vertigo examined the prevalence of migraine and compared the prevalence of vestibular disturbances in migraineurs and nonmigraineurs.

Methods.—The study group was drawn from a database at the National Hospital for Neurology and Neurosurgery. Eligible patients had symptoms that included an illusion of movement; excluded were patients with alternobaric vertigo, Tullio's phenomenon, and hyperventilation. Migraine was defined according to the Classification and Diagnostic Criteria for the Diagnosis of Migraine, with modifications to allow for vertigo as a migraine aura and an extension of the duration of aura. All patients had a standardized neurologic assessment, a full medical history and examination, audiovestibular investigations, electro-oculographic assessment, bithermal caloric testing, and blood tests.

Results.—There were 116 migraineurs (32%) among the 363 patients with vertigo. Migraine with aura had a prevalence of 24.5%. Other identifiable pathologic conditions were present in 17 of the 116 migraineurs and 122 of the 247 nonmigraineurs. Idiopathic vertigo was present significantly more often in migraineurs (85%) than in nonmigraineurs (51%). Migraineurs and nonmigraineurs also differed significantly in the proportion without a demonstrable vestibular disturbance (47% vs. 6%, respectively), in the proportion with an idiopathic central vestibular disturbance (6% vs. 0.8%), in the proportion with an idiopathic combined central and peripheral vestibular disturbance (9% vs. 0%), and in the proportion with an idiopathic peripheral vestibular disturbance (37% vs. 94%) (Table 2).

Discussion.—Although there have been many reports of an association and a possible pathophysiologic relationship between vertigo and migraine, the issue remains controversial. Approximately one third of these patients with vertigo also had migraine, indicating a definite association between the 2 disorders. The combination of central and peripheral vestibular signs was a feature of migraine with aura.

▶ This valuable study confirms what most headache specialists already know, namely, that a high percentage of patients with migraine complain of vertiginous symptoms. The study also demonstrates 2 important findings: vertigo is frequently a migraine aura and migraineurs have a high prevalence of central and peripheral vestibular disturbances. In addition, complaints of dizziness and vertigo *unassociated* with headache are considerably more frequent in migraineurs than in nonmigrainous individuals. A syndrome designated benign paroxysmal vertigo is considered by some to be a definite migraine equivalent. It occurs as an autonomous event in children and in younger adults who have migraine headaches or it may be the first manifestation of migraine. Vertigo may be intense and associated with nausea, vomiting, and hyperhidrosis, but cochlear symptoms such as tinnitus or focal neurologic symptoms do not occur. Positional or spontaneous nystagmus may be seen. Migraine should be kept in mind when patients with vertigo are seen, and a course of antimigraine medication should be considered for such patients.

R.A. Davidoff, M.D.

Relationship Between Balance and Abnormalities in Cerebral Magnetic Resonance Imaging in Older Adults
Tell GS, Lefkowitz DS, Diehr P, et al (Univ of Bergen, Norway; Bowman Gray School of Medicine, Winston-Salem, NC; Univ of Washington, Seattle)
Arch Neurol 55:73–79, 1998   10–3

Introduction.—Falls among older adults are associated with significant disability and morbidity. Since poor balance is a primary cause of frequent falls, it is important to be able to assess balance and its risk factors. A positive Romberg test has historically been used as a predictor of falls. Cerebral changes detectable on MRI may be related to balance. The relationship between cerebral atrophy identified on MRI and balance was assessed in a community-based sample of ambulatory adults over age 65.

Methods.—Participants were recruited from the Cardiovascular Health Study, an observational cohort investigation of cardiovascular diseases among 700 community-dwelling older men and women, black and white, in four United States communities. Balance examination included posturography, functional reach, Romberg test, tandem stand, and 1-foot stand. The cerebral MRI evaluation included ventricular size, sulcal widening, white matter disease, and ischemic infarctions. Cardiovascular disease and hypertension were assessed and taken into account during analysis.

Results.—Mean ages of the 452 females and 323 males were 74.1 and 74.9, respectively. Participants with even mild degrees of cerebral atrophy had more balance problems than individuals without cerebral changes. The strongest correlations between balance and MRI findings were observed for white matter disease and ventricular size. All except the ischemic infarction variable remained significantly correlated with balance after adjustment for sex, race, age, cardiovascular disease, and hypertension.

Conclusion.—Findings support an association between cerebral MRI abnormalities and postural instability. Since balance is related to the risk of falling, these findings contribute to the understanding of a significant cause of morbidity and mortality in elderly adults.

▶ Identification of the cause of chronic imbalance and falls in the elderly (over 65 years of age) can be challenging, once sensory deficits (vestibular and proprioception), motor weakness, spasticity, ataxia, apraxia, basal ganglia disease, and arthritis have been ruled out. Cerebral MRI scans may be helpful in this group of patients. Several articles have correlated imbalance with ventricular enlargement or leukoaraiosis (white matter changes in corona radiata). These studies are limited in that they contain 30 or fewer subjects and usually did not critically assess balance. The article by Tell et al. describes the most comprehensive study to date. This study examined a battery of functional balance tests, dynamic posturography, and MRI scans in 775 community-dwelling elderly subjects recruited from the Cardiovascular Health Study. Cardiovascular disease and hypertension were controlled for in the analysis. Both leukoaraiosis and ventricular enlargement correlated with imbalance. When results were adjusted for age, ventricular size was the most significant factor. Poor tandem stance was the most common balance defect found among patients with increased ventricular size. Two obvious questions were not addressed. This study did not examine whether the MRI results correlated with subjective reports of poor balance or falls. In addition, it did not examine whether ventricular enlargement leads to a form of gait apraxia.

R.J. Tusa, M.D., Ph.D.

A Double-Blind Controlled Study of Gabapentin and Baclofen as Treatment for Acquired Nystagmus
Averbuch-Heller L, Tusa RJ, Fuhry L, et al (Case Western Reserve Univ, Cleveland, Ohio; Bascom Palmer Eye Inst, Miami, Fla; Ludwig-Maximilians Univ, Munich; et al)
Ann Neurol 41:818–825, 1997   10–4

Introduction.—The symptoms of acquired nystagmus may be alleviated if the ocular oscillations are reduced or abolished, but few reliable clinical therapies are available. A double-blind, crossover trial compared gabapentin to baclofen as therapy for acquired nystagmus.

Methods.—Fifteen patients had acquired pendular nystagmus (APN) and 6 had jerk nystagmus that was either downbeat or torsional downbeat. Several had tried a variety of other medications, with only minor or temporary relief. Treatment consisted of gabapentin (up to 900 mg/day) and baclofen (up to 30 mg/day). Experimental studies suggest that γ-aminobutyric acid (GABA) plays an important role in the mechanism by which gaze is held steady during visual fixation, and both gabapentin and baclofen involve GABAergic mechanisms. Visual acuity and nystagmus were measured before and at the end of 2 weeks of treatment by each agent.

Results.—Twenty patients completed both 2-week test periods. The 2 patient groups differed in their responses to each agent. Only gabapentin significantly improved visual acuity in patients with APN; median eye speed was significantly reduced in all 3 planes with gabapentin, but baclofen affected only the vertical plane. Eight patients with APN elected to continue gabapentin treatment. With both therapies, patients with downbeat or torsional downbeat nystagmus had less consistent changes in median slow-phase eye speed. Only 1 of 6 patients had consistent reduction in median eye speed, and the 2 drugs were similarly effective in this case.

Conclusion.—Gabapentin proved to be an effective therapy for most patients with APN. Visual acuity was improved and all components of the nystagmus were reduced. Ataxia may be worsened, however, and care should be taken to avoid falls. Both gabapentin and baclofen may benefit some patients with downbeat nystagmus.

▶ Nystagmus that occurs in primary position or down-gaze that produces oscillopsia has been most difficult to manage with medications. The authors present preliminary evidence that gabapentin may be effective in the treatment of patients with APN by decreasing amplitude frequency and frequency of the nystagmus and by improving visual acuity. This treatment should be considered in all patients with APN with visual symptoms.

N.J. Schatz, M.D.

11 Neuro-ophthalmology

Recurrent Optic Neuromyelitis With Endocrinopathies: A New Syndrome
Vernant J-C, Cabre P, Smadja D, et al (Hôpital Pierre Zobda-Quitman, Fort de France, Martinique; Centre Médico-Chirurgical Foch, Suresnes, France; Hôpital Lariboisière, Paris; et al)
Neurology 48:58–64, 1997

11–1

Background.—Sometimes the classification of a demyelinating disease is a challenge. These authors report a new variant, recurrent optic neuromyelitis with endocrinopathies, that differs from both multiple sclerosis and Devic's syndrome.

Methods.—A demyelinating disease involving only the spinal cord and optic nerves developed in 8 Antillean women 17 to 53 years of age. Each experienced recurrent optic (either monocular or binocular) and/or spinal cord (either acute or subacute) symptoms, hence the name "recurrent optic neuromyelitis." Furthermore, each also had amenorrhea, galactorrhea, diabetes insipidus, hypothyroidism, and/or hyperphagia that failed to respond to therapy.

Findings.—Sarcoidosis, myringomyelia, brain tumor, lupus erythematosus, human T-cell lymphotropic virus type 1 infection, multiple sclerosis, and Devic's syndrome were carefully ruled out. All but 1 patient had CSF leukocytosis, and all but 2 had elevated levels of IgG. Magnetic resonance imaging studies of the spinal cord showed cavitation in 3 patients. The visual symptoms were worse in those with endocrinopathies of hypothalamic origin. All but 2 of the patients died within 2 to 6 years; autopsy in 1 showed demyelinizing lesions of the cervical spinal cord and thick-walled blood vessels but no inflammation. One of the survivors is tetraplegic, and the other is blind and paraplegic.

Conclusion.—Careful rule-out of the systemic manifestations of other demyelinating diseases indicates that a new entity is needed to describe these patients' courses. Symptoms are limited to the optic nerve and spinal cord, and recurrence is typical. Although the neuromyelitis is probably caused by a previous infection, no explanation can be given for the endocrinopathies (primarily amenorrhea and galactorrhea).

▶ This article adds a new dimension to a variant of Devic's syndrome. The patients were meticulously studied. The endocrine manifestations are distinctly unique, with hyperprolactinemia, amenorrhea, and hypothalamic dysfunction, an otherwise unrecognized entity. The spinal cord syndrome with bandlike dissociated sensory loss was a characteristic and, pathologically, MRI showed cavitation. The isolated involvement of optic nerves and spinal cord suggests classic neuromyelitis optica (Devic's syndrome), but, as the authors suggest, the multiphasic course makes this a new entity.

In the setting of the "classic" Devic's syndrome, either monophasic or multiphasic forms, it is clear that a careful pursuit of associated endocrinopathy may have been overlooked in the past. To the authors' credit, they have excluded other known etiologies. These cases do not represent multiple sclerosis, human T cell lymphotropic virus type 1 disease, or sarcoidosis.

N.J. Schatz, M.D.

Oculomotor Nerve and Muscle Abnormalities in Congenital Fibrosis of the Extraocular Muscles

Engle EC, Goumnerov BC, McKeown CA, et al (Harvard Med School, Boston; Tufts Univ, Boston; Univ of Kentucky, Lexington)
Ann Neurol 41:314–325, 1997   11–2

Purpose.—Congenital fibrosis of the extraocular muscles (CFEOM) is inherited in autosomal dominant fashion. Patients with CFEOM have bilateral ptosis, restrictive external ophthalmoplegia with the eyes partially or completely fixed in an infraduced strabismic position, and markedly limited and aberrant residual eye movements. These clinical manifestations are traditionally thought to result from myopathic fibrosis of the extraocular muscles. A clinicopathologic study of several members of 1 family with classic CFEOM is reported.

Patients.—The study included 5 members of 1 family with CFEOM, the gene for which is mapped to chromosome 12. All living members underwent ophthalmologic and neurologic examinations; neuropathologic examination was performed 20 hours after death in 1 member. Two patients underwent extraocular muscle biopsy.

Results.—The 2 children examined showed congenital bilateral ptosis and near-complete external ophthalmoplegia, with mildly delayed gross motor milestones. Their affected parents had static congenital ptosis and ophthalmoplegia with mild bifacial weakness. All patients had a chin-up posture with profound bilateral ptosis and almost no levator palpebrae superioris function. Extraocular movements were significantly limited, especially in upgaze. Forced duction tests showed strikingly restricted globe movement in all directions beyond voluntary gaze (Fig 1). No patients had diplopia. All patients had anomalously directed eye movements, often dysconjugate, including synergistic convergence and divergence, aberrant downward movement on attempted horizontal gaze, and globe retraction into the orbit.

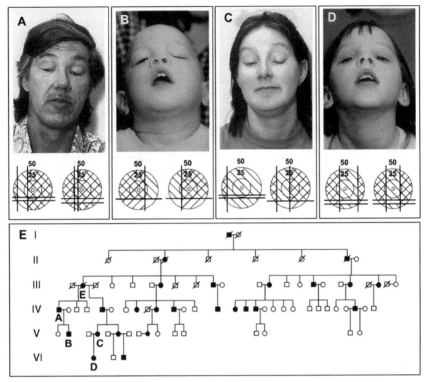

FIGURE 1.—Four affected patients and their family pedigree. **A–D**, below each individual's photograph is a diagram of the range of motion of each globe. The normal pupil location is indicated by the *central circle*, and 25 and 50 degrees of movement are indicated by *concentric circles* (normal globe movement is approximately 50 degrees in any direction). *Backward slashes* indicate areas of no vertical movement, and *forward slashes* indicate areas of no horizontal movement. The *clear areas without slashes* indicate areas of globe movement. **E**, family pedigree in which *circles* indicate females, *squares* indicate males, and *blackened symbols* indicate individuals affected with congenital fibrosis of extraocular muscles. Affected individuals referred to in the text as patients A, B, C, D, and E are indicated by the appropriate letter beneath their symbol. (Courtesy of Engle EC, Goumnerov BC, McKeown CA, et al: Oculomotor nerve and muscle abnormalities in congenital fibrosis of the extraocular muscles. *Ann Neurol* 41:314–325, 1997.)

The pathologic studies showed absence of the superior division of the oculomotor nerve and its alpha motor neurons. There were also abnormalities of the levator palpebrae superioris and rectus superior, which are innervated by the superior division of the oculomotor nerve. The other extraocular muscles showed increased numbers of internal nuclei with central mitochondrial clumping. These findings suggest that the pathologic abnormalities did not involve just the muscles innervated by the superior division of cranial nerve III.

Conclusions.—The clinical and pathologic findings in 5 family members with CFEOM are presented. This condition appears to arise from an abnormality in the development of the lower motor neuron system of the extraocular muscles. It is still unknown whether the cause of CFEOM involves a primary brain stem or primary extraocular muscle process; however, the normal CFEOM gene product appears to play at least a transient role in normal development or function of the skeletal muscle.

▶ The authors have described an important finding in the syndrome of CFEOM. In the autosomal dominant disease that maps to the locus on chromosome 12, autopsy material, although the midbrain and pons were well formed, has been identified to have absent or markedly abnormal caudal central alpha motor neurons of the ocular motor nucleus, with complete absence of the superior division of the third nerve innervating the superior rectus and levator palpebral muscles. This pathologic study provides important evidence that the anatomic abnormality in CFEOM is in the motor neuron axons and superior division of the ocular motor nerve.

N.J. Schatz, M.D.

12 Miscellaneous Conditions

Cohort Study of Multiple Brain Lesions in Sport Divers: Role of a Patent Foramen Ovale

Knauth M, Ries S, Pohimann S, et al (Univ of Heidelberg, Germany; Univ of Frankfurt, Germany)

BMJ 314:701–705, 1997

12–1

Background.—Multiple brain lesions are more frequent in scuba divers than in nondivers. These lesions may be caused by arterial gas embolism, with emboli perhaps entering arterial circulation through a patent foramen ovale.

Methods.—In 87 sport divers with at least 160 scuba dives, multiple brain lesions were looked for with cranial MRI and existence (and size) of patent foramen ovale were determined by echocontrast transcranial Doppler US.

Results.—Of 25 subjects with a right-to-left shunt, 13 had a hemodynamically relevant patent foramen ovale. In all, 41 lesions were found in 11 subjects: 7 lesions in 7 subjects without a shunt and 34 lesions in 4 subjects with right-to-left shunt. The only cases of multiple brain lesions were in 3 divers with a large patent foramen ovale ($P = 0.004$). Brain lesions were seen even when decompression sickness was not reported.

Conclusions.—Paradoxical gas embolism is a likely pathologic mechanism for multiple brain lesions, and a patent foramen ovale may be an important risk factor for development of such lesions. Because about a quarter of all sport divers have a patent foramen ovale, discussion is needed regarding how this condition affects dive fitness. Different decompression tables could be developed for such divers.

▶ This fascinating study is of great interest vis-a-vis the potential neurologic complications of sport diving. It indicates that those divers having a patent foramen ovale with right-to-left shunt of high hemodynamic relevance are particularly likely to show multiple small brain lesions on MR imaging. By contrast, single lesions were found in 7 of 62 divers without a right-to-left shunt and in 1 of 25 divers with a shunt. These findings serve to raise caution as to the enhanced possibility of paradoxical gas embolism in sport divers having large, hemodynamically significant patent foramen ovale. The potential clinical relevance of the lesions, however, is not clarified by this report.

M.D. Ginsberg, M.D.

Neurological Effects of Microwave Exposure Related to Mobile Communication
Hermann DM, Hossmann K-A (Max-Planck-Inst, Cologne, Germany)
J Neurol Sci 152:1–14, 1997   12–2

Background.—With the burgeoning growth of mobile communication systems comes concern about the possible effects of electromagnetic radiation on the brain. Because mobile telephones are held to the ear, they are associated with relatively high specific absorption rates (SAR) to the brain. To date, there are no conclusive data on the possible association between microwave exposure and the occurrence of malignant tumors. Studies of the effects of microwave radiation on the brain were reviewed.

Discussion.—Several studies have evaluated the electrophysiologic, biochemical, and morphologic effects of continuous or pulsed microwave radiation on the brain. Both in vitro and in vivo studies have been performed in animals and humans. Microwave exposure has been reported to affect neuronal electrical activity, cellular calcium homeostasis, energy metabolism, genomic responses, neurotransmitter balance, and blood-brain barrier permeability. However, some of these effects have not been replicated in further experiments, whereas others have been attributed to procedural side effects. In sum, there are few data to suggest that pulsed or continuous microwave exposure associated with mobile communications systems poses any threat to the health of the brain.

Summary.—Experimental evidence suggests that microwave exposure related to mobile communication may have biological effects on the brain. However, at the power levels and frequencies used in mobile phones, there is no evidence of increased health risks related to mobile communication systems. Given the public health importance of this issue, further studies of the possible neurologic effects of microwave exposure—including strict positive and negative control conditions—will be needed.

▶ There has been a great deal of recent concern about the role of electromagnetic radiation in causing cancer.[1] A few epidemiologic studies have suggested that ionizing electromagnetic fields may play a role in the production of brain tumors and leukemia. There has also been recent concern that cellular telephones might cause brain tumors. Most reports provide little evidence to support these fears. A recent article in *The New England Journal of Medicine* on residential exposure to magnetic fields dispels the notion that such exposure can increase the risk of acute lymphocytic leukemia.[2] A review of electronic industry workers shows "no meaningful association" between video display terminal development workers and brain tumor mortality; a statistical association in 1 subgroup probably resulted from chance.[3]

A U.S. Federal Panel of scientists concluded that "no conclusive evidence" exists linking exposure to electromagnetic fields with cancer, reproductive and developmental abnormalities, or learning and behavioral problems. These findings are part of a report released by the National Academy of Sciences, National Research Council commissioned by Congress in 1993.

The International Agency for Research on Cancer (IARC) has launched a study of possible consequences of exposure to weak radiofrequency radiation (300 Hz to 300 GHz), particularly that emanating from mobile telephones. Such telephones have probably been on the market too short a time to be implicated in the apparent increase in brain cancer, particularly in the elderly. Furthermore, there is no evidence that the incidence of left temporal lobe tumors, the site that would receive the most electromagnetic radiation (by individuals who normally use the telephone in their left ear), is increasing.

J.B. Posner, M.D.

References

1. Salvatore JR, Weitberg AB, Mehta S: Nonionizing electromagnetic fields and cancer: A review. *Oncology* 10:563–570, 1996.
2. Linet MS, Hatch EE, Kleinerman RA, et al: Residential exposure to magnetic fields and acute lymphoblastic leukemia in children. *N Engl J Med* 337:1–7, 1997.
3. Beall C, Delzell E, Cole P, et al: Brain tumors among electronics industry workers. *Epidemiology* 7:125–130, 1996.

Homozygosity for an Allele Carrying Intermediate CAG Repeats in the Dentatorubral-Pallidoluysian Atrophy (DRPLA) Gene Results in Spastic Paraplegia
Kurohara K, Kuroda Y, Maruyama H, et al (Saga Med School, Japan; Hiroshima Univ, Japan)
Neurology 48:1087–1090, 1997   12–3

Background.—Mutations in the gene encoding for dentatorubral-pallidoluysian atrophy (DRPLA) can also cause Huntington's disease, spinocerebellar ataxia 1, Machado-Joseph disease, and X-linked spinal and bulbar muscular atrophy. All but the last of these diseases are inherited in an autosomal dominant manner. This report describes 2 sisters with spastic paraplegia who had a novel DRPLA genotype and who inherited the defect in an autosomal recessive manner.

Methods.—Both sisters (37 and 35 years old) were products of a consanguineous marriage in which both parents and 2 other sisters were neurologically normal. Both sisters had spastic paraplegia with truncal ataxia and slurred speech but no convulsions or other psychomotor problems. Blood samples were drawn for isolation of DNA and amplification of CAG repeats by polymerase chain reaction. For comparison, patients with DRPLA have between 49 and 88 CAG repeats in the DRPLA gene locus, and those with normal chromosomes have between 6 and 35 CAG repeats. CAG repeats between 36 and 48 would be considered of intermediate size.

Findings.—Both parents carried 1 intermediate allele and 1 normal allele in the gene; the mother had 41 and 18 CAG repeats and the father had 41 and 11. One normal sister had 18 and 11 CAG repeats and the other had 41 and 11. But 1 of the affected sisters had 41 and 41 repeats, and the other had 41 and 40 repeats. Therefore, both patients were homozygous for an intermediate allele that was inherited in an autosomal recessive fashion.

Conclusion.—Patients with DRPLA do not typically have spastic paraplegia. Yet these 2 patients who were homozygous for an intermediate allele in the DRPLA gene locus did have spastic paraplegia. Furthermore, inheritance was likely in an autosomal recessive fashion, which differs from the autosomal dominant pattern typical of most disorders associated with the DRPLA gene locus.

▶ Gene cloning for neurologic diseases now occurs at a frenzied pace. We might expect this epic period to end early in the next century as all our genes are mapped and cloned. But it is not that simple, as this and other recent papers illustrate. Phenotypic variation from allelic mutations complicates matters. Here we see a *dominant* disease gene for DRPLA, when mutated somewhat differently, producing a *recessive* spastic paraplegia. And remember the SCA6 gene, which produces dominant ataxia, episodic ataxia, or hemiplegic migraine. And, of course, a given phenotype might come from a multitude of genes. In this article, at least 5 other spastic paraplegia gene localizations are sited; for epilepsy the count is over 20!

D.A. Stumpf, M.D., Ph.D.

Familial Episodic Ataxia: Clinical Heterogeneity in Four Families Linked to Chromosome 19p
Baloh RW, Yue Q, Furman JM, et al (Univ of California, Los Angeles; Univ of Pittsburgh, Pa)
Ann Neurol 41:8–16, 1997   12–4

Background.—Familial episodic ataxia is an uncommon neurologic disorder characterized by episodes of ataxia with minimal interictal neurologic findings. Two distinct forms have been identified: (1) familial episodic ataxia with interictal myokymia (EA-1) and (2) familial periodic ataxia with interictal nystagmus (EA-2), which is characterized by longer episodes of ataxia. Both have autosomal dominant inheritance patterns and respond to acetazolamide treatment. EA-2 has been linked to the same region of chromosome 19p as hemiplegic migraine. This report describes the linkage of 4 EA-2 families to chromosome 19p.

Study Design.—Family members were interviewed and examined. Affected individuals were identified by reports of intermittent vertigo and/or ataxia with or without associated symptoms of nausea, vomiting, slurred speech, headache, extremity weakness or numbness, visual symptoms, auditory symptoms, and consciousness decrease. Other features that supported a diagnosis of EA-2 were nystagmus, truncal instability, and response to acetazolamide. Peripheral blood DNA was obtained and typed for a series of microsatellite markers on chromosome 19p.

Findings.—The strongest linkage evidence was for D19S221. Significant linkage was also observed for D19S413 and D19S226/S415. These results indicate that the gene for EA-2 is located within an 11-cm region flanked by D19S413 and D19S226/S415. Most affected participants reported that ataxia episodes were triggered by stress and exertion. The age of onset varied from 3 to 44 years, but without evidence of anticipation. Most patients responded to acetazolamide. About half reported headaches that met the criteria for migraine. Interictal nystagmus was common. Saccade overshoot dysmetria occurred in more than half of those affected.

Conclusions.—This report describes the linkage of EA-2 in 4 families to a region on chromosome 19p. This syndrome is variable in onset and symptoms. Episodes were often triggered by stress or exercise and could be relieved by acetazolamide. Vertigo, nausea, vomiting, and headache were commonly associated symptoms. The mechanism of phenotypic variation in these families with EA-2 linked to chromosome 19p is not known.

▶ Episodic ataxia has gotten very interesting! Two forms are recognized. EA-1 results from a mutation in a brain potassium channel (KCNA-1), and kinesogenic choreoathetosis occurs in occasional family members. *Allelic mutations* of the brain-specific P/Q-type Ca^{2+} channel $\alpha 1$-subunit gene (CACNL1A4) produce hemiplegic migraine, episodic ataxia (EA-2), or both.[1] A CAG repeat expansion at this same locus produces slowly progressive SCA6, dominant ataxia.[2] Finally, mutations of the homologous locus (tg) in mice produce absence seizures. There is a lot of neurologic action at one locus!

There are some other lessons. Episodes of ataxia leave patients with residual deficits, leading to a stepwise decline. Acetazolamide prevents episodic attacks as well as the stepwise progression in episodic ataxia. Might it do the same in SCA6? We can anticipate channel defects in other familial migraine syndromes and the elucidation of further channelopathies producing epilepsy.

D.A. Stumpf, M.D., Ph.D.

References

1. Ophoff RA, Terwindt GM, Vergouwe MN, et al: Familial hemiplegic migraine and episodic ataxia type-2 are caused by mutations in the CA2+ channel gene CACNL1A4. *Cell* 87:543–552, 1996.
2. Zhuchenko O, Bailey J, Bonnen P, et al: Autosomaldominant cerebellar atatia (SCAG) associated with small polyglutamine expansions in the alpha 1A-voltage-dependent calcium channel. *Nat Genet* 15:62–69, 1997.

X Linked Adrenoleukodystrophy: Clinical Presentation, Diagnosis, and Therapy

van Geel BM, Assies J, Wanders RJA, et al (Univ of Amsterdam)
J Neurol Neurosurg Psychiatry 63:4–14, 1997   12–5

Background.—X-linked adrenoleukodystrophy (X-ALD) involves atrophy of the adrenal cortex and diffuse cerebral sclerosis. It can occur in childhood, adolescence, or adulthood. It usually occurs in males but has been documented in females as well. Although X-ALD is rare, early identification is crucial for instituting steroid hormone therapy. Thus, clinicians should be aware of its clinical presentations and the diagnostic and therapeutic options available.

Presentation.—Six variants of X-ALD have been identified (Table); childhood cerebral ALD and adrenomyeloneuropathy (AMN) account for about 80% of all cases. Extensive periventricular demyelination and cavitation occur in the occipital white matter in 80% of patients with childhood cerebral ALD. Spinal cord and peripheral nerve involvement is typical of AMN. Addison's disease is present in about two thirds of male patients with neurologic dysfunction, and almost all males have testicular insufficiency and scanty scalp hair.

Diagnosis.—Levels of very long chain fatty acids (VLCFAs) are elevated in skin fibroblasts, plasma, and blood cells and can be detected by biochemical tests. Deoxyribonucleic acid linkage analysis can be used to identify heterozygotes. Prenatal diagnosis by measuring levels of VLCFAs in amniotic fluid and chorionic villus cells and by mutational analysis has also been reported. To avoid false negative results, when X-ALD is suspected, plasma levels of VLCFAs should be measured by repeat assays. The exclusion of peroxisomal disorders with neonatal onset indicates a biochemical profile consistent with X-ALD, at which point mutational analysis is warranted.

Therapy.—It is crucial that the underlying adrenocortical insufficiency be treated with steroid hormone therapy. Dietary therapy with "Lorenzo's oil" (glyceroltrioleate and glycerol trierucate oils) will normalize hexacosanoic acid (C26:0) concentrations within 1 month but has not halted the neurologic progression in patients with a cerebral form of the disease. In fact, these authors no longer recommend Lorenzo's oil for patients with childhood cerebral ALD, newly diagnosed patients with AMN, or symptomatic female carriers. Bone marrow transplant has been successful in treating the childhood and adolescent forms. Other therapies have included plasmapheresis, clofibrate, L-carnitine, immunosuppression (none of which have worked), IV immunoglobulins (mixed results), and β-interferon (trials underway).

Conclusion.—Although rare, X-ALD can be identified on the basis of biochemical and mutational factors and, in the childhood cerebral form, by periventricular white matter damage. Given the debilitating and poten-

TABLE.—Clinical Characteristics of the Different Phenotypes of X-ALD in Hemizygotes

	Pre- or asymptomatic ALD	CCALD	AdolCALD	ACALD	AMN	Addison only
Relative frequencies (%)	4–10	31–57		1–3	25–46	8–14
Age at onset of neurological symptoms	—	< 10	10–21	> 21	> 18; frequent 3rd–4th decade	> 2
Behavioural disturbances	—	+	+	+	—	—
Impaired cognition	—	+	+	Frequent	—	—
Pyramidal tract involvement	—	Eventually, not initially	Eventually, not initially	Frequent	Present by definition	—
Cerebral MRI abnormalities	Absent or mild*	Extensive in occipital or frontal myelin	Extensive in occipital or frontal myelin	Extensive in occipital or frontal myelin	Internal capsule, basal ganglia, mesencephalon, pons	Absent or mild*
Polyneuropathy	—	—	Rare	Possible	Sensorimotor, mostly axonal	—
Abnormal evoked potentials	—	VEP, BAEP (not initially) sometimes SEP	VEP, BAEP (not initially)	VEP (not initially), BAEP sometimes SEP	BAEP, SEP	Sometimes BAEP
Impaired endocrine function	—	AD in most	AD in most	AD in most	AD and hypogonadism in most	AD by definition
Abnormal neuropsychological examination	—	+	+	Frequent	—	—
Progression	—	Rapidly, rarely slowly	Rapidly, rarely slowly	Rapidly, sometimes slowly	Slowly, sometimes rapidly	—

— = Absent, + = present; * = depending on definition; CCALD = childhood cerebral ALD; AdolCALD = adolescent cerebral ALD; ACALD = adult cerebral ALD; AMN = adrenomyeloneuropathy; VEP = visual evoked potential; BAEP = brainstem auditory evoked potential; SEP = somatosensory evoked potential; AD = adrenocortical insufficiency (Addison's disease).
(Courtesy of van Geel BM, Assies J, Wanders RJA, et al: X Linked adrenoleukodystrophy: Clinical presentation, diagnosis, and therapy. *J Neurol Neurosurg Psychiatry* 63:4-14, 1997.)

tially fatal nature of the disease, gene therapy holds much promise for treating these patients.

▶ Recent years have brought an increasing molecular understanding of neurodegenerative disease. Because of this explosion of new information, it has become possible, in many instances, to distinguish at a molecular level the different clinical phenotypes of some diseases previously thought to be a single entity, and to group other diseases thought to be distinct into a class of molecular lesions. Adrenoleukodystrophy is 1 disorder for which the clinical and molecular information available have begun to complement one another, and genotype may allow prognostication and the identification of asymptomatic carriers of the disease. This article does an excellent job of synthesizing the basic science and clinical information available (much of it having come to fruition in the past 5 years) and reviewing the current state of experimental clinical therapies for this disorder.

D.A. Stumpf, M.D., Ph.D.

The Stiff Leg Syndrome
Brown P, Rothwell JC, Marsden CD (Inst of Neurology, Queen Square, London)
J Neurol Neurosurg Psychiatry 62:31–37, 1997   12–6

Background.—The stiff man syndrome is well characterized, consisting of chronic axial rigidity, reflex, and action-induced spasms and continuous

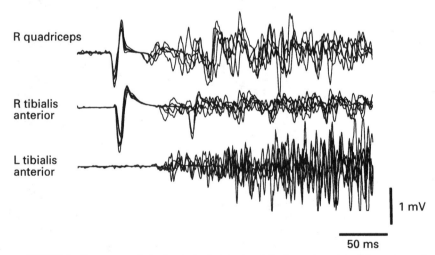

FIGURE 3.—Responses to single electric shocks in patient 1. Each record consists of 5 superimposed unrectified single trials, beginning at the time of each shock to the tibial nerve at the right ankle. A very short latency and highly synchronous response is recorded in R (right) quadriceps and R tibialis anterior at about 34 msec and 39 msec, respectively. A spasm follows this in both legs, with an onset latency of about 70 msec. (Courtesy of Brown P, Rothwell JC, Marsden CD: The stiff leg syndrome. *J Neurol Neurosurg Psychiatry* 62:31–37, 1997.)

motor unit activity at rest (CMUA). In some patients, the same features are confined to one or both legs, and corticobasal degeneration, focal lesions of the spinal cord, and encephalomyelitis must be excluded. Four patients were seen with a chronic progressive disorder characterized by painful involuntary spasms, stiffness, and CMUA limited to the legs, with no evidence of cerebral, brain stem, extrapyramidal, pyramidal, or sensory dysfunction.

Patients and Findings.—The patients were 2 women, both aged 35 years, and 2 men, aged 52 and 60 years, respectively. Their duration of illness ranged from 20 months to 16 years. Stiffness and painful spasms were present in the legs. Spasms were spontaneous and reflex, induced by voluntary movement. Rigidity and abnormal postures were noted in 1 or both legs. No truncal rigidity or exaggerated lumbar lordosis was present. None of the patients had signs or symptoms of brain stem, pyramidal, or sensory dysfunction. In 1 patient, sphincter disturbance developed after many years. No cause could be identified after extensive evaluation. There were no anti-GAD antibodies. Baclofen and diazepam resulted in some relief of painful spasms, but the condition continued to be disabling. Four core electrophysiologic features were documented: continuous motor unit activity was noted at rest in at least one limb muscle; spasms tended to involve the repetitive grouped discharge of motor units; cutaneomuscular reflexes were abnormal; and little or no electrophysiologic evidence of long tract disturbance was noted (Fig 3).

Conclusions.—These patients' signs and symptoms comprise a characteristic syndrome that is separate from the stiff man syndrome and also distinguishable from encephalomyelitis with rigidity. This condition may result from a chronic spinal interneuronitis.

▶ Brown et al. describe 4 patients with long-standing, chronic and progressive, spontaneous and stimulus-sensitive, painful, involuntary muscle spasms and stiffness together with continuous motor-unit activity at rest restricted to the lower extremities without evidence to support a diagnosis of either stiff-man syndrome or encephalomyelitis with rigidity. Of interest, truncal muscles were spared. Patients responded only partially to baclofen alone or in combination with diazepam. The authors postulate a localized dysfunction of spinal interneurons. Confirmation of this clinical entity (termed "stiff-leg syndrome") and further clarification of possible pathophysiologic mechanisms are awaited.

J.H. Noseworthy, M.D.

13 Neurorehabilitation

A Functional MRI Study of Subjects Recovered From Hemiparetic Stroke
Cramer SC, Nelles G, Benson RR, et al (Harvard Med School, Boston; Beth Israel-Deaconess Med Ctr, Boston)
Stroke 28:2518–2527, 1997   13–1

Introduction.—Hemiparesis is the most frequent deficit after stroke; recovery varies widely. The process of brain recovery after stroke is unclear. This is particularly true in the case of cortical stroke, about which there are limited data. Functional MRI was used to assess brain-activation patterns in patients who had recovered from hemiparetic stroke as compared with normal controls.

Methods.—The study included 10 patients who had recovered well from nonhemorrhagic, hemiparetic stroke. The defect was deep in 5 patients and cortical in 5. Nine control patients were studied for comparison. Both groups underwent functional MRI, with brain activation achieved by finger tapping. Activated brain volume in 5 bilateral motor regions was compared with the distribution of activation volumes in control subjects.

Results.—Finger tapping led to the activation of the same motor regions in patients and controls, although activation often occurred in a larger brain volume in patients. Six of nine stroke patients showed increased sensorimotor cortex activation in the unaffected hemisphere, compared with controls. The patients also showed increased activation in the contralateral cerebellar hemisphere and the ipsilateral premotor cortex, as well as in supplementary motor areas. The affected hemisphere in stroke patients rarely showed activation greater than that in controls, although foci of activation around the infarct were noted in 3 of 5 patients who had cortical strokes. The stroke patients usually did not show increased activation during finger tapping on the unaffected side. However, they did show decreased activation in the sensorimotor cortex on the unaffected side, suggesting increased responsiveness to the ipsilateral hand and decreased responsiveness to the contralateral hand. The findings were similar when different activation thresholds were used.

Conclusions.—In patients who have recovered from hemiparetic stroke, functional MRI shows activation of the same motor regions in response to finger tapping as in control subjects. However, the extent of activation is greater in controls, especially in the unaffected hemisphere. Motor recovery after stroke may depend heavily on these motor areas. Further functional MRI studies are needed to clarify the process related to recovery of neurologic function after stroke.

▶ This study used functional MRI to document that motor areas not damaged by a stroke are recruited during recovery from the stroke. As the authors point out, this evidence agrees with previous studies carried out by a number of methods and with mechanisms proposed by Denny-Brown in 1950. Of particular interest in this study are the variations among the ten subjects in the extent to which different brain regions are activated. This finding agrees with the existence of significant brain-to-brain variations among humans, not only in areas affected by strokes but also in areas involved in functional recovery from stroke.

J.P. Blass, M.D., Ph.D.

Mapping of Motor Cortical Reorganization After Stroke: A Brain Stimulation Study With Focal Magnetic Pulses
Traversa R, Cicinelli P, Bassi A, et al (Universitá "Tor Vergata" Rome; Ospedale Fatebenefratelli Isola Tiberina, Rome)
Stroke 28:110–117, 1997   13–2

Background.—Focal transcranial magnetic stimulation (TCS) is a noninvasive method for mapping the somatotopical organization of the motor cortex. To assess the reorganization of hand maps during rehabilitation after vascular monohemispheric lesion, TCS mapping of motor cortical output to the abductor digiti minimi (ADM) muscle was followed by evaluation of motor evoked potentials (MEPs). The results were compared to those of the unaffected contralateral side and to healthy controls.

Study Design.—Ten men and 5 women, age 30–80 years, who had experienced a first monohemispheric stroke were enrolled in this study. Motor maps were constructed 2 months after the vascular event by recording MEPs from the ADM muscle by focal TCS in the affected hemisphere (AH) and the unaffected hemisphere (UH) at baseline and after 8–10 weeks of neurorehabilitation. Clinical improvement was measured with the Barthel Index and Canadian Neurological Scale. These results were compared with those of 15 healthy age- and sex-matched controls.

Findings.—The MEP excitability threshold was significantly higher in the AH of stroke patients than it was in the UH or in normal controls. There was no significant difference between the UH and normal controls. In the AH, MEPs were significantly delayed in latency before and after rehabilitation therapy, with a significant decrease of the extenuation motor output area to the ADM muscle before therapy, compared with the UH or the controls. This area was significantly larger after rehabilitation therapy and included anomalous sites, not normally associated with ADM activation. The MEPs amplitude both at rest and during voluntary contraction was significantly lower than normal in AH before rehabilitation. After rehabilitation therapy, it was significantly increased during relaxation, but remained significantly smaller than normal during voluntary contraction. There were significant improvements in both Barthel Index and Canadian Neurological Scale scores during the course of rehabilitation therapy. Central conduction time remained prolonged in the stroke patients.

Conclusions.—These neurophysiologic data are consistent with ongoing rearrangement of the motor cortical output area 2–4 months after a monohemispheric stroke. This reorganization is reflected in the enlargement of the excitable brain area and increased MEP amplitude during this time. This enlargement also may include anomalous sites not normally associated with activation. These neurophysiologic modifications are significantly associated with the clinical improvement of disability.

▶ A greater or lesser degree of recovery commonly follows acute stroke. Studies using positron emission tomography suggest that one of the mechanisms of recovery is neurons taking over functions previously carried out by cells destroyed by the stroke. In this article, results are reported using an electrophysiologic technique to document that such "plastic rearrangements" of cortical functions are still occurring 2–4 months after an acute stroke. The persistence and the degree of neurologic plasticity, even months after a stroke, provide a biological rationale for stroke rehabilitation. Because the brains of stroke victims retain the capacity to reorganize themselves during a prolonged recovery period, it is reasonable to assume that manipulations can be developed that increase not only the rate but also the extent of such reparative reorganization.

J.P. Blass, M.D., Ph.D.

Hemineglect in Acute Stroke—Incidence and Prognostic Implications: The Copenhagen Stroke Study
Pedersen PM, Jørgensen HS, Nakayama H, et al (Bispebjerg Hosp, Copenhagen)
Am J Phys Med Rehabil 76:122–127, 1997   13–3

Background.—Hemineglect is the failure to respond to meaningful stimuli presented to the side opposite a brain lesion. The incidence of hemineglect in stroke patients and its prognostic implications were investigated in a large community-based group of stroke patients.

Study Design.—From January 1992 to September 1993, 1,014 community-based stroke patients were recruited to the Copenhagen Stroke Study. Patients who were unconscious, unable to cooperate, or who were not admitted to the hospital until more than 1 week after onset were excluded. The remaining 602 patients were younger, had a lower mortality, less neurologic impairment, and were more likely to be male, than the excluded patients. At admission, patients were examined for stroke severity, stroke history, anosognosia, and hemineglect. Computed tomographic scans were inspected to determine lesion type, size, and localization. Activities of daily living (ADL) were evaluated by the Barthel Index (BI). In-hospital rehabilitation was by the Bobath technique.

Findings.—Hemineglect was detected in 23% of the 602 stroke patients in the study group. Anosognosia was present in 73% of patients with hemineglect and in 6% of those without hemineglect. Hemineglect was associated with stroke severity, age, lesion in right hemisphere, larger lesion, and parietal lobe involvement. Hemineglect had no independent influence on admission BI, discharge BI, length of hospital stay, mortality, or discharge to independent living.

Conclusions.—In this study population, hemineglect had no independent, negative prognostic effect on functional outcome. Many of the patients with hemineglect also had anosognosia. The overall outcome of patients with anosognosia was much worse than that of patients with hemineglect.

▶ The Copenhagen Stroke Study continues to provide useful, epidemiologically based information on stroke and stroke outcome. This study reports that hemineglect (neglect of a side) does not worsen the functional outcome of stroke, whereas anosognosia (failure to recognize the existence of defect) does. Hemineglect and anosognosia often occur together, which may explain the widespread impression that hemineglect is a risk factor for poorer recovery after strokes. This study therefore suggests a way to make the neurologic examination in patients recovering from stroke a more precise predictor of functional outcome.

J.P. Blass, M.D., Ph.D.

Walking Ability of Stroke Patients: Efficacy of Tibial Nerve Blocking and a Polypropylene Ankle-Foot Orthosis
Beckerman H, Becher J, Lankhorst GJ, et al (Academisch Ziekenhuis Vrije Universiteit Amsterdam; Univ of Nijmegen, The Netherlands)
Arch Phys Med Rehabil 77:1144–1151, 1996   13–4

Background.—Percutaneous radiofrequency thermocoagulation has been used for relief of local spasticity. An ankle–foot orthosis (AFO) in a 5-degree dorsoflexion position also can be used to inhibit the spastic position of the foot. A placebo-controlled, randomized clinical trial was performed to test the efficacy of both thermocoagulation of the tibial nerve and an AFO on the walking ability of stroke patients with spastic equinus or equinovarus foot. The impact of these procedures was assessed by the Sickness Impact Profile (SIP), a self-assessment health status instrument.

Methods.—A placebo-controlled, randomized clinical trial with a 2 × 2 factorial design was carried out. Sixty primary stroke patients between the ages of 18 and 75 years, with walking problems caused by spastic equinus or equinovarus position of the foot, were eligible to participate 4 months after stroke occurrence. Each patient had a temporary nerve block to eliminate those whose standing and walking were dependent on extensor

TABLE 5.—Adjusted Treatment Effects: Comparison of Complier Analysis (n = 30) With Full Analysis (n = 57)

Outcome Measure	Adjusted Effect Total Group	95% CI	Adjusted Effect Compliers	95% CI
Improvement SIP ambulation (%)				
Effect$_{thermocoagulation}$	.56	−3.01/4.13	4.28	−.04/8.59
Effect$_{AFO}$	2.72	−.94/6.38	−1.69	−6.54/3.17
Walking speed (m/sec)				
Comfortable with shoes				
Effect$_{thermocoagulation}$	−.02	−.06/.02	.00	−.07/.07
Effect$_{AFO}$	.01	−.03/.06	.02	−.05/.10
Maximal safe, with shoes				
Effect$_{thermocoagulation}$	−.02	−.07/.03	.02	−.06/.11
Effect$_{AFO}$	.04	−.01/.10	.10	.02/.19

Effects adjusted for baseline differences with respect to age, period poststroke, and quadriceps' strength. Positive signs indicate improvement from baseline; negative signs indicate a decline from the baseline scores.

(Courtesy of Beckerman H, Becher J, Lankhorst GJ, et al: Walking ability of stroke patients: Efficacy of tibial nerve blocking and a polypropylene ankle-foot orthosis. *Arch Phys Med Rehabil* 77:1144–1151, 1996.)

spasticity. Patients were randomized to placebo, thermocoagulation (TH), AFO, or both treatments. The primary outcome measure was walking ability as measured by the SIP at baseline and then after 12 weeks. Measurements were conducted in a blinded fashion.

Results.—With respect to the walking ability of these stroke patients, there was little effect of either treatment intervention or of both interventions together. When the analysis was performed only on compliant participants, the efficacy of TH increased, but the efficacy of AFO decreased (Table 5). The changes in comfortable and maximum safe walking speed over the study period were not significant.

Conclusions.—This article describes the results of the first randomized clinical trial of the effects of thermocoagulation and an AFO on the walking ability of stroke patients. This trial found no benefit of either intervention on the walking ability of these patients.

▶ This careful, placebo-controlled, randomized clinical trial tested the clinical value of interventions that improve a variety of physiologic parameters in the gait of poststroke patients on the ability of the patients to walk. Despite previously reported improvements in measurements such as stride length, stance symmetry, and heel-contact time in hemiplegic patients, the patients did not walk better or faster. This study again demonstrates that physiologic measurements are only surrogates for the clinical variables that matter to the patients. Whether or not clinically important improvements occur with a treatment can only be determined by appropriately structured, placebo-controlled clinical tests of the relevant functions in the patients themselves, including asking the patients in the treated and placebo groups how they feel.

J.P. Blass, M.D., Ph.D.

The Effect of Robot-assisted Therapy and Rehabilitative Training on Motor Recovery Following Stroke

Aisen ML, Krebs HI, Hogan N, et al (Burke Rehabilitation Hosp, White Plains, NY; Massachusetts Inst of Technology, Cambridge)
Arch Neurol 54:443–446, 1997   13–5

Background.—Recent evidence suggests that neurologic function may be restorable after stroke. Rehabilitation may play a role in this recovery. The MIT-Manus is a robot developed to provide interactive, goal-directed motor activity for clinical neurologic applications. Whether robotic manipulation of the impaired limb affects motor recovery in patients with hemiplegia was determined.

Methods and Findings.—Twenty patients with hemiplegia after stroke were enrolled in a standard rehabilitation program supplemented by robot-aided or sham robot-aided treatment. Both groups experienced a decrease in impairment and disability between hospital admission and discharge. Patients receiving robot-aided therapy had a greater degree of improvement on all 3 measures of motor recovery. The change in motor status measured in the proximal upper limb musculature was significant. Robot-assisted therapy produced no adverse effects.

Conclusion.—Robotic manipulation of the impaired limb may favorably influence recovery after stroke. Robotics may be a new source of strategies for neurologic rehabilitation. Further research is needed to confirm the results of this pilot study.

▶ The pilot experiment described in this article uses one of the new technologies—robotics—to train people who have had strokes to perform better. It is an intriguing and original use of modern technology for increasing the effectiveness while reducing the labor costs of stroke rehabilitation. Determining the true clinical utility of this approach will, of course, require much more extensive study of many more patients.

J.P. Blass, M.D., Ph.D.

Randomised Controlled Trial to Evaluate Early Discharge Scheme for Patients With Stroke

Rudd AG, Wolfe CDA, Tilling K, et al (St Thomas's Hosp, London)
BMJ 315:1039–1044, 1997   13–6

Background.—Some authorities argue for stroke care that is more balanced between the hospital and community. The clinical efficacy of an early discharge policy using a community-based rehabilitation team for stroke victims was studied.

Methods.—Three hundred thirty-one patients with stroke were enrolled in a randomized, controlled study comparing conventional care with the early discharge policy. The patients were medically stable, lived alone and were able to transfer independently, or lived with a caregiver who could help them transfer. One hundred sixty-seven patients received specialist community rehabilitation for up to 3 months, and 164 patients continued with conventional hospital and community care.

Findings.—Clinical outcomes did not differ significantly between the groups 1 year after randomization. The community therapy group expressed greater satisfaction with hospital care than did the conventional-care group. Length of stay in the 2 groups was 12 and 18 days, respectively. Impaired patients were more likely to receive treatment in the community therapy group.

Conclusions.—Early discharge with specialist community rehabilitation after stroke is as clinically effective as conventional care and acceptable to patients. The early discharge policy results in marked reductions in the use of hospital beds.

▶ Stroke is common, and the cost of caring for patients with stroke is large. This British study suggests that early discharge from hospital and specialty care at home is as effective as prolonged hospital stay for medically stable patients who were able to transfer at home. The study was done in London, a metropolis with good public transport; whether the results would generalize to more rural areas needs to be answered by an independent study. Per-day hospital costs in the United States are high, suggesting that early discharge of appropriate patients with stroke could be very cost-effective here.

J.P. Blass, M.D., Ph.D.

A Randomized Controlled Trial of Rehabilitation at Home After Stroke in Southwest Stockholm
Holmqvist LW, von Koch L, Kostulas V, et al (Huddinge Univ, Sweden; Carlos III Inst of Health, Madrid)
Stroke 29:591–597, 1998   13–7

Background.—In Sweden, 95% of patients with acute stroke are hospitalized, and the cost of hospital care, outpatient care, and social services constitute 76% of the cost of stroke. It has been reported that specialized rehabilitation programs can achieve better and faster functional outcomes than general medical units, and it has been suggested that home rehabilitation should be emphasized. The best combination of inpatient, outpatient, and home rehabilitation services has not been determined for patients with strokes.

Methods.—Of 81 patients with acute stroke, 41 (50.6%) were randomly assigned to home rehabilitation and 40 (49.4%) were assigned to routine rehabilitation in a hospital, day care facility, or as an outpatient. Eligible patients had impaired motor function and/or aphasia 1 week after stroke, but were continent, could feed themselves, and had normal mental function. Home rehabilitation was managed by 2 physical therapists, 2 occupational therapists, and 1 speech therapist. The home rehabilitation program was task-oriented and context-oriented, and activities were based on each patient's needs. Follow-up was 3 months. Outcome was evaluated by the Frenchay Social Activity Index, Extended Katz Index, Barthel Index, Lindmark Motor Capacity Assessment, Nine-Hole Peg Test, walking speed greater than 10 m, reported falls, and subjective dysfunction on the Sickness Impact Profile. The patient's use of hospital and home rehabilitation services was determined, as was patient satisfaction with the rehabilitation program.

Results.—No significant differences in patient outcome were seen between the 2 rehabilitation programs. For patients in the home rehabilitation group, multivariate logistic regression analysis showed a systematic positive effect in social activity, ADL, motor capacity, manual dexterity, and walking. There was a substantial difference in use of resources during the 3-month period. A 52% decrease in hospitalization was seen in patients who had home rehabilitation (14 days) compared with patients who had routine rehabilitation (29 days). Patients who had home rehabilitation were more satisfied with their care, especially with being able to assist in planning their rehabilitation program. No decrease in outcome in the first 3 months was seen in most of these moderately disabled patients who had early supported discharge and home rehabilitation after acute stroke compared with patients who had routine rehabilitation.

Conclusions.—If follow-up at 6 and 12 months confirms this suggested effectiveness and reduced use of health care services, then home rehabilitation may be considered an alternative to routine rehabilitation after acute stroke.

▶ A pressing issue in stroke rehabilitation is the triage of poststroke patients into the form of rehabilitation that is most useful for the patients while still being cost-effective. This Swedish study indicates that rehabilitation at home is about as effective as other forms of rehabilitation, for patients moderately disabled after stroke. Moderate disability was defined as motor and/or speech impairments in patients who were continent, able to feed themselves, and reasonably intact mentally (Mini-Mental State Exam score of 23). What is missing in this trial (for understandable reasons) is a test of the null hypothesis, that is, whether these moderately-disabled patients needed rehabilitation at all. Although further studies are clearly needed, this carefully constructed trial does suggest that there are a population of patients in whom early discharge after stroke combined with home rehabilitation is as clinically effective and more cost effective than other forms of care.

J.P. Blass, M.D., Ph.D.

The Impact of Inpatient Rehabilitation on Progressive Multiple Sclerosis

Freeman JA, Langdon DW, Hobart JC, et al (Inst of Neurology, London)
Ann Neurol 42:236–244, 1997   13–8

Introduction.—Progressive disability is experienced by most patients with multiple sclerosis (MS). The socioeconomic impact on patients and their families is considerable. There is a great need to address the disability and handicap in both the provision and evaluation of health and social service interventions in patients with MS. The effectiveness of a short period of multidisciplinary inpatient rehabilitation was evaluated in patients with MS in the progressive phase of the disease.

Methods.—Patients were stratified according to disease severity (mild, moderate, or severe), then randomly assigned to immediate treatment or placed on a waiting list with no rehabilitation intervention. Patients in both groups were evaluated using validated measures of impairment at the start and end of the rehabilitation program. The rehabilitation program was based on a model of comprehensive care that emphasized achievement of the best possible quality of life within the limits of the disease.

Results.—Of 70 patients recruited for treatment, 34 were randomly assigned to immediate treatment, 36 acted as controls, and 4 withdrew before the second assessment. There were no between-group changes in impairment at a 6-week evaluation. The treatment group had significant improvements in motor domain, self-care, transfers, and sphincter control

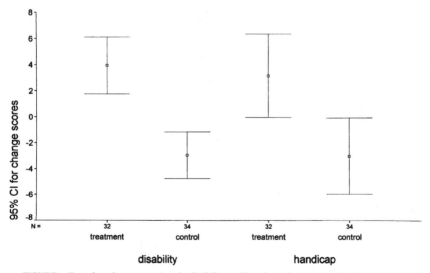

FIGURE.—Error-bar chart comparing the disability and handicap change scores in the treatment and the control groups. *Abbreviation: CI,* confidence interval: (Reprinted from Freeman JA, Langdon DW, Hobart JC, et al: The impact of inpatient rehabilitation on progressive multiple sclerosis. *Ann Neurol* 42:236–244, 1997, by permission of Little, Brown and Company, copyright ANA.)

compared to controls (Fig). There were no between-group differences in walking and wheelchair locomotion.

Conclusion.—The disability and handicap were significantly diminished, despite unchanged neurologic impairment in treatment and control groups of patients in the progressive phase of MS. Rehabilitation is beneficial and effective in decreasing the handicap and disability in patients with progressive MS.

▶ Neurologists and physiatrists routinely recommend inpatient rehabilitation for patients severely disabled by MS. This randomized study provides some evidence that disability (neurologic function) and handicap (disadvantages identified in activities of daily living and self care) may be improved by this procedure, although impairment (abnormalities in the neurologic examination) was less responsive to inpatient rehabilitative measures. The authors acknowledge some methodological shortcomings of this work, particularly those related to evaluator and patient blinding. In addition, they noted that delay in enrollment was followed by continued progression in the control group. Nonetheless, this is the first carefully designed study to begin to assess inpatient rehabilitation in patients with progressive MS with moderately severe impairment. Further work of this nature from this and other academically oriented units is needed to clarify the utility of rehabilitation measures, particularly as currently available therapies have not convincingly shown arrest or delay in eventual progression of impairment in this illness.

J.H. Noseworthy, M.D., F.R.C.P.C.

14 Infectious Disease of the Nervous System

Dendritic Injury Is a Pathological Substrate for Human Immunodeficiency Virus–related Cognitive Disorders
Masliah E, Heaton RK, Marcotte TD, et al (Univ of California, San Diego; Veterans Affairs Med Ctr, San Diego, Calif; Presbyterian Univ, Pittsburgh, Pa)
Ann Neurol 42:963–972, 1997   14–1

Introduction.—Neuropsychologic deficits occur in nearly 55% of patients with AIDS who have no opportunistic diseases of the brain. Dendritic loss may be an important neuropathologic substrate for HIV-related cognitive changes. Twenty patients with AIDS were examined before their death, and antemortem neuropsychologic performance was related to postmortem indicators of HIV encephalitis, viral burden, and presynaptic and postsynaptic neuronal injury.

Methods.—Median interval between last neurobehavioral assessment and death was 4.8 months. Patients underwent neuropsychologic testing and were classified using 4 clinical levels of neurocognitive functioning: unimpaired, subsyndromical neuropsychological impairment (NPI), minor cognitive/motor disorder (MCMD), and HIV-associated dementia (HAD). Postmortem neuropathologic evaluation and analysis of brain tissue were performed to assess for neuronal damage.

Results.—Eleven patients (55%) had either syndromic or subsyndromic NPI, with impairment being mild or mild to moderate in 9 patients. Clinical classifications of impaired patients were 5 NPI, 5 MCMD, and 1 HAD. Nine patients had normal neurocognitive evaluations. There was a strong relationship between degree of neurocognitive impairment and amount of dendritic simplification with microtubule-associated protein 2 immunohistochemical staining (Fig 1). This relationship was somewhat less noticeable when a semiquantitative viral burden score was based on numbers of HIV gp41-immunoreactive cells, and much less so to the presence of multinucleated giant cells or microglial nodules.

Conclusion.—Loss of dendritic complexity may be the strongest correlate of HIV-associated neurocognitive impairment. Further investigation should define the specific subsets of neurons that are vulnerable to the damage, identify the mechanisms by which dendrites are injured, and

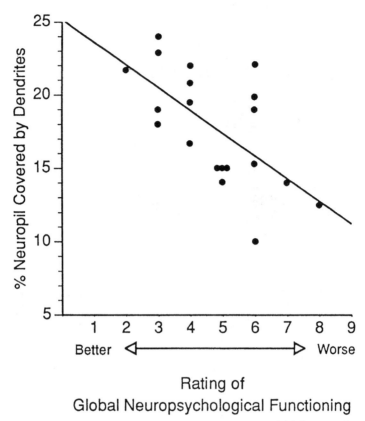

FIGURE 1.—Relationship of midfrontal dendritic complexity to rating of global cognitive functioning. (Reprinted from *Annals of Neurology* courtesy of Masliah E, Heaton RK, Marcotte TD, et al: Dendritic injury is a pathological substrate for human immunodeficiency virus-related cognitive disorders. *Ann Neurol* 42:963–972, 1997, by permission of Little, Brown and Company, Inc., copyright ANA.)

examine the impact of antiretroviral and other mechanism-specific treatments on preservation of cognitive function and its neuroanatomical substrates.

▶ Dr. Masliah and colleagues elegantly demonstrate that pruning of the dendritic branches correlates very well with progressive HIV-associated neurocognitive impairment. Additionally, they demonstrate that the viral burden of HIV in the brain correlates inversely with the dendritic complexity observed. However, the former was believed to be insufficient by itself to be responsible for the HIV-associated neurocognitive disorders. These findings complement those of other investigators who have demonstrated a significant loss of cortical neurons accompanying HIV dementia. It is not unlikely that HIV-dementia is not only the consequence of the structural changes of neuronal loss and decreased dendritic branching, but also the consequence of impaired neuronal function due to viral proteins or inflammatory products.

J.R. Berger, M.D.

Relationship Between Human Immunodeficiency Virus–associated Dementia and Viral Load in Cerebrospinal Fluid and Brain

McArthur JC, McClernon DR, Cronin MF, et al (Johns Hopkins Univ, Baltimore, Md; Glaxo-Wellcome Inc, Research Triangle Park, NC; Organon Teknika Corp, Durham, NC)

Ann Neurol 42:689–698, 1997   14–2

Introduction.—Human immunodeficiency virus dementia (HIV-D) develops with immunodeficiency. Its prevalence is low during the asymptomatic phase of HIV infection and rises to 15% to 20% in patients with symptomatic disease. The relationship between viral load and dementia severity, immune status, and markers of immune activation were assessed in 207 seropositive patients.

Methods.—All patients underwent lumbar puncture and venipuncture for determination of CSF viral RNA and serum HIV RNA and CD4 counts, respectively. Of 207 patients evaluated, 37 had HIV plus dementia, 77 had HIV plus minor neurologic signs (HIV-MCMD), and 93 had HIV

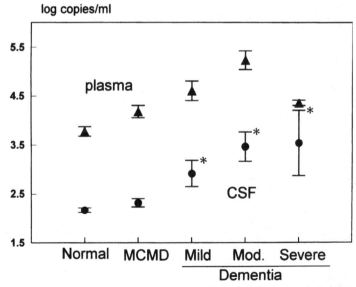

FIGURE 2.—Mean ± SEM CSF and plasma HIV RNA levels in different neurologic groups. Significantly higher CSF levels in subjects with HIV dementia compared with HIV-NML and MCMD, after controlling for CD4 counts. Plasma levels are only of borderline significance. *Abbreviations*: MCMD, minor cognitive/motor disorder; *Mod.*, moderate. (Reprinted from *Annals of Neurology* courtesy of McArthur JC, McClernon DR, Cronin MF, et al: Relationship between human immunodeficiency virus–associated dementia and viral load in cerebrospinal fluid and brain. *Ann Neurol* 42:689–698, 1997, by permission of Little, Brown and Company, Inc. Copyright ANA.)

and were neurologically normal (HIV-NML). The HIV-1 viral load was assessed by the Nucleic Acid Sequence-Based Amplification (NASBA) assay. The NASBA assay limit of detection was 100 copies per milliliter.

Results.—The mean CSF log HIV RNA levels were significantly higher in patients with dementia after adjusting for CD4 count and were correlated with dementia severity (Fig 2). The plasma levels did not distinguish comparably immunosuppressed patients with or without dementia. The CSF and plasma RNA levels were significantly intercorrelated for patients with CD4 counts of less than 200/mm^3 and inversely correlated with CSF β_2-microglobulin. The CSF RNA levels were independent of both CSF pleocytosis and antiretroviral exposure. Brain RNA levels were consistently higher than CSF levels but correlated with CSF values in patients with dementia.

Conclusion.—The NASBA assay may be used reliably to detect HIV RNA levels in CSF, brain, and plasma samples. The correlation with brain levels suggests that CSF HIV RNA is a surrogate marker for brain infection. The association between plasma HIV RNA and CSF levels of HIV and β_2-microglobulin indicates that both viral load and CNS immune activation are important determinants of neurologic disease.

▶ These 2 studies from the Baltimore and San Diego groups (Abstracts 14–1 and 14–2) address the presence of HIV RNA levels in the CNS and dementia. The former group demonstrated that there is a correlation between the level of the virus in the CSF and that in the brain, indicating the value of the former as a surrogate marker for brain infection. The San Diego group notes a close correlation between the HIV RNA level in the CSF and that in the serum before the development of AIDS. In their study, this correlation ceased to exist at the time of disease progression to AIDS.

Both groups of investigators indicate that there is a relationship between active viral infection in the CNS and the presence of neurocognitive abnormalities. The contribution of immunomediators to the pathogenesis of dementia is suggested by the presence of β_2-microglobulin in the CSF. It is not unlikely that a wide variety of cytokines and chemokines generated in the brain during HIV infection contribute to the dementia.

J.R. Berger, M.D.

Levels of Human Immunodeficiency Virus Type 1 RNA in Cerebrospinal Fluid Correlate With AIDS Dementia Stage

Brew BJ, Pemberton L, Cunningham P, et al (Univ of New South Wales, Sydney, Australia)
J Infect Dis 175:963–966, 1997   14–3

Introduction.—Patients with advanced HIV-1 infection may be affected by a subacute dementing illness known as *AIDS dementia complex* (ADC). Several studies report a relationship between severity of ADC and a number of markers of inflammation in CSF. A study of patients with HIV-1 infection examined the relationship of CSF viral load to the presence and severity of ADC and CNS opportunistic infections.

Methods.—Samples of CSF from patients who had been assessed neurologically for ADC and other CNS complications were selected from a clinical CSF data bank. Plasma samples, when available, were also analyzed. All patients had fewer than 200 CD4 cells /µL. The CSF samples were assessed for levels of HIV-1 RNA, cryptococcal antigen, cytology, and a number of other factors.

Results.—Twenty-five patients had ADC with varying degrees of severity: 6 were at stage 0 (normal function), 8 were at stage 1 (mild symptoms or signs), and 11 were at stages 2 or 3 (mild or moderate symptoms or signs). Plasma samples were available for 10 patients, 4 with ADC stage 1, 5 with stage 2, and 1 with stage 3. Also studied were 10 patients with CNS opportunistic infections but no evidence of ADC. Among patients with ADC, there was a significant relationship between increasing CSF viral burden and severity of ADC. No relationship was found, however, between plasma burden and ADC severity. The median concentrations of HIV-1 RNA in the CSF ranged from 323 copies/ml in ADC stage 0 to 93,000 copies/ml in ADC stage 3. Patients without ADC but with cryptococcal meningitis also exhibited elevated levels of CSF HIV-1 RNA.

Discussion.—There was a correlation between CSF concentrations of HIV-1 RNA and severity of ADC in these patients, but plasma concentrations did not show the same relationship. Patients without dementia but with cryptococcal meningitis also had elevated CSF HIV-1 RNA concentrations. Once other CNS opportunistic infections are excluded, however, a CSF HIV-1 RNA load greater than 1000 copies/ml has a high specificity (83%) and reasonable sensitivity (58%) for suspected ADC.

▶ The pathogenesis of ADC remains controversial. Several mechanisms for neuronal injury in the face of HIV infection have been proposed, including neuronal toxicity from virus itself or viral proteins, neuronal toxicity from immune mediators elaborated from infected brain macrophages or other resident inflammatory cells, alterations in the blood-brain barrier, the induction of an autoimmune process, and infectious or metabolic cofactors. These Australian investigators demonstrate a highly significant direct correlation between the level of CSF HIV-1 RNA (determined by polymerase chain reaction) and the stage of AIDS dementia complex. This observation suggests that high local viral titers are an important requisite for the development of ADC and strongly supports the importance of suppressing viral replication in the brain in this disorder.

J.R. Berger, M.D.

Evaluation of Human Immunodeficiency Virus (HIV) Type 1 RNA Levels in Cerebrospinal Fluid and Viral Resistance to Zidovudine in Children With HIV Encephalopathy

Sei S, Stewart SK, Farley M, et al (Natl Cancer Inst, Bethesda, Md; SRA Technologies Inc; Walter Reed Army Inst of Research, Rockville, Md)
J Infect Dis 174:1200–1206, 1996   14–4

Purpose.—Patients with advanced HIV disease—particularly children—may develop HIV encephalopathy. The mechanism of action of this condition is unknown but may involve active HIV-1 infection of macrophages or microglia within the CNS. Zidovudine is a beneficial treatment for this condition; however, the neurologic response is variable. It is uncertain whether viral replication in the CNS is increased in patients with HIV encephalopathy. Children with HIV encephalopathy were studied to assess the amount of HIV-1 RNA in CSF and plasma and to look for the mutation conferring viral resistance to zidovudine.

Methods.—The study included 41 children (median age, 2 years) with HIV-1 infection. Thirty-two had moderate-to-severe encephalopathy, whereas 9 had no encephalopathy. Serum and CSF levels of HIV-1 RNA were assessed, as was the presence of a codon 215 mutation that indicates zidovudine resistance. The effect of zidovudine resistance on the neurologic outcome of zidovudine treatment was evaluated as well.

Results.—Ninety-one percent of children with HIV encephalopathy had HIV-1 RNA in their CSF, compared with 22% of those without encephalopathy. Plasma HIV-1 RNA levels were similar among groups, and the CSF and plasma HIV-1 RNA levels were unrelated to each other. Total cell counts and protein concentrations were higher and glucose levels were lower in CSF samples with more than 1,000 HIV-1 RNA copies/mL. Samples positive for HIV-1 p24 antigen had more HIV-1 RNA copies than samples negative for this antigen. Patients treated with zidovudine had lower levels of HIV-1 RNA in CSF than those not treated with zidovudine, but there was no difference in their plasma HIV-1 RNA levels. Children with the mutant codon 215 in CSF were more likely to have progressive encephalopathy while receiving zidovudine therapy. At follow-up CSF evaluation, the extent of HIV-1 RNA reduction was not directly correlated with improvement in neuropsychometric test scores.

Conclusions.—Children with HIV encephalopathy are more likely to have HIV-1 RNA in their CSF than HIV-infected children without encephalopathy. The results suggest that HIV turnover in the CNS may be independent of that in the peripheral blood. Active viral replication may be necessary for HIV encephalopathy to develop; however, the quantity of virus is not necessarily the only factor affecting the pathophysiologic changes in the brain. Progressive encephalopathy may occur without effective suppression of viral replication in the CNS compartment.

▶ This study from the National Institutes of Health demonstrates 3 important findings in HIV-infected children, namely, (1) a direct correlation between CSF levels of HIV-1 RNA and the degree of encephalopathy; (2) the absence of a correlation between CSF and plasma levels of HIV-1 RNA; and (3) a poor response to zidovudine therapy for encephalopathy in children whose CSF harbored HIV with a codon 215 mutation (a mutation frequently observed in the setting of zidovudine resistance). Although some investigators contend that the CSF provides, at best, an inexact picture of the events occurring within brain parenchyma in HIV infection, it is the only practical source of virus for studying issues related to neuropathogenesis and treatment.

Despite controversy surrounding the issue of a correlation between CSF and plasma levels of HIV, the findings from this study in children are likely generalizable to the adult population. Neurologists caring for large numbers of patients with AIDS have noted a decline in frequency of HIV dementia and, in some instances, the remarkable resolution of symptoms of this illness after the institution of aggressive antiretroviral therapy which includes a protease inhibitor.

The findings of Dr. Sei and colleagues highlights the potential of the brain as a source of viral sequestration and the need to suppress viral replication in the CNS to treat HIV dementia. Accomplishing the latter may require the use of aggressive therapy that decreases the likelihood of the development of antiviral-resistant strains of HIV.

J.R. Berger, M.D.

Proton MRS and Quantitative MRI Assessment of the Short Term Neurological Response to Antiretroviral Therapy in AIDS
Wilkinson ID, Lunn S, Miszkiel KA, et al (Univ College London)
J Neurol Neurosurg Psychiatry 63:477–482, 1997   14–5

Introduction.—Human immunodeficiency virus-associated dementia complex (HADC), a common neurological complication of HIV infection, results in cognitive dysfunction and may be accompanied by motor dysfunction and behavioral change. Previous reports suggest that quantitative imaging techniques can be used to monitor changes in cognitive function after therapy for HADC. Five patients with AIDS and HADC were studied with MRI and proton MR spectroscopy (MRS) before and during antiretroviral therapy.

Methods.—All patients were seen with a subacute encephalopathy consistent with HADC, a diagnosis confirmed by clinical evaluation and psychometric testing. Three markers of neurological response were evaluated: cerebral spinal fluid/intracranial volume (CSF-ICV) ratio; T2-weighted signal ratio between parieto-occipital white and subcortical gray matter; and metabolite ratios from long echo time (TE=135 ms) single voxel proton spectra of parieto-occipital white matter. All MR data from the patients were compared with the means from a control group made up of 17 homosexual men who were HIV-seronegative but at high risk for HIV infection.

Results.—During zidovudine therapy all 5 patients demonstrated an increase in CSF/ICV ratio, irrespective of clinical response. In 4 of 5 patients, spectroscopic changes indicated initial increases in N-acetyl/(N-acetyl + choline + creatine) ratio [NA/(NA+Cho+Cr)] and progression of atrophy after antiretoviral therapy was started. Subsequent neurological deterioration in 2 of 5 patients was accompanied by a decline in the NA/(NA+Cho+Cr) ratio.

Conclusion.—Proton MRS was able to mirror both clinical improvement and clinical deterioration after the initiation of antiretroviral therapy in patients with HADC. Despite initial clinical improvement after treatment, atrophy progressed in 4 of 5 patients. The remaining patient exhibited a small increase in CSF/IVC. Quantitative MRI and spectroscopy may be useful in assessing the neurological effects of new combination therapies.

▶ Dr. Wilkinson and colleagues correctly assert that there need to be objective measures to assess progression or improvement in the course of the dementia associated with HIV. Although the number of patients studied is small, and the course of their disease seems to be one of progression despite antitretroviral therapy, the authors demonstrate the potential utility of MRS and quantitative MRI in this population.

J.R. Berger, M.D.

Regression of HIV Encephalopathy and Basal Ganglia Signal Intensity Abnormality at MR Imaging in Patients With AIDS After the Initiation of Protease Inhibitor Therapy
Filippi CG, Sze G, Farber SJ, et al (Yale–New Haven Hosp, Conn; Royal London Hosp at Whitechapel)
Radiology 206:491–498, 1998   14–6

Introduction.—The pathophysiology of HIV encephalopathy is not well understood. The pathologic findings in milder infections include astrogliosis and myelin pallor that involves deep gray nuclei, basal ganglia, and deep white matter. Findings in patients with severe HIV encephalitis include presence of multinucleated cells located primarily in the white matter or less frequently in the gray matter. Magnetic resonance images (MRI) were examined to determine if protease inhibitors cause regression of periventricular white matter signal intensity abnormalities in patients with HIV encephalopathy and whether the changes on MRIs correlate with cognitive improvement.

Methods.—The MRIs of 16 adult patients with HIV encephalopathy were assessed retrospectively and prospectively. White matter and basal ganglia signal intensity abnormalities on initial long repetition time (TR) images were compared with those on subsequent long TR images in patients who did and did not take protease inhibitors. Images and clinical findings were correlated.

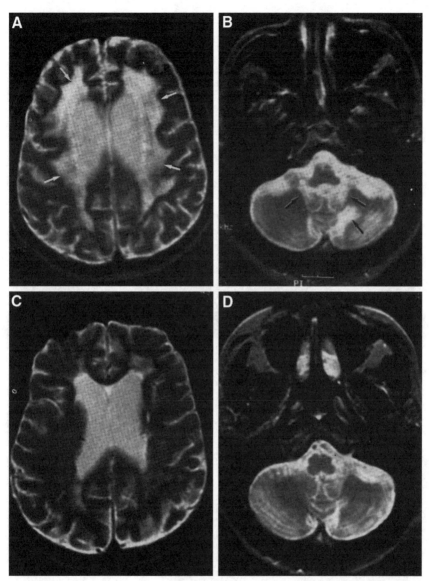

FIGURE 1.—Long TR axial MR images (2,000/80) in a 49-year-old man with HIV leukoencephalopathy being treated with zidovudine and lamivudine. **A**, before the initiation of protease inhibitor therapy, image demonstrates symmetric confluent areas of hyperintensity (*arrows*) within the periventricular white matter. **B**, image of the cerebellum obtained at the same time as **A** shows hyperintense signal abnormalities within the brachium pontis bilaterally and within the left cerebellar hemisphere (*arrows*). **C**, 7 months after protease inhibitor therapy with saquinavir was added to the patient's reverse transcriptase regimen, image demonstrates a considerable decrease in the amount of periventricular white matter disease, which correlated with cognitive improvement. **D**, image obtained at the same time as **C** shows complete resolution of the previously noted hyperintense signal abnormality within the cerebellum. (Courtesy of Filippi CG, Sze G, Farber SJ, et al: Regression of HIV encephalopathy and basal ganglia signal intensity abnormality at MR imaging in patients with AIDS after the initiation of protease inhibitor therapy. *Radiology* 206:491–498, 1998. Radiological Society of North America.)

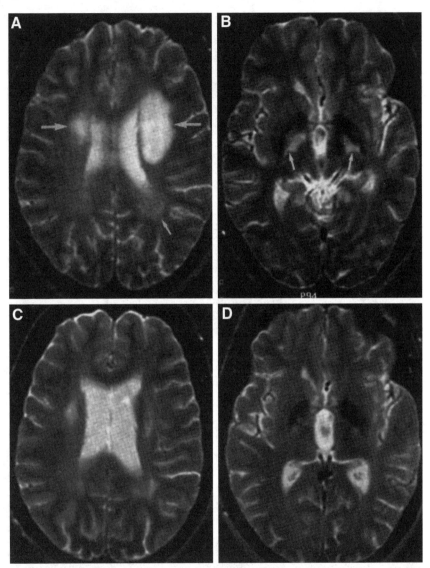

FIGURE 2.—Long TR axial MR images (2,000/80) in a 33-year-old woman with AIDS and HIV leukoencephalopathy being treated with a single nucleoside analogue (zidovudine). **A,** before the initiation of protease inhibitor therapy, image demonstrates confluent hyperintense signal abnormalities within the periventricular white matter, in the frontal areas (*large arrows*) more than in the parieto-occipital areas (*small arrow*), and on the left side more than on the right side. **B,** image obtained at the same time as **A** demonstrates symmetric hyperintensity (*arrows*) within the posterior limb of the internal capsule and the medial aspects of the globus pallidus bilaterally. **C,** 3 months after the addition of the protease inhibitor ritonavir to this patient's regimen, there is a dramatic reduction in the signal intensity abnormalities previously noted within the periventricular white matter, which correlated with improvements in the patient's memory and cognitive function. **D,** image obtained at the same time as **C** shows a substantial interval decrease in the hyperintense signal abnormalities within the posterior limb of the internal capsule and the medial aspects of the globus pallidus bilaterally. (Courtesy of Filippi CG, Sze G, Farber SJ, et al: Regression of HIV encephalopathy and basal ganglia signal intensity abnormality at MR imaging in patients with AIDS after the initiation of protease inhibitor therapy. *Radiology* 206:491–498, 1998. Radiological Society of North America.)

Results.—Four of 9 patients taking protease inhibitors had nearly complete regression, 4 had interval stability, and 1 had slight progression. The 8 patients (89%) with either stability or improvement in white matter disease also had cognitive improvement. In 7 patients not taking protease inhibitors, 6 had marked progression with a decline in cognitive function, and 1 had no interval change. Changes between those who did and did not take protease inhibitors were significant. Of 2 patients with basal signal intensity abnormalities who were taking protease inhibitors, 1 had resolution (Fig 1) and 1 had nearly complete resolution (Fig 2).

Conclusion.—Protease inhibitors may cause regression of periventricular white matter and basal ganglia signal intensity abnormalities in HIV encephalopathy and may be important in treatment.

▶ Although no studies of sufficient magnitude addressing the value of highly active antiretroviral therapy (HAART) in the treatment of HIV encephalopathy have yet been performed, anecdotal evidence suggests that HIV encephalopathy may regress with HAART. Dr. Filippi and colleagues demonstrate not only clinical improvement but also improvement in the cranial MRIs of patients with HIV encephalopathy treated with protease inhibitors. Additionally, they draw attention to an interesting finding, namely, basal ganglia hyperintensity in two of their patients, which resolved completely or substantially following treatment. Abnormalities of the basal ganglia (chiefly calcification) are usually a feature of HIV encephalopathy in children.

J.R. Berger, M.D.

Diagnosis of AIDS-related Focal Brain Lesions: A Decision-making Analysis Based on Clinical and Neuroradiologic Characteristics Combined With Polymerase Chain Reaction Assays in CSF
Antinori A, Ammassari A, De Luca A, et al (Catholic Univ, Rome; Natl Statistical Inst, Rome)
Neurology 48:687–694, 1997   14–7

Purpose.—In patients with HIV infection, focal brain lesions (FBL) can be difficult to diagnose. Toxoplasmic encephalitis (TE) is the major cause of FBL, though this problem will decline with the use of anti-*Toxoplasma* prophylaxis. Other causes of FBL are emerging; their exact frequency is difficult to determine. A prospective study of the disease patterns of FBL-causing conditions is presented, including a decision-making strategy for differential diagnosis of FBL.

Methods.—The 4-year, single-center study included 136 consecutive HIV-infected patients with a confirmed diagnosis of FBL-causing disorder. All patients received empiric anti-*Toxoplasma* therapy. Brain biopsy specimens were obtained in patients who had progressive or stable disease after 3 weeks. Cerebrospinal fluid specimens were obtained from 66 patients for polymerase chain reaction (PCR) amplification of Epstein-Barr virus (EBV)-, JC virus (JCV)-, and *Toxoplasma gondii*-DNA. Diagnoses were made by histopathologic examination of biopsy or autopsy material for all conditions and by resolution of FBL after anti-*Toxoplasma* therapy. Bayes' theorem was used to determine the probabilities of various CNS disorders. These calculations used clinical variables (mass effect at CT or MRI, the results of serologic studies for *Toxoplasma*, and anti-*Toxoplasma* therapy) and the results of the PCR assays.

Results.—Imaging studies were unable to differentiate between TE and primary CNS lymphoma. Patients who were seropositive for *Toxoplasma*, had a mass effect, and were not receiving anti-*Toxoplasma* prophylaxis had an 87% probability of TE. For those receiving anti-*Toxoplasma* prophylaxis, this probability dropped to 59%. Patients who were seronegative for *Toxoplasma* and had a mass effect had a 74% probability of primary CNS lymphoma. The probability that primary CNS lymphoma or TE was present jumped to >96% for patients who tested positive for EBV- or *T. gondii*-DNA. Toxoplasmic encephalitis could not be ruled out by a negative test for *T. gondii*-DNA.

Patients with FBL but no mass effect had an 81% probability of progressive multifocal leukoencephalopathy. If they tested positive for JCV-DNA, this probability jumped to 99%. Brain biopsy was 93% sensitive; associated morbidity was 12%, and mortality 2%.

Conclusions.—Clinical information is insufficient to diagnose HIV-related FBL. Thus PCR testing of CSF is important in the differential diagnosis, particularly seeking EBV- and JCV-DNA. Polymerase chain reaction assays are particularly important for patients who have FBL without a mass effect or who have a mass effect but are seronegative or are receiving anti-*Toxoplasma* prophylaxis. Patients who are EBV-DNA positive or who are seronegative with FBL and a mass effect should undergo brain biopsy. For patients who have FBL without mass effect and are positive for JCV-DNA, brain biopsy may be avoidable. The authors recommend an advanced approach to the diagnosis of FBL. The combination of clinical data and PCR testing can promptly identify those patients who require brain biopsy or treatment for a specific diagnosis.

▶ This Italian study is the first prospectively designed study to address the frequently encountered issue of the diagnosis of FBL in association with HIV infection. The study incorporated the use of CSF PCR for a variety of AIDS-related neurologic diseases (*T. gondii*, EBV, JC virus) in the diagnostic algorithm. The authors conclude that clinical and radiologic data, when combined with the results of CSF PCR, are frequently sufficient to allow the rapid institution of specific therapy. However, patient management in the United States is often dissimilar from that in Europe. The performance of a lumbar puncture in patients with mass lesions of the brain due to toxoplasmosis or primary CNS lymphoma is not likely to be widely accepted in the United States. The performance of CSF PCR in patients with non–mass-producing lesions, such as those related to progressive multifocal leukoencephalopathy, is being widely adopted in lieu of brain biopsy, although the sensitivity of this test is probably somewhere between 60% and 90%.

J.R. Berger, M.D.

Myelopathy Among Brazilians Coinfected With Human T-cell Lympho-tropic Virus Type I and HIV
Harrison LH, Vaz B, Taveira DM, et al (Johns Hopkins Univ, Baltimore, Md; Federal Univ of Rio de Janeiro, Brazil; NIH, Bethesda, Md)
Neurology 48:13–18, 1997   14–8

Introduction.—Both human T-lymphotropic virus type I (HTLV-I) and HIV cause a myelopathy characterized by spastic paraparesis. The HTLV-I–associated myelopathy and vacuolar myelopathy are clinically similar but different histopathologically. A prospective study was designed to determine whether patients coinfected with HTLV-I and HIV have a higher frequency of myelopathy than those singly infected with HIV.

Methods.—The study setting was a university hospital outpatient HIV clinic in Rio de Janeiro. All participants were HIV seropositive by enzyme-linked immunosorbent assay and Western blot and were screened for HTLV infection. Patients who were singly infected served as controls; up to 4 controls were selected for each case of coinfection. Neurologic evaluations were performed by a neurologist unaware of the patients' HTLV serologic status. Patients with at least 2 pyramidal signs were defined as having myelopathy.

Results.—Thirty-one patients with coinfection and 118 controls were eligible for the study; 77 were enrolled. In the enrolled group, 15 patients were HTLV-I seropositive and 62 were seronegative for both HTLV-I and HTLV-II. The coinfected and singlely infected groups were similar in mean age, gender distribution, World Health Organization HIV stage, and mean CD4+ percentage. There was evidence of myelopathy in 11 coinfected patients (73%), but in only 10 patients (16%) with HIV single infection. The association between myelopathy and coinfection remained after adjustment for HIV transmission risk group and when only patients with significant myelopathy (based on the Kurtzke Functional Disability Scale) were counted as having myelopathy. Peripheral neuropathy was also more common in coinfected patients (40%) than in controls (16%).

Discussion.—Patients coinfected with HIV and HTLV-I have a higher frequency of myelopathy than similar patients with HIV single infection. The relative contributions of the 2 diseases in the pathogenesis of coinfection-associated myelopathy is uncertain. An unexpected finding was the lack of an association between the CD4+ lymphocyte count and myelopathy.

▶ Although the increased likelihood of myelopathy occurring in the setting of coinfection with HTLV-I and HIV had been previously reported, in this sizeable series from Brazil, Harrison and colleagues were able to demonstrate that nearly three quarters of all coinfected patients had a myelopathy. This percentage is substantially higher than the frequency of myelopathy that occurs with either virus independently. Unfortunately, the clinical features of HIV-associated vacuolar myelopathy do not permit distinction from those of HTLV-I associated myelopathy/tropical spastic paraparesis, precluding a definitive statement regarding the underlying etiology of this myelopathy. Both viral illnesses may also be associated with a peripheral neuropathy, which was detected in 40% of the patients in this study.

A definitive assessment of the underlying etiology of the myelopathy will require pathologic examination of the spinal cord. However, in light of the frequency with which latent viruses are reactivated and result in clinical illness in the face of HIV infection, it is not unlikely that the myelopathy and peripheral neuropathy seen in the face of coinfection is the direct consequence of HTLV-I infection.

J.R. Berger, M.D.

Clinical and Neuropathological Study of Six Patients With Spastic Paraparesis Associated With HTLV-I: An Axomyelinic Degeneration of the Central Nervous System
Cartier LM, Cea JG, Vergara C, et al (Univ of Chile, Santiago; Regional Hosp of Antofagasto, Chile)
J Neuropathol Exp Neurol 56:403–413, 1997   14–9

Introduction.—Tropical spastic paresis/human T-lymphotropic virus type-I (HTLV-I)–associated myelopathy (TSP/HAM), a dorsal myelopathy, has been reported in patients from Japan, Jamaica, South Africa, and Brazil. The CNS lesions in this condition may have an inflammatory or immunologic pathogenesis, as indicated by the observation of perivascular T-lymphocytic infiltrates, abnormal immunologic findings, and immunocytochemistry studies. The finding of axomyelinic degeneration may require another hypothesis, however. Six cases of TSP/HAM from Chile are reported.

Patients.—The patients were 3 women and 3 men, average age 57 years. They had had paraparesis for a mean of 7 years; pseudobulbar signs were present in 2 patients. Other causes of spastic paresis were excluded. Postmortem examination was performed in each patient.

Findings.—Macroscopic atrophy of the spinal cord was apparent in 3 of the 6 patients. Pyramidal tract lesions were observed in all patients. Four patients had somatotopic lesions of Goll's tracts, which showed a "dying back" ascendant and descendant distribution. Two patients with intellectual decline showed demyelination of the subcortical and parathalamic areas, but no U-fiber involvement. The spinal cord, brain stem, midbrain, and meninges all showed abnormal blood vessels with macroscopic adventitial thickening, often with lymphocytic cuffs. These findings were unrelated to the parenchymal lesions, however. Patients in whom the posterior column was affected showed neuronal changes, with proliferation of satellite cells in the dorsal ganglia. Histologic examination revealed sialoadenitis in all patients, but inflammatory muscle changes in none.

Discussion.—The clinical and neuropathologic findings of TSP/HAM are presented in detail. The extent of the pathologic changes clearly influences the clinical severity. Neuraxial lesions occur in a systemic axial fashion, as they do in degenerative diseases. These pathologic changes seem unrelated to vascular or inflammatory abnormalities. The inflammatory findings in TSP/HAM could result from factors disturbing the ability of axons to maintain their distal architecture, regardless of the observed immunologic changes.

▶ Detailed neuropathologic studies of TSP/HAM are few. In this pathological study from Chile of 6 patients with TSP/HAM, the authors suggest that the CNS findings were most compatible with a neurodegenerative condition rather than an infectious or inflammatory disorder, on the basis of histologic findings consistent with dying back observed chiefly in the pyramidal tracts and fasciculus gracilis. Their suggestion challenges the widely accepted hypothesis regarding the etiopathogenesis of this disorder relating it to an inflammatory/immunologic disorder and raises the possibility of parallels to HIV-associated myelopathy that has been proposed by some investigators to be the consequence of a nutritional-metabolic disturbance affecting cobalamin (vitamin B_{12}) metabolism. Parenthetically, another interesting observation from this study was the appearance of demyelination in subcortical and parathalamic areas in 2 of their patients who exhibited cognitive abnormalities. Discrete abnormalities of cerebral white matter on MR images have been well described in TSP/HAM but generally are thought to be of little clinical consequence. This study implies that they may be clinically important.

J.R. Berger, M.D.

Herpes Simplex Encephalitis (HSE) and the Immunocompromised: A Clinical and Autopsy Study of HSE in the Settings of Cancer and Human Immunodeficiency Virus-Type 1 Infection
Schiff D, Rosenblum MK (Mem Sloan-Kettering Cancer Ctr, New York)
Hum Pathol 29:215–222, 1998   14–10

Introduction.—Herpes simplex encephalitis (HSE) can occur in immunocompromised patients. Although HSE is not considered an opportunistic infection, previous reports suggest that immunodeficient patients with HSE have distinct clinical and neuropathologic features. The clinical and pathologic findings of 3 immunocompromised patients with HSE are reported.

Patients.—The patients were 3 women, aged 24–35. Two had cancer: 1 had lymphoma with suspected underlying HIV-1 infection, and the other had glioblastoma multiforme. The third patient was HIV-1 seropositive. Two patients were taking dexamethasone when their HSE began. Clinical findings included fever, altered mental status, and new or worsened focal neurologic deficits. Cerebrospinal fluid samples showed absent or minimal pleocytosis. Computed tomography provided no useful information. None of the patients were suspected on clinical grounds of having HSE. Only 1 patient received acyclovir, which was given for mucocutaneous herpes.

Herpes simplex encephalitis was a major contributor to death in all patients. At autopsy, the patients were found to have an unusual noninflammatory, pseudoischemic histologic presentation. The viral antigens persisted in higher numbers, even though the patients survived beyond the clinical stage at which inflammatory responses peak and brain infection wanes.

Conclusions.—Herpes simplex encephalitis in immunocompromised patients may be more frequent than is generally thought. The diagnosis may be difficult to make because of preexisting neurologic disease, noninflammatory CSF findings, and negative CT results, even though the clinical presentation is typical. The diagnosis may be based on a high index of clinical suspicion, MRI scanning, and polymerase chain reaction analysis of CSF for evidence of herpes simplex virus. Patients may have the catastrophic neurologic injury characteristic of HSE, despite the lack of an intact immune response.

▶ HSE in the immunocompromised patient may present in an insidious fashion, failing to display the typical manifestations that suggest the correct diagnosis. These cases, as well as others previously reported, illustrate the important contribution of the immune system to the stereotypic appearance of HSE. Acute, hemorrhagic, necrotizing lesions of the orbital frontal and medial temporal lobes may not be observed with HSE in the face of disorders affecting cell-mediated immunity. In immunocompromised patients with altered mental status, focal neurologic findings, and fever, HSE must be considered. Diagnostic measures should include CSF polymerase chain reaction for HSV, and consideration should be given to prompt treatment with acyclovir.

J.R. Berger, M.D.

Detection of 14-3-3 Protein in the Cerebrospinal Fluid Supports the Diagnosis of Creutzfeldt-Jakob Disease
Zerr I, Bodemer M, Gefeller O, et al (Georg-August-Universität, Göttingen, Germany; Neurologische Klinik, Marienkrankenhaus, Hamburg, Germany)
Ann Neurol 43:32–40, 1998   14–11

Introduction.—The 14-3-3 protein has been described as a useful CSF marker for the in vivo diagnosis of Creutzfeldt-Jakob disease (CJD). False negative and false positive results of 14-3-3 analysis have been reported. No data have been presented regarding the stability of 14-3-3 protein in CSF; instability could cause false readings. The predictive values for detecting 14-3-3 protein in CSF for the clinical diagnosis of CJD was assessed.

Methods.—Four hundred eighty-four patients from the German national CJD surveillance trial with clinically suspected CJD underwent clinical examinations and were evaluated for presence of 14-3-3 protein using a modified western blot technique.

Results.—The 14-3-3 protein was detected in 95.4% and 92.8% of definitive and probable CJD, respectively. Two patients who were classified clinically as not having CJD had positive 14-3-3 and were later proved to have definite CJD. The positive and negative predictive values were 94.7% and 92.4%, respectively. False positive results in a single CSF analysis were observed in patients with herpes simplex encephalitis, hypoxic brain damage, atypical encephalitis, intracerebral metastases of a bronchial carcinoma, metabolic encephalopathy, and progressive dementia of unknown cause. Western blot analysis for 14-3-3 protein was positive in 5 of 10 patients with familial forms of spongiform encephalopathies.

Conclusion.—Only patients who have met the clinical criteria for "possible CJD" and who are positive for 14-3-3 protein should be considered as having laboratory-supported CJD. Until there are ways to identify reliably the pathologic agent of transmissible spongiform encephalopathies in clinical samples, the presence of 14-3-3 protein in CSF should be considered a characteristic and highly suggestive but nonspecific marker for CJD that must be interpreted within the context of clinical differential diagnosis.

▶ This study from Germany confirms the findings of Hsich and colleagues[1] regarding CSF 14-3-3 published in 1996. A positive CSF 14-3-3 in the appropriate clinical setting is virtually diagnostic of CJD and precludes the need for brain biopsy. Unfortunately, it does not appear to have the same sensitivity in familial CJD.

J.R. Berger, M.D.

Reference

1. Hsich G, Kenney K, Gibbs CJ, et al: The 14-3-3 brain protein in cerebrospinal fluid as a marker for transmissible spongiform encephalopathies. *N Engl J Med* 335:924–930, 1996.

Neurologic Manifestations in *Staphylococcus aureus* Endocarditis: A Review of 260 Bacteremic Cases in Nondrug Addicts
Røder BL, Wandall DA, Espersen F, et al (Rigshospitalet, Copenhagen)
Am J Med 102:379–386, 1997   14–12

Background.—Infective endocarditis can cause CNS complications ranging from altered level of consciousness to sudden death from intracranial hemorrhage or ischemic stroke. The incidence and severity of neurologic complications of *Staphylococcus aureus* infective endocarditis may be changing. A 10-year experience with neurologic complications of *S. aureus* infective endocarditis was reviewed.

Methods.—The investigators analyzed the medical records of all 8,514 patients with *S. aureus* bacteremia reported to a Danish central laboratory from 1982 to 1991. Records for patients suspected of having infective endocarditis were reviewed and classified according to Durack's new proposed diagnostic criteria for endocarditis. Drug addicts were excluded. The neurologic manifestations of *S. aureus* bacteremia in 260 cases from 63 hospitals were reviewed, with focus on the clinical presentation, epidemiologic findings, and mortality.

Results.—Neurologic manifestations of *S. aureus* infective endocarditis occurred in 91 patients (35%). Neurologic complications were an initial sign in 61 patients and developed a median of 10 days later in the rest. Forty-five percent of patients had unilateral hemiparesis, the most common neurologic complication. Neurologic manifestations were seen in 42% of female patients vs. 30% of male patients. They occurred in 44% of patients with infection of a native mitral valve, compared with 29% of patients with other valvular involvement. The difference was significant only in comparison with patients having native aortic valve infection (31%). Neurologic manifestations were present in just 2 patients with tricuspid valve infections and no patients with congenital heart disorders.

Thirty-five percent of cases with vegetations detected on echocardiograms were associated with neurologic manifestations, compared with 26% of cases without vegetations. Seventy-four percent of patients with major neurologic manifestations died, compared with 56% of those without neurologic complications. Among patients with neurologic complications, 80% of those treated with antibiotics only died, compared with 20% of those treated surgically.

Conclusions.—Among non–drug users with *S. aureus* infective endocarditis, the risk for neurologic complications is higher in association with native mitral valve infection. Echocardiographic evidence of vegetations does not appear to be a risk factor for neurologic manifestations, though only half of the patients in this study underwent transthoracic echocardiography. Most neurologic manifestations are noted at presentation or shortly thereafter. They carry a low risk for recurrent embolism but an increased risk for death. Surgery may offer better outcomes for patients with neurologic complications of *S. aureus* infective endocarditis.

▶ In this Danish study of *S. aureus* endocarditis in a non–drug abusing population, one third of all patients developed neurologic disease. Among the latter, two thirds presented with neurologic manifestations. The neurologic sequelae were classified into 3 groups: thromboembolic events (57%), meningitis (22%), and "toxic confusion" (24%). At autopsy, nearly 50% of patients with neurologic sequelae of *S. aureus* endocarditis had infarcts, 14% had hemorrhages, and 14% had brain abscesses. These observations underscore the importance of considering endocarditis in the differential diagnosis of any patient with a heart murmur presenting with a stroke or meningitis. Blood culture is an essential component of the diagnostic evaluation, because echocardiograms in 44% of those patients with neurologic sequelae failed to demonstrate vegetations.

J.R. Berger, M.D.

Whipple's Disease: Staging and Monitoring by Cytology and Polymerase Chain Reaction Analysis of Cerebrospinal Fluid

von Herbay A, Ditton H-J, Schuhmacher F, et al (Univ of Heidelberg, Germany)
Gastroenterology 113:434–441, 1997   14–13

Introduction.—The intestinal tract is most commonly affected in patients with Whipple's disease, but the CNS can also be involved and carries a much less favorable prognosis. Samples of CSF from 24 patients with Whipple's disease were examined to determine the value of polymerase chain reaction (PCR) analysis and its application in staging and monitoring of the disease.

Methods.—The study group consisted of 21 men and 3 women with a mean age of 50.9 years at diagnosis. Diagnosis was established by intestinal histology in 23 patients and by brain biopsy in 1. Five of the patients

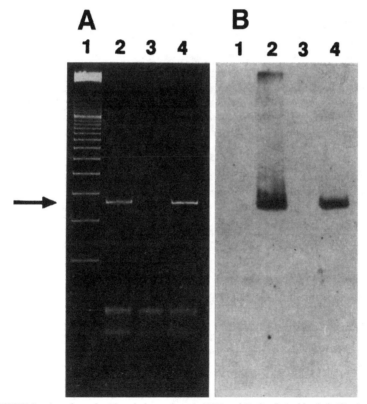

FIGURE 2.—**A,** polyacrylamide gel electrophoresis (8%) and **B,** Southern blot hybridization after polymerase chain reaction testing. *Lane 1,* 100–base pair DNA marker; *lane 2,* positive control prepared from the intestinal biopsy specimen of patient 12 with Whipple's disease (diluted 10^{-4}); *lane 3,* negative control; and *lane 4,* CSF from patient 4 with symptomatic cerebral Whipple's disease. (Courtesy of von Herbay A, Ditton H-J, Schuhmacher F, et al: Whipple's disease: Staging and monitoring by cytology and polymerase chain reaction analysis of cerebrospinal fluid. *Gastroenterology* 113:434–441, 1997.)

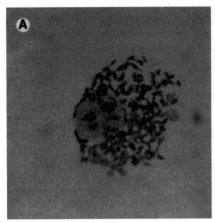 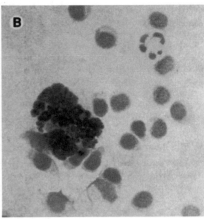

FIGURE 1.—**A,** typical sickleform particle–containing (SPC) cell from CSF observed at diagnostic staging of patient 12 with intestinal Whipple's disease but no neurologic symptoms. **B,** cell with large periodic acid-Schiff (PAS)–positive material in the cytoplasm that does not resemble that of typical SPC cells. This indeterminate finding was observed during monitoring of patient 4 while undergoing therapy; both cells, PAS stain; original magnification: A, ×196 and B, ×158. (Courtesy of von Herbay A, Ditton H-J, Schuhmacher F, et al: Whipple's disease: Staging and monitoring by cytology and polymerase chain reaction analysis of cerebrospinal fluid. *Gastroenterology* 113:434–441, 1997.)

had neurologic symptoms characteristic of Whipple's disease. Two had cerebral disease at diagnosis, 1 with and 1 without intestinal disease. Neurologic symptoms developed during the course of the disease in the remaining 3 patients. Thirty-two of the 39 CSF samples were examined by PCR for *Tropheryma whippelii* and 20 samples were examined by cytology. The 2 brain biopsy specimens were analyzed histologically. Also tested by PCR were 25 control CSF samples. The specificity of all PCR products was confirmed by hybridization (Fig 2).

Results.—Cytology showed periodic acid-Schiff–positive sickleform particle–containing (SPC) cells in the CSF of all 3 tested patients with neurologic symptoms and in 4 of 5 patients without neurologic symptoms (Fig 1). All 25 control CSF samples were negative for *T. whippelii* when tested by PCR. Fourteen of the 32 CSF samples from patients with Whipple's disease were positive and 18 were negative for *T. whippelii*. Follow-up examinations were performed on 2 patients with and 4 without neurologic symptoms. After 12 to 26 months of continuous antibiotic treatment, 3 patients showed conversion of PCR from positive to negative; positive results persisted in 1 patient with neurologic symptoms and in 1 who was neurologically asymptomatic. Both brain biopsy specimens showed SPC cells.

Discussion.—Even in patients without neurologic symptoms of Whipple's disease, CSF testing yields a high rate of positive results. And although PCR analysis of CSF can be added to diagnostic criteria for Whipple's disease of the CSF, cerebral disease can be present without diagnostic findings in the CSF.

▶ Whipple's disease is the consequence of an actinomycete, *Tropheryma whippelii*, that cannot be cultured by any of the methods currently used. In 1959, Sieracki first recognized that the CNS could be involved by Whipple's disease when he demonstrated the presence of PAS stain–positive organisms, both intracellularly and extracellularly, in the cerebral tissues of a patient. Cerebral Whipple's disease may result in a wide variety of neurologic manifestations. The classic clinical triad of the disease includes dementia, myoclonus, and an external ophthalmoplegia with pupillary sparing.

Until recently, the diagnosis of cerebral Whipple's was dependent on brain biopsy. However, in this article, von Herbay and colleagues show that PCR for *T. whippelii* performed on CSF may prove quite effective in detecting the organism. Furthermore, they demonstrate a high frequency with which the CSF PCR is positive for *T. whippelii* in the absence of clinically apparent neurologic disease. This raises important therapeutic questions regarding the optimal therapy for Whipple's disease that will undoubtedly require additional study.

J.R. Berger, M.D.

15 Multiple Sclerosis

Genetic Epidemiology of Multiple Sclerosis
Compston A (Univ of Cambridge, England)
J Neurol Neurosurg Psychiatry 62:553–561, 1997   15–1

Background.—There have been many studies of the epidemiology of multiple sclerosis in an attempt to discover the causes, to assess the need for services on a local basis, and to define the natural history of the disease. This article reviews data on the epidemiology of multiple sclerosis, including the evidence for environmental and genetic causes.

Epidemiology of Multiple Sclerosis.—Large-scale studies of the epidemiology of multiple sclerosis have suggested bands of high, low, and medium prevalence. High-prevalence areas include the northern parts of Europe and North America and southern Australia; southern Europe, the southern United States, and northern Australia are medium-risk areas, whereas Asia and South America are low-risk areas. Studies of migrating populations have suggested that multiple sclerosis is an acquired, exogenous disorder. Environmental factors may even override genetic susceptibility; however, the age of exposure appears to be critical. Some authors have suggested that point source epidemics of multiple sclerosis exist. However, others maintain that these result from the arrival of specialist medical services in island communities, rather than a true change in incidence. Most studies have found that women are affected twice as often as men. Several factors have been studied for their effect on the clinical course, such as age at onset, early attack rate, trauma, anesthesia, and pregnancy.

The familial recurrence rate of multiple sclerosis is about 15%. This could result from coinheritance of susceptibility factors, or from common childhood exposure to environmental factors. Risk varies by genetic relationship, from 1 in 200 for children of affected parents, to 1 in 17 for children of conjugal pairs, to 1 in 3 for monozygotic twins (Fig 5). Various studies have attempted to identify markers of genetic susceptibility to multiple sclerosis; meta-analysis of these studies may strengthen the cause of some of the provisional areas of linkage identified so far.

Discussion.—Extensive research into the epidemiology of multiple sclerosis has been performed. The evolving epidemiologic pattern has led to the creation of elaborate explanatory hypotheses. Besides infective causes, climatic, dietary, geomagnetic, and toxic causes have been proposed. From

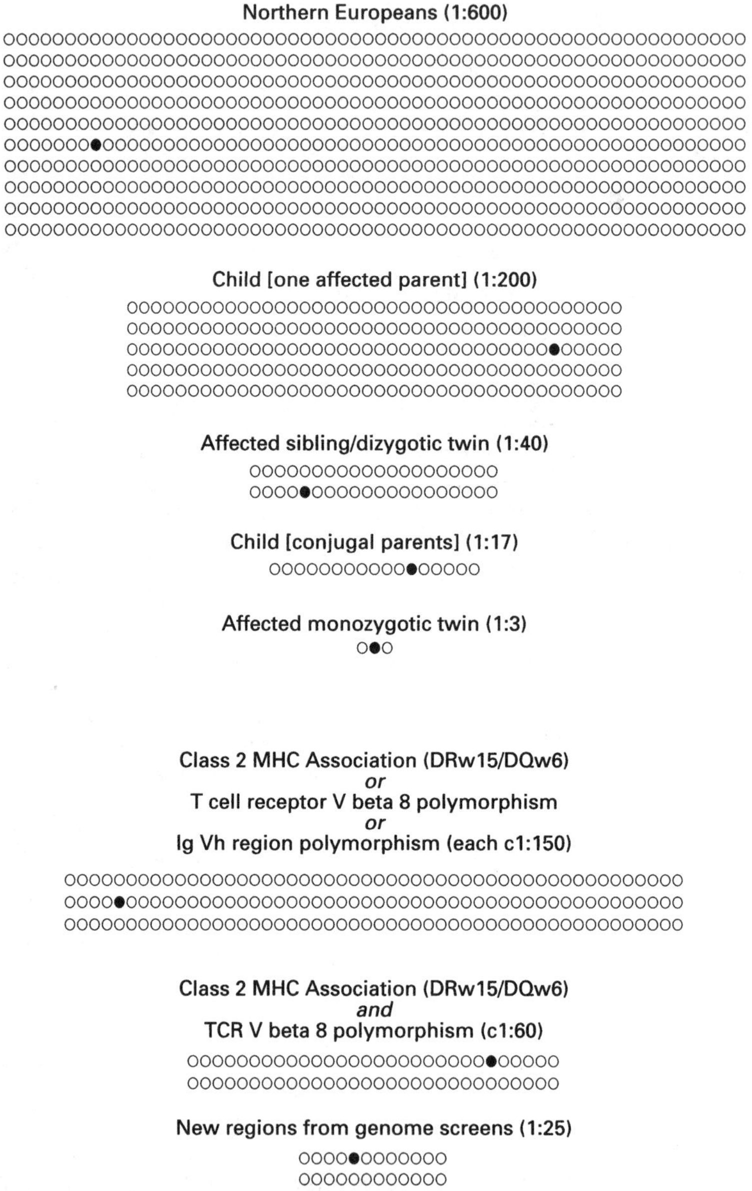

Northern Europeans (1:600)

ooooooooooooooooooooooooooooooooooooooooooooooooooooooooooooo
ooooooooooooooooooooooooooooooooooooooooooooooooooooooooooooo
ooooooooooooooooooooooooooooooooooooooooooooooooooooooooooooo
ooooooooooooooooooooooooooooooooooooooooooooooooooooooooooooo
ooooooooooooooooooooooooooooooooooooooooooooooooooooooooooooo
ooooooo●oooooooooooooooooooooooooooooooooooooooooooooooooooooo
ooooooooooooooooooooooooooooooooooooooooooooooooooooooooooooo
ooooooooooooooooooooooooooooooooooooooooooooooooooooooooooooo
ooooooooooooooooooooooooooooooooooooooooooooooooooooooooooooo
ooooooooooooooooooooooooooooooooooooooooooooooooooooooooooooo

Child [one affected parent] (1:200)

ooooooooooooooooooooooooooooooooooooooooooooo
ooooooooooooooooooooooooooooooooooooooooooooo
ooooooooooooooooooooooooooooooooooooo●ooooo
ooooooooooooooooooooooooooooooooooooooooooooo
ooooooooooooooooooooooooooooooooooooooooooooo

Affected sibling/dizygotic twin (1:40)

oooooooooooooooooooooo
ooooo●oooooooooooooooo

Child [conjugal parents] (1:17)

oooooooooooo●ooooo

Affected monozygotic twin (1:3)

o●o

Class 2 MHC Association (DRw15/DQw6)
or
T cell receptor V beta 8 polymorphism
or
Ig Vh region polymorphism (each c1:150)

oooooooooooooooooooooooooooooooooooooooooooooooooooooo
ooooo●ooooooooooooooooooooooooooooooooooooooooooooooooo
oooooooooooooooooooooooooooooooooooooooooooooooooooooo

Class 2 MHC Association (DRw15/DQw6)
and
TCR V beta 8 polymorphism (c1:60)

oooooooooooooooooooooooooooo●ooooo
ooooooooooooooooooooooooooooooooooo

New regions from genome screens (1:25)

ooooo●ooooooo
oooooooooooo

FIGURE 5.—Scheme to show the reduction in crude risk for multiple sclerosis depending on relation to the proband and the presence of defined susceptibility factors. Comparable age-adjusted figures are: children of single affected parents 1 in 50; siblings 1 in 30; children of conjugal pairs 1 in 5; and monozygotic twins 1 in 2. (Courtesy of Compston A: Genetic epidemiology of multiple sclerosis. *J Neurol Neurosurg Psychiatry* 62:553–561, 1997.)

a genetic standpoint, the disease seems to follow the spread of northern European genes. Markers of genetic susceptibility show a geographic pattern similar to that of the disease itself. In the meantime, there remains a considerable body of circumstantial evidence to suggest environmental factors as the predominant cause of multiple sclerosis.

▶ Compston reviews the evidence that environmental agents and genetic factors influence both the development of multiple sclerosis (MS) and the course of the disease. Compston surveys the environmental literature (global distribution, migration data, outbreaks) and reminds the reader of the absence of evidence for a specific environmental agent despite exhaustive efforts in this area. He argues that recently completed studies of familial MS (multiplex families, identical twins, adoptive families, conjugal pairs) strongly suggest an important genetic influence on disease susceptibility. The failure of 3 recent international surveys of multiplex families to identify a common group of potential susceptibility genes does not deter Professor Compston from suggesting that genetic influences are more likely to predominate in this long-debated controversy over the relative strength of environmental agents and genetic factors.

J.H. Noseworthy, M.D., F.R.C.P.C.

Primary Progressive Multiple Sclerosis
Thompson AJ, Polman CH, Miller DH, et al (Inst of Neurology, London; Vrije Universiteit Hosp, Amsterdam; Centre Hospitalier Universitaire, Bordeaux, France, et al)
Brain 120:1085–1096, 1997   15–2

Purpose.—The classical clinical pattern of multiple sclerosis is a relapsing remitting course, eventually leading to progressive disability. However, some patients have a progressive course from the start—with no relapses or remissions—often with predominant involvement of the spinal cord. In these cases, the disease can be difficult to diagnose, monitor, and treat; there is a particular need for approaches to rule out other conditions. Available information on primary progressive multiple sclerosis was reviewed, including its diagnosis.

Diagnosis.—The definite diagnosis of multiple sclerosis requires demonstration of a multiplicity of lesions in time and space. In patients with primary progressive multiple sclerosis, this may be done by evoked potentials or MRI. Clinical examination or investigation may be done to demonstrate the development of new lesions over time. A 2-year duration of symptoms is recommended to demonstrate dissemination and exclude relapses. The differential diagnosis should include chronic progressive myelopathy, as progressive paresis is the most common presenting symptom of primary progressive multiple sclerosis. Some patients will not show lesion dissemination in space, even with long-term follow-up. Reported estimates of the frequency of multiple sclerosis that is progressive from onset range from 11% to 37%. In 1 study, when only patients seen from their initial presentation were included, the frequency decreased to 8%.

Characteristics.—Patients with primary progressive multiple sclerosis have a later age at presentation than those with relapsing remitting disease—37 vs. 29 years—in 1 study. The primary progressive type may affect a greater proportion of men than the relapsing remitting form. There is some evidence that patients with primary progressive multiple sclerosis have a smaller cerebral lesion load on MRI. Although multiple sclerosis has been linked to the haplotype A3-B7-DR2(15)-DQw6, this association is mainly with the relapsing remitting type. No consistent genetic relationships with primary progressive multiple sclerosis have been identified. One pathologic study suggested less marked inflammation in patients with primary progressive multiple sclerosis than in those with the secondary progressive type. Outcome studies have suggested that development of disability is the only significant predictive factor in patients with primary progressive disease.

Studies with MRI have confirmed that cranial abnormalities are relatively sparse in primary progressive multiple sclerosis, with few new lesions appearing over time. The evidence supports the hypothesis that the primary progressive type may be a less inflammatory form of multiple sclerosis. The mechanism remains unknown. However, newer MRI techniques focusing on intrinsic change in normal-appearing white matter and assessment of atrophy, suggest an important role of axonal loss. Primary progressive and relapsing remitting multiple sclerosis are often found in the same family, suggesting a spectrum of disease rather than distinct disease entities. In the absence of data on the mechanisms of progressive disability, it is difficult to choose treatment approaches.

Discussion.—More information on the less-frequent, primary progressive form of multiple sclerosis is needed. A multicenter European study group has been formed, with the goal of studying 200 patients for 2 years, including clinical, cognitive, and MRI data. This will provide a valuable database for use in treatment trials.

▶ In a recent article, Lublin and Reingold[1] used the results of an international survey to suggest guidelines for classifying the course of multiple sclerosis (MS) for clinical research and therapeutic trials. There has been a need, however, for a comprehensive review of so-called "primary progressive MS." Is this a form of MS or an unrelated illness? This clinical entity (most often a slowly progressive myelopathy developing after age 40) is generally excluded from randomized controlled trials because of a degree of uncertainty about the nosology of this condition and alleged apparent therapeutic unresponsiveness to immunosuppressive and anti-inflammatory therapies. Thompson and colleagues use clinical, genetic, immune, neurophysiologic, pathologic, and MRI evidence to argue that primary progressive MS is a distinct form of MS and not a separate disease entity.

J.H. Noseworthy, M.D., F.R.C.P.C.

Reference

1. Lublin FD, Reingold SC: Defining the clinical course of multiple sclerosis: Results of an international survey. *Neurology* 46:907–911, 1996.

Western Versus Asian Types of Multiple Sclerosis: Immunogenetically and Clinically Distinct Disorders
Kira J-i, Kanai T, Nishimura Y, et al (Kyushu Univ, Fukuoka, Japan; Kumamoto Univ, Japan)
Ann Neurol 40:569–574, 1996   15–3

Background.—Studies of Japanese patients with multiple sclerosis (MS) have found no statistically significant association of any HLA class II antigens or alleles with the disease. Asian patients with MS may present with disseminated signs, similar to those in occidental patients, or with a distinctive predilection for severe optic-spinal involvement. Combined HLA-DRB1, HLA-DRB3, and HLA-DRB5 gene typing and MRI were performed to document the distinct subtypes of MS among Japanese patients.

Methods.—Fifty-seven Japanese patients were included. Clinically, 23 patients had selective involvement of the optic nerve and spinal cord. This group was classified as having Asian-type MS. The remaining 34 had disseminated CNS involvement, classified as Western-type MS.

Findings.—Asian-type MS was associated with fewer brain lesions on MRI but more gadolinium-enhanced spinal cord lesions than Western-type MS. The DR2-associated DRB1*1501 allele and DRB5*0101 allele were associated with Western-type MS, occurring in 41.2% of this group, but not with Asian-type MS, present in 0. These alleles were found in 14.2% of a healthy control group (not statistically significant).

Conclusions.—Despite the low prevalence of MS in Japanese populations, there is a significant association between the HLA-DRB1*1501 and DRB5*0101 alleles and Western-type but not Asian-type disease. Thus immunogenetic background appears to play a critical role in the development and manifestations of MS. Multiple sclerosis in Asians may represent 2 distinct diseases with different clinical and MRI features. Alternatively, an HLA-linked gene may affect the clinical and MRI features in a single disease.

▶ It has long been recognized that the optospinal variant of MS is more commonly seen in Asians than in Northern Europeans and North Americans. This study presents the first attempt to delineate the immunogenetics and MRI characteristics of this variant of MS, as well as the more typical clinical pattern of Western-type MS in a cohort of 57 Japanese patients. Patients with single episodes of neuromyelitis optica and acute disseminated encephalomyelitis were excluded. This study suggests that Asian-type MS may differ from Western-type MS (e.g., not associated with the DR 2-associated

DRB1*1501 or DRB5*0101 allele). Asian-type MS may differ as well in clinical (later age of onset, more frequently a relapsing-remitting course, higher CSF cell count, and total protein concentration) and MRI behavior (e.g., spinal predominance).

J.H. Noseworthy, M.D., F.R.C.P.C.

Indictment of the Microglia as the Villain in Multiple Sclerosis
Sriram S, Rodriguez M (Vanderbilt Med Ctr, Nashville, Tenn; Mayo Med School, Rochester, Minn)
Neurology 48:464–470, 1997   15–4

Introduction.—A current theory holds that multiple sclerosis (MS) is an autoimmune disease that may be triggered by an infectious agent, such as a virus, in susceptible individuals. Investigations of this hypothesis focus on the role of autoreactive CD4+ T cells in CNS demyelination. The model of CNS demyelination proposed by these authors suggests that microglial activation is a central element and that the target is the oligo-dendrocyte-myelin unit.

Background.—The role of autoreactive T cells in autoimmune disease has been difficult to demonstrate, in part because T cell reactivity to autoantigens is present in the normal healthy population. The assumption that MS is a T cell–mediated autoimmune disease is based upon 3 obser-vations: similarities between MS and experimental allergic encephalitis (EAE); a predominant T cell inflammatory response at the end organ; and an association with genes of the major histocompatibility complex (MHC). Dissimilarities between EAE and MS, however, suggest that al-ternative immunopathogenic mechanisms may be involved in MS.

Comparison of Multiple Sclerosis and Experimental Allergic Encepha-litis.—Various lines of evidence indicate important differences between MS and EAE. Some patients with MS have had leakage of the retinal vein and perivenous mononuclear inflammation. Yet, because the retina does not have myelin, the vascular damage, in such cases, could not be caused by T cells recognizing myelin antigens. Deletion of CD4+ cells is able to prevent and treat virtually every known animal model of autoimmune disease. The effects of T cell suppression and depletion on EAE have not been dupli-cated in MS. Differences are also suggested by the role of MHC class II antigens in the 2 disorders.

Proposed Model of CNS Demyelination.—The autoreactive CD4+ T–cell model of MS is questionable, for a virus specific for MS has never been isolated and conventional immunosuppressive agents are ineffective against the disease. In contrast, the model (Figure) based upon microglial activation is likely to explain the varied clinical presentation and disease course of MS. Immunotherapy would attempt to reduce the activity of macrophages rather than targeting T cells.

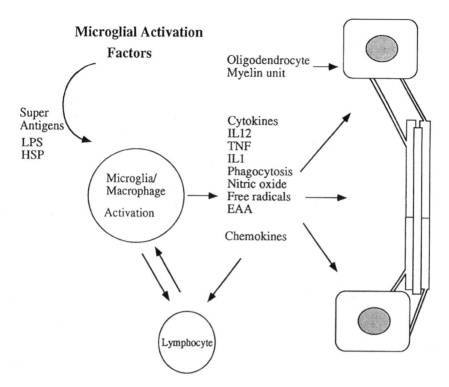

Lymphocyte recruitment

FIGURE.—Schematic model of CNS demyelination initiated by microglial activating factors. Activated microglia secrete cytokines, organic molecules, excitatory amino acids, and chemokines that sustain inflammation and demyelination. *Abbreviations*: *HSP*, heat shock protein; *EAA*, excitatory amino acid; *LPS*, lipopolysaccharide; *TNF*, tumor necrosis factor. (Reprinted from *Neurology*, from Sriram S, Rodriguez M: Indictment of the microglia as the villain in multiple sclerosis. *Neurology* 48:464–470, 1997, copyright American Academy of Neurology. Used with permission of Lippincott-Raven Publishers.)

▶ Although the mechanism of injury in MS is unknown, the most commonly held hypothesis focuses on the role of autoreactive CD4+ T cells to CNS myelin antigens. In this article, Sriram and Rodriguez develop an alternative hypothesis, namely that CNS microglia activation is the essential element underlying the pathogenesis of MS and that the oligodendrocyte-myelin unit is the target of myelinotoxic factors released by microglia cells (oxidative free radicals, excitatory amino acids, proinflammatory cytokines, etc.).

The authors marshal a series of compelling reasons why EAE in general and the T cell–mediated autoimmune hypothesis specifically may not be tenable. They suggest that future trials focus on downregulating microglia activation in the CNS. This provocative article will be of considerable interest to all involved in MS research and treatment.

J.H. Noseworthy, M.D., F.R.C.P.C.

Cell Death and Birth in Multiple Sclerosis Brain

Dowling P, Husar W, Menonna J, et al (New Jersey Health Care System, East Orange; UMDNJ, Newark, NJ; Saint Vincent's Hosp, New York)
J Neurol Sci 149:1–11, 1997   15–5

Purpose.—White matter plaques, the key pathologic lesions of multiple sclerosis (MS), are characterized by myelin destruction and oligodendrocyte loss. The recently developed in situ terminal deoxynucleotidyl transferase-mediated dUTP-biotin nick end labeling (TUNEL) technique, which can detect nuclear DNA fragmentation associated with cell death within tissue sections, offers the first opportunity to identify cells undergoing programmed cell death in the MS brain. This technique was used to investigate the role of apoptosis in the development of MS lesions.

Findings.—In contrast to normal brain sections, most specimens of MS brain showed significantly increased numbers of labeled cells (Fig 2). In acute MS lesions, the TUNEL technique identified patchy areas with massive numbers of inflammatory and glial cells undergoing apoptosis. Chronic MS lesions also showed punched-out areas with labeled glial cells, demonstrating that the MS attack was not a single event. Fourteen percent to 40% of dying cells were myelin-sustaining oligodendroglial cells, according to immunocytochemical studies using glial specific marker co-

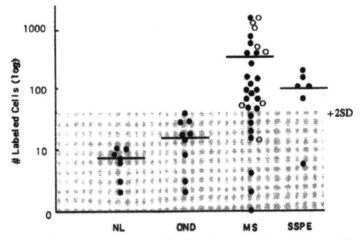

FIGURE 2.—Log value of TUNEL positive cells in the 4 frozen cerebral cortex test groups. The control range shown is derived from the other neurologic disease group (OND) mean value (18 cells + 2SD = 44 cells). The MS group (*closed circles*) is significantly different from all other groups by the Kruskal-Wallis 1-way analysis of variance $p = 0.001$, and also significantly different from the OND group ($p - 0.004$ (Mann-Whitney U test). The MS column also contains additional values from a subset of 8 untreated MS patients (*open circles*); mean value is 477. The untreated MS subset is also significantly different from the OND control group ($p = 0.004$). Mean values for the other groups: NL, 6.7; OND, 18; MS, 199; subacute sclerosing panencephalitis (SSPE), 92 cells. To be certain that the section area of experimental groups was comparable, the area of each cryosection was measured by image analysis, and the mean values in square millimeters for each group (NL, 23.9; OND, 22.3; MS, 20.2; SSPE, 21.5) are not significantly different. (Courtesy of Dowling P, Husar W, Menonna J, et al: Cell death and birth in multiple sclerosis brain. *J Neurol Sci* 149:1–11, 1997.)

labeling. When examined by confocal microscopy with fluorescein labeling, the nuclei of TUNEL-positive cells showed the morphologic characteristics of apoptosis. On electrophoresis of MS brain DNA, a laddering pattern characteristic of apoptotic DNA cleavage was observed. This confirmed that many, but not necessarily all, of the labeled cells were dying as a result of apoptosis rather than necrosis. Further studies using a marker for cell proliferation in MS lesions showed large numbers of perivascular inflammatory cells and parenchymal glial cells in the cell proliferation cycle.

Conclusions.—The results offer insight into the role of apoptosis in the development of MS lesions. The pathology of MS is marked by the opposing glial cell responses of ongoing cell death and brisk cellular proliferation. However, glial cell loss ultimately prevails. Apoptosis may be the critical mechanism of myelin depletion in MS.

▶ The important issue of oligodendrocyte cell death and regeneration in the MS lesion has been addressed by Osawa et al.[1] and Bruck et al.[2] In this elegant and thorough article (23 patients with treated MS, and 8 with untreated MS, 6 patients with subacute sclerosing panencephalitis, 16 with other neurologic diseases, and controls, as well as additional experiments with allergic encephalomyelitis), Dowling and colleagues provide additional support for the concept that apoptosis may be an important mechanism in oligodendrocyte cell death in both the acute and chronic MS lesion. In addition, Dowling and colleagues have shown rather extensive evidence for glial cell proliferation, suggesting an important balance between cell death and "cell birth" in the dynamic MS plaque. Although others[3] have suggested that oligodendrocytes do not undergo apoptosis, Dowling's extensive studies in patients with MS and suitable controls appears convincing. As such, the concepts presented by Dowling enhance our understanding of disease pathogenesis and may assist in planning treatment strategies.

J.H. Noseworthy, M.D., F.R.C.P.C.

References

1. Osawa K, Suchanek G, Bristschopf H, et al: Patterns of oligodendroglial pathology in multiple sclerosis. *Brain* 117:1311–1322, 1994.
2. Bruck W, Schmeid M, Suchanek G, et al: Oligodendrocytes in the early course of multiple sclerosis. *Ann Neurol* 35:65–73, 1994.
3. Bonetti B, Raine CS: Multiple sclerosis: Oligodendrocytes display cell death-related molecules in situ but do not undergo apoptosis. *Ann Neurol* 42:74–84, 1997.

Axonal Damage in Acute Multiple Sclerosis Lesions

Ferguson B, Matyszak MK, Esiri MM, et al (Oxford Univ, England; Radcliffe Infirmary, Oxford, England)
Brain 120:393–399, 1997   15–6

Background.—One histologic characteristic of early multiple sclerosis (MS) lesions is primary demyelination, marked by myelin destruction and relative sparing of axons. However, axonal loss is known to occur in, and appears to be responsible for, the permanent disability that characterizes the subsequent, chronic progressive stage of MS. At which disease stage of the disease axonal damage (in addition to demyelination) occurs was investigated.

Methods.—Brain tissue was obtained after death from 18 subjects who had had MS and from 5 who had not. Tissue blocks were fixed in 10% formalin and embedded in paraffin wax. An antibody against amyloid precursor protein (APP)—known to be a sensitive marker of axonal damage in several other contexts—was used in the immunocytochemical experiments.

Findings.—Acute lesions had the highest number of APP-positive (APP+) axons and macrophages. The correlation between the number of macrophages and the extent of axonal damage was good. The mean density of APP+ elements in acute lesions was comparable to that at the border of active chronic lesions. In active chronic lesions, APP staining was seen primarily at the border and correlated well with the number of macrophages in these areas. However, significantly less staining was noted in the center of these lesions.

Conclusion.—The expression of APP in damaged axons was documented in acute MS lesions and in the active borders of less acute lesions. These data may have implications for the design and timing of treatment—1 goal of which is to reduce permanent disability.

▶ It is being increasingly recognized that progressive axonal damage underlies disability progression in MS and limits the success of current therapeutic strategies. Advanced MRI and MR spectroscopy techniques are now beginning to address this important aspect of this disease. Using an antibody to APP, Ferguson et al. have correlated the degree of axonal loss in acute, active chronic (center and border zone regions), and chronic MS lesions with the number of lesional macrophages in formalin-fixed paraffin embedded sections of postmortem brain tissue.

Evidence from this work suggests that axonal damage occurs at sites of acute, active, inflammatory demyelination (e.g., acute plaques and active chronic plaques), although this study cannot determine that this damage is irreversible. If confirmed, these findings would support arguments for initiating effective therapies early in the course of the disease, if therapies that prevent axonal loss and are suitable for chronic administration are identified.

J.H. Noseworthy, M.D.

Axonal Transection in the Lesions of Multiple Sclerosis

Trapp BD, Peterson J, Ransohoff RM, et al (Cleveland Clinic Found, Ohio; Haukeland Hosp, Bergen, Norway)
N Engl J Med 338:278–285, 1998   15–7

Objective.—The cause of multiple sclerosis (MS) is unknown, although environmental factors and genetic factors play a role in susceptibility. At the onset of MS, MRI may show breakdown of the blood-brain barrier. Even with anti-inflammatory or immunosuppressive therapy, progressive neurologic deterioration—perhaps reflecting axonal loss—occurs in most patients with this condition. One report suggested axonal accumulation of the amyloid precursor protein in MS lesions, possibly related to irreversible axonal damage. The pathologic changes of the axons in MS were analyzed by 3-dimensional imaging of brain sections.

Methods.—The study included autopsy specimens of brain from 11 patients with MS and 4 subjects without brain disease. A total of 14 active MS lesions and 33 chronic active lesions (Fig 2) were examined for demyelination and other abnormalities, together with samples of normal-appearing white matter. The finding of terminal axonal ovoids was used as an indicator of axonal transection.

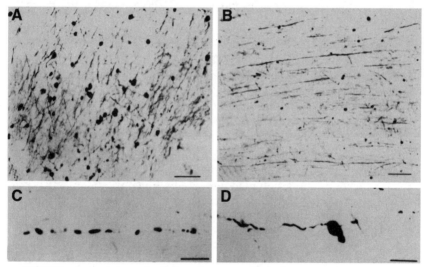

FIGURE 2.—Patterns of axonal pathologic changes in multiple sclerosis lesions. In active lesions **A,** SMI-32–positive ovoids and axons are abundant. At the edges of chronic active lesions **B,** nonphosphorylated neurofilament–positive axons and ovoids are less abundant and the ovoids are smaller. Most nonphosphorylated neurofilament–positive axons in multiple sclerosis have a normal appearance (**A** and **B**). Some have discontinuous staining for nonphosphorylated neurofilaments **C,** which is characteristic of axonal degeneration. Other axons have constrictions, dilatations, or large swellings **D.** The scale bars in **A** and **B** represent 60 μm; the scale bars in **C** and **D** represent 52 μm. (Reprinted by permission of *The New England Journal of Medicine* courtesy of Trapp BD, Peterson J, Ransohoff RM, et al: Axonal transection in the lesions of multiple sclerosis. *N Engl J Med* 338:278–285, copyright 1998, Massachusetts Medical Society.)

Results.—Multiple sclerosis lesions were consistently associated with transected axons. The more severe the inflammation within the lesions, the greater the frequency of transected axons.

Conclusion.—Axonal transection consistently follows demyelination in MS lesions in the brain. The axons appear to be a major target of disease in MS. The findings strengthen the rationale for early anti-inflammatory treatment, as axonal transection is most frequent in inflamed areas. The ramifications of reduced N-acetyl aspartate in MS lesions need to be clarified, and new approaches to monitoring and treating the axonal pathologic changes are needed.

▶ This article and the accompanying editorial have sparked considerable interest. It has long been recognized that the MS lesion is associated with "relative" axonal preservation. These authors have elegantly demonstrated that axonal transection occurs at various stages of the MS lesion. It remains to be decided, however, whether axonal transection is a common or important finding early in the illness in patients with classical relapsing-remitting MS. Most subjects studied in this article had primarily long-standing, progressive MS (primary progressive and secondary progressive disease; duration, 5–27 years); 1 had the acute, fulminating Marburg variant (duration, 2 weeks). Nonetheless, this study highlights the need to consider the evolving underlying pathologic process as one designs future treatment strategies for this disease.

J.H. Noseworthy, M.D., F.R.C.P.C.

---

¹H Magnetic Resonance Spectroscopy of Chronic Cerebral White Matter Lesions and Normal Appearing White Matter in Multiple Sclerosis
Davie CA, Barker GJ, Thompson AJ, et al (Inst of Neurology, London)
J Neurol Neurosurg Psychiatry 63:736–742, 1997   15–8

Introduction.—The clinical course of multiple sclerosis (MS) has various patterns. There is poor correlation between degrees of disability in patient subgroups and lesion load measured with conventional MRI. Proton MR spectroscopy (MRS) has the potential to detect axon loss noninvasively. The normal proton spectrum is dominated by N-acetyl (NA) derived groups. Loss of neurons may cause persistent reduction of N-acetyl aspartate (NAA), an amino acid of unknown function that has been shown in neonatal rats to be contained almost exclusively within neurons. The apparent concentration of NA was compared in patients with MS to determine if irrecoverable neurologic deficit in MS is associated with axon loss.

Methods.—Thirty-one patients with clinically definite MS underwent ¹H MRS. Patients with relapsing-remitting, secondary progressive, primary progressive, or benign MS underwent MRS to determine the apparent concentration of NA [NA], the sum of NAA (a neuronal marker) and N-acetylaspartylglutamate.

Results.—Compared with controls, there was a highly significant decrease in [NA] from an area of high signal in the 9 patients with relapsing-remitting disease, 10 patients with secondary progressive disease, and 6 patients with primary progressive disease. There was no significant difference in [NA] from an area of high signal or from an area of normal appearing white matter in patients with benign disease, compared with controls. In patients with primary progressive disease, there was a significant decrease in [NA] from an area of normal appearing white matter, compared with controls. A significant inverse correlation was observed between [NA] from lesions in patients with MS and disability, as determined by the Kurtzke Expanded Disability Scale score (EDSS).

Conclusion.—These findings indicate that axonal loss is important in the development of disability in patients with MS. A less destructive pathologic process was observed in patients with benign MS who had preservation of NA from lesions and normal appearing white matter. Patients with primary progressive MS had low [NA] from lesions and reduction of [NA] from normal appearing white matter, suggesting a more pathologic process in this subgroup. It is important to find a reliable means of predicting clinical outcome at an early disease stage in patients with MS.

▶ The authors clearly demonstrate differences between lesional pathology and normal-appearing white matter between controls and those with benign relapsing-remitting, secondary progressive, and primary progressive MS. In general, patients with benign MS (and a few relatively minimally disabled patients with relapsing-remitting disease) behaved much more like controls than do patients with more advanced levels of MS. Their observations that [NA] in benign MS patients is relatively preserved both in lesions and in normal appearing white matter appears to distinguish this patient group from those with relapsing-remitting, secondary progressive, or primary progressive MS. This may lend support to the published observations of Lucchinetti et al.[1] that there may be important differences in pathologic mechanisms between cases and that pathologic patterns may remain constant throughout the course of a patient's illness. As such, it may be possible to identify patients with relatively "benign" pathology and clinical course early in the illness. This remains to be tested. Similarly, the difference in [NA] between patients with benign MS and those destined to progress quickly to more marked disability lends additional supportive evidence to this concept. The correlation between [NA] and EDSS is modest, but again supportive that these findings are biologically relevant and possibly clinically useful.

This study is timely, given the recent attention being paid to axonal pathology in the MS lesion, and will be useful in ongoing efforts to identify prognostic variables, deciding the timing of treatment (treat early or treat late?), and the specifics of new treatment strategies (e.g., remyelination, axonal preservation).

J.H. Noseworthy, M.D., F.R.C.P.C.

Reference

1. Lucchinetti CF, Bruck W, Rodriguez M, et al: Distinct patterns of multiple sclerosis pathology indicates heterogeneity in pathogenesis. *Brain Pathol* 6:259–274, 1996.

Imaging Axonal Damage of Normal-appearing White Matter in Multiple Sclerosis

Fu L, Matthews PM, De Stefano N, et al (McGill Univ, Montreal; Univ of Oxford, England)
Brain 121:103–113, 1998   15–9

Introduction.—Magnetic resonance imaging (MRI) can detect macroscopic lesions associated with multiple sclerosis (MS), but it lacks sensitivity for underlying pathologic processes, such as inflammation, demyelination, or axonal loss. Magnetic resonance spectroscopy (MRS) is a potentially useful method for characterization of pathology in MS because it provides chemical indices associated with relatively specific pathologic changes. It can also detect axonal damage or loss in normal-appearing white matter. Serially collected magnetic resonance spectroscopic imaging (MRSI) data from 28 patients with MS were collected to determine the relative distribution of reductions of N-acetylaspartate (NAA), a marker of axonal damage, between lesions. Data were also collected for normal-appearing white matter of patients with established MS and to search for associations between changes in the ratio of NAA to creatine/phosphocreatine (NAA:Cr) in those compartments and changes in disability.

Methods.—Of 28 patients with MS, 11 had relapsing/remitting and 17 had secondary progressive disease. Patients underwent physical examination, MRSI, and conventional MRI examinations at 6- 8-month intervals. Associations between proton MRSI, MRI, lesion volume, and clinical data were tested by means of general linear models.

Results.—The NAA:Cr ratio was lower in lesions than in normal-appearing white matter in patients with MS (-15.3% in relapsing/remitting MS and -8.8% in secondary progressive MS). The lower NAA:Cr ratio per unit lesion volume observed earlier for secondary progressive relative to patients with relapsing/remitting MS was determined to result from a significantly lower ratio (8.2%) in the normal-appearing white matter rather than from any differences within lesions. The importance of changes in the normal-appearing white matter was accentuated further with the observation that the NAA:Cr ratio in normal-appearing white matter was responsible for most of the observed significant 15.6% reduction in the NAA:Cr ratio in the brains of patients with relapsing/remitting disease over the trial period. There was a strong association between decrease in the NAA:Cr in normal-appearing white matter and changes in disability in the relapsing/remitting subgroup.

Conclusion.—These findings add to the data suggesting that axonal damage or loss may be responsible for functional impairments in patients with MS. The accumulation of secondary axonal damage in the normal-appearing white matter may be key to understanding chronic disability in MS.

▶ There have now been a series of recent studies (reviewed in the YEAR BOOK OF NEUROLOGY AND NEUROSURGERY) which have addressed the issue of subclinical MS disease activity, in general, and axonal loss, specifically, in MS plaques and normal-appearing white matter. This study by Fu et al. contributes additional information to the ongoing awareness that normal appearing white matter is frequently the site of MS pathology (in this case, likely axonal loss) in patients with relapsing-remitting and secondary-progressive disease. The NAA:Cr ratio in the relapsing-remitting patients correlated with increasing levels of neurologic impairment in this small series. The MS research community is now increasingly attentive to this concept that MS is often, if not usually, a continually active disease and, therefore, repeated or continuous therapy is likely to be needed unless short-term administration of treatment can be shown to have a prolonged lasting effect. The sensitive measurements of monitoring disease progression described by Fu et al. may be useful in measuring the effectiveness of MS therapies in future studies.

J.H. Noseworthy, M.D.

The Application of Multifactorial Cluster Analysis in the Staging of Plaques in Early Multiple Sclerosis: Identification and Characterization of the Primary Demyelinating Lesion
Gay FW, Drye TJ, Dick GWA, et al (Anglia Polytechnic Univ, Cambridge, England; Radcliffe Infirmary, Oxford, England)
Brain 120:1461–1483, 1997   15–10

Objective.—In multiple sclerosis and other primary demyelinating diseases, the myelin sheath is believed to be targeted specifically for CD4+ T cell–mediated damage. However, the specific autoimmune T cell target and the mechanism of demyelination remain to be determined. A sample of early cases of multiple sclerosis (MS) were analyzed in an attempt to define the primary demyelinating lesion.

Methods.—Autopsy specimens from 13 subjects with very early MS were studied using various histologic and immunocytochemical techniques. The hope was to study initial MS lesions and their immediate derivatives before secondary complications occurred. The data were analyzed by multifactorial cluster analysis in an attempt to define important stages in lesional maturation. Also studied were specimens from subjects with other early demyelinating and inflammatory conditions.

Findings.—On cluster analysis, 5 distinct groups of lesions were identified. The initial histologic finding was simple microglial lesions, which predominated in the earliest cases. These "type I" lesions, present in both white and gray matter, were not associated with histologic signs of fibrinogen leakage. The type I lesions progressed to complex, hypercellular, fully demyelinated plaques, found mainly after MS had been present for an intermediate time. All disease stages showed quiescent lesions with evidence of remyelination. Cases of longer duration showed hypocellular, inactive plaques in addition.

The findings suggested that activated resident microglia were the cause of the initial demyelination effect. The initial event appeared to be envelopment of undegraded myelin by membranes with fixed complexes of immunoglobulin and complement. In specimens of perivenous encephalopathy, T cell infiltration was the dominant feature of demyelination. In MS lesions of comparable duration, however, humoral immune reactions were present. As plaques matured, parenchymal CD4+ T cell infiltration occurred. No complement or immunoglobulin was found on the myelin sheath or in the myelinic debris. However, C3d/IgG complexes bound to the microglial membranes were seen.

Conclusions.—Clinically early MS lesions can be classified into distinct types using histologic and immunocytochemical data. Five distinct lesional types, which seem to represent key stages in plaque morphogenesis, were identified. The findings underscore the need to stage MS lesions when the tissues are being used for study of pathogenic mechanisms. Future attempts to identify the primary provoking antigens of MS should focus on the oligoclonal B-cell response.

▶ T cell-mediated immune responses are thought possibly to be of primary pathogenic importance in some models of experimental allergic encephalomyelitis (e.g., the MOG EAE model is primarily B cell-mediated) and acute postinfectious disseminated encephalomyelitis. Some workers have suggested this is also the case in MS. In this study, Gay and colleagues have addressed the nature of the early pathologic events in MS. Using their database consisting of autopsies predominantly from acute fulminant forms of MS, the authors have shown evidence for abundant humoral immune activity and microglia activation with deposition of IgG and complement bound to microglia membranes with little evidence for fibrinogen leakage. The authors suggest that the earliest events in the MS lesion may involve activation of microglia by factors crossing pial membranes and the glia limitans from perivascular spaces before there is major disruption to the blood-brain barrier. These authors also provide additional evidence supporting the findings of others that active remyelination is commonly seen in the majority of early MS lesions. It must be realized, however, that it is by no means certain that their findings are generalizable to patients with more typical forms of MS. It is not entirely apparent that their lesional groups I–IV are readliy distinguishable; it appears that types I and V are clearly different. Nonetheless, these findings, if confirmed, have particular relevance for the development of therapeutic strategies designed to abort the development of the established MS lesion.

J.H. Noseworthy, M.D., F.R.C.P.C.

Daily Urinary Neopterin Excretion as an Immunological Marker of Disease Activity in Multiple Sclerosis

Giovannoni G, Lai M, Kidd D, et al (Inst of Neurology, London)
Brain 120:1–13, 1997

15–11

Background.—In multiple sclerosis (MS), macrophage activity is strongly enhanced by gamma interferon (IFN-γ), a major T-cell proinflammatory cytokine that induces relapses. Neopterin, a product of IFN-γ-activated macrophages, may be used to measure IFN-γ and IFN-γ-induced macrophage activity levels indirectly. The production of neopterin is augmented by tumor necrosis factor-alpha. Cells of the monocyte lineage are the main producers of neopterin, resulting from a functional block in the pathway synthesizing tetrahydrobiopterin, an essential co-factor for the inducible form of nitric oxide synthase. Neopterin was assessed as a possible surrogate marker of inflammation in patients with MS.

Methods.—Urinary neopterin to creatinine ratios (UNCRs) were measured daily in a group of patients with MS and control subjects for up to 14 weeks. The patient group consisted of 10 patients with primary progressive disease, 10 with relapsing remitting MS, and 11 with secondary progressive disease. Fourteen healthy control subjects were also tested.

Findings.—After infection-related measures were excluded, the median of individuals' average UNCRs was significantly greater in patients than in controls. The median UNCRs were 187 for the primary progressive group, 187 for the relapsing-remitting group, 218 for the secondary progressive group, and 134 for the control group. Patients also had a higher median proportion of days with UNCR exceeding normal values and a greater number of peaks in serial UNCR measures. During the study, 9 patients had a total of 9 relapses, all of which were associated with increased neopterin excretion, which tended to be greater than that on days not associated with a relapse. Three relapses were preceded by an upper respiratory tract infection. Eight of 13 patients with infections during the study had increased neopterin excretion for up to 6 weeks after the infection, which was significantly longer than that after infections in controls.

Conclusions.—Urinary neopterin excretion, increased in patients with progressive and relapsing MS, is a potential surrogate marker of the inflammatory component of disease activity. The current data provide further evidence of the pivotal role of IFN-γ in the pathogenesis of MS and confirm that infection is a potent inducer of symptomatic and asymptomatic disease activity in MS.

▶ There is no adequate laboratory marker of ongoing inflammatory demyelination or subclinical disease activity in MS. Despite innumerable studies, serum, urine, and CSF measurements of immunologic products have failed to find their place as adequate surrogates for longitudinal studies of natural history and response to experimental therapies in this disease. In this article, Giovannoni and colleagues present the first longitudinal assessment of urinary neopterin, a product of interferon-γ–activated macrophages, and provides evidence suggesting that this test may be useful as a longitudinal marker of clinical and subclinical immune-mediated injury in patients with relapsing-remitting and progressive MS. These preliminary studies suggest that urinary neopterin levels are highest in patients most likely to be experiencing active immune-mediated injury either spontaneously (secondary progressive MS) or in response to symptomatic infections; IV corticosteroid administration was associated with suppression of these levels. Serial studies with MRI monitoring are anxiously awaited to determine whether this assay detects subclinical MS disease activity and whether it will be useful in following the course of the disease in response to treatment.

J.H. Noseworthy, M.D., F.R.C.P.C.

Acute Myelitis Associated With HyperIgEemia and Atopic Dermatitis
Kira J-i, Yamasaki K, Kawano Y, et al (Kyushu Univ, Fukuoka, Japan)
J Neurol Sci 148:199–203, 1997   15–12

Background.—The causes of myelitis include a variety of infectious agents as well as an autoimmune mechanism. There have been no previous reports of hyperIgEemia or atopic disorders in association with myelitis. Four adults with cervical myelitis as well as hyperIgEemia and atopic dermatitis were seen.

Patients and Findings.—The patients were 3 women and 1 man, aged 20–47 years. All had paresthesia in the distal parts of all limbs. HyperIgEemia was also documented in all patients. Two had full-blown atopic dermatitis at the time of neurologic illness, and the other 2 had a history of atopic dermatitis. In all patients, high-signal intensity lesions were demonstrated at the C3 or C4 segment, which primarily affected the posterior column on the T2-weighted spinal cord MRI. Specific IgE antibodies to 2 mite antigens were documented in all patients, and myelitis onset coincided with the seasonal increase of mite antigens.

Conclusions.—Atopic conditions with hyperIgEemia may have contributed to the development of myelitis in these patients. Cervical MRI in atopic patients with either paresthesia or dysesthesia in the distal parts of all 4 limbs should be performed to establish the correct diagnosis.

▶ Kira et al. describe an apparent relationship between atopic dermatitis (alone or in combination with high levels of IgE to mite antigens) and cervical myelitis in 4 patients. The onset of this syndrome was in June and September, suggesting a relationship with contact with mites. The apparent pattern of the cervical myelitis (lesions appearing to extend from the submeningeal regions to the more central regions) suggests that mast cells may be involved. It is unclear whether this is simply an association or a causal relationship. Confirmation is needed from other investigators, but this ob-

servation raises the possibility that atopy to common environmental antigens may influence blood-brain barrier permeability.

J.H. Noseworthy, M.D.

**A Multicenter, Randomized, Double-Blind, Placebo-controlled Trial of
Influenza Immunization in Multiple Sclerosis**
Miller AE, Morgante LA, Buchwald LY, et al (State Univ of New York, Brook-
lyn; Mt Auburn Hosp, Cambridge, Mass; Thomas Jefferson Univ, Philadel-
phia; et al)
Neurology 48:312–314, 1997   15–13

Background.—The Advisory Committee on Immunization Practices rec-
ommends annual influenza immunization for those at risk for disease
complications. However, in multiple sclerosis (MS) patients, influenza
vaccination is controversial, because it has been reported to exacerbate MS
attacks. A multicenter, double-blind, randomized, placebo-controlled trial
of influenza immunization was conducted among relapsing-remitting MS
patients during the influenza season of 1993.

Methods.—During autumn 1993, 104 patients from 5 MS centers were
randomized to receive either standard influenza immunization or placebo
injection. These 2 patient groups did not differ significantly in age, gender,
or disability. Patients were monitored for 6 months for neurologic evaluation and for the occurrence of influenza. Influenza was defined as a fever
of at least 38°C in the presence of coryza, cough, or sore throat at a time
when the disease was known to be in the community. Patients were
examined by a blinded neurologist at 1 and 6 months after inoculation and
were contacted by phone at 1 week and 3 months. They also were examined at times of attacks.

Results.—There was no significant difference in the number of attacks
experienced by the 2 groups following vaccination. Exacerbation rates for
both groups were no more than those expected from published series.
There was no difference in attack rate or disease progression in the first
month or over the entire 6-month flu season between these 2 groups.

Conclusions.—This large, prospective, multicenter, double-blind, randomized, placebo-controlled study examined the effect of influenza immunization on relapsing-remitting MS patients throughout the 1993 influenza
season. These results confirm that influenza immunization is safe for MS
patients and is not associated with an increased risk of disease exacerbation. Influenza immunization should be recommended for MS patients.

▶ There has long been a concern that immunization may exacerbate MS.
This concern has been supported by isolated anecdotal experiences with a
variety of vaccines. In this landmark study, Miller et al. have demonstrated
definitively that influenza immunization is well tolerated and is not associated with an increased attack rate or a short-term increase in disease
progression in patients with relapsing-remitting MS. This study essentially

settles the important concern regarding influenza immunization of MS patients.

J.H. Noseworthy, M.D., F.R.C.P.C.

Randomised Placebo-controlled Trial of Monthly Intravenous Immuno-globulin Therapy in Relapsing-Remitting Multiple Sclerosis

Fazekas F, for the Austrian Immunoglobulin in Multiple Sclerosis Study Group (Karl-Franzens Univ, Graz, Austria; Leopold-Franzens Univ, Innsbruck, Austria; CIS Clinical Investigation Support GmbH & Co KG, Vienna; et al)
Lancet 349:589–593, 1997   15–14

Background.—Multiple sclerosis (MS) is a common central nervous system demyelinating disorder, characterized by episodes of neurologic dysfunction with variable remission. Autoimmune mechanisms appear to play a role in pathogenesis of MS. Intravenous immunoglobulin (IVIg) has been used to successfully treat other autoimmune neurologic disorders. This randomized, double-blind, placebo-controlled, multicenter study examined the effect of monthly IVIg treatment on the clinical course of relapsing-remitting MS.

Methods.—Between 1992 and 1996, 148 patients with relapsing-remitting MS from 13 Austrian neurologic centers were enrolled in this study. Of these 148 patients, 75 were randomly assigned to IVIg treatment, and

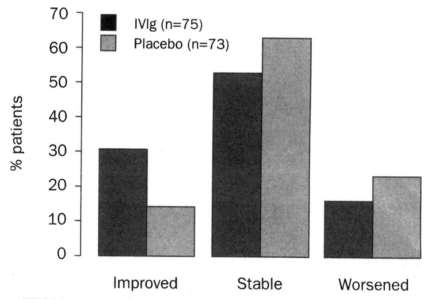

FIGURE 2.—Proportion of patients with change in clinical disability (1≥ 1.0 grade EDSS score) by intention to treat. (Courtesy of Fazekas F, for the Austrian Immunoglobulin in Multiple Sclerosis Study Group: Randomized placebo-controlled trial of monthly intravenous immunoglobulin therapy in relapsing-remitting multiple sclerosis. *Lancet* 349:589–593, 1997. Copyright by the Lancet Ltd., 1997.)

TABLE 3.—Acute Relapses

	IVIg (n=75)	Placebo (n=73)	p
Number of relapses	62	116	
Relapse-free patients	40 (53%)	26 (36%)	0·03
Mean (95% CI) annual relapse rates			
Prestudy	1·30 (1·09–1·51)	1·41 (1·21–1·61)	0·4
Study period	0·52 (0·32–0·72)	1·26 (0·75–1·77)	0·0037
Year 1	0·49 (0·29–0·69)	1·30 (0·79–1·81)	0·011
Year 2*	0·42 (0·24–0·60)	0·83 (0·59–1·07)	0·006
Characteristics of relapses†			
Mean (range) days to first relapse	237 (4–659)	151 (2–719)	0·35
Mean (range) days between relapses	720 (83–744)	362 (28–738)	0·026
Mean (95% CI) change in EDSS score during relapse	1·00 (0·78–1·22)	1·26 (1·04–1·48)	0·22

*IVIg (n=65), placebo (n=63). †IVIg (n=35), placebo (n=47).
(Courtesy of Fazekas F, for the Austrian Immunoglobulin in Multiple Sclerosis Study Group: Randomised placebo-controlled trial of monthly intravenous immunoglobulin therapy in relapsing-remitting multiple sclerosis. *Lancet* 349:589–593, copyright 1997, by The Lancet Ltd.)

73 were assigned to IV placebo monthly for 2 years. Patients were examined at the start and then every 6 months until the end of the study by a blinded neurologist. Clinical disability was measured by the Hurtzke's expanded disability status score (EDSS) and the functional systems scale. Primary outcome measures were the between-group difference in EDSS change and in the proportion with improved, stable, or worse clinical disability. Secondary outcome measures were relapse number, annual relapse rate, proportion of relapse-free patients, and the time to first relapse. The primary analysis was by intention to treat.

Results.—Intention to treat analysis revealed that EDSS decreased in the IVIg-treated patients and increased in the placebo group. The percentage of IVIg patients improved was 31; stable, 53; and worse, 16. The percentage of placebo patients improved was 14; stable, 63; and worse, 23 (Fig 2). There were half the number of confirmed relapses in the treatment group as there were in the placebo group (Table 3). The interval between relapses was significantly longer for the patients in the treatment group than it was for the placebo group. No side effects were linked to the treatment.

Conclusions.—Intravenous immunoglobulin appears to be a beneficial option for the treatment of relapsing-remitting MS. Monthly IVIg administration appears to be as effective as interferon or copolymer 1 treatment and has fewer adverse effects associated with it. The optimum treatment strategy for relapsing-remitting MS has not yet been defined.

▶ This multicenter Austrian study provides some evidence that relapsing-remitting multiple sclerosis patients treated with monthly courses of IVIg fare better than placebo-treated patients over a 2-year interval. The evidence includes a higher proportion of patients with reduced clinical impairment and a lower proportion with clinical worsening. The magnitude of this change (the primary outcome measure was the between-group difference in the absolute EDSS) was modest. However, IVIg-treated patient's EDSS improved by 0.23 points, and placebo-treated patient's EDSS scores worsened by 0.12 points. The difference between the treated groups was less than that recordable by the EDSS scale (e.g., 0.5 points). The authors did not use a "confirmed" measurement of worsening (e.g., repeat clinical evaluation at 3 or 6 months after the first evidence of EDSS worsening). Other comparable trials have used a 1.0 EDSS point worsening for patients with baseline EDSS of ≤5.5. Deterioration of EDSS by 1 point or greater occurred in similar numbers of patients in both groups (11 in the IVIg group [17%] vs. 13 in the placebo group [23%]). However, IVIg-treated patients experienced a more dramatic benefit in terms of relapse-frequency reduction (secondary outcome measure). Improvement of at least 1.0 EDSS point was seen in a slightly greater proportion of IVIg-treated patients at 2 years (31%) than was seen in the North American trials of interferon-β 1a (Avonex) and Copolymer 1 (Copaxone, 18% to 25%). Confirmatory trials with serial MRI studies, evaluating "confirmed" worsening and the success of evaluatory blinding would be welcome.

J.H. Noseworthy, M.D.

Interferon Beta Results in Immediate Reduction of Contrast-enhanced MRI Lesions in Multiple Sclerosis Patients Followed by Weekly MRI
Calabresi PA, Stone LA, Bash CN, et al (NIH, Bethesda, Md; Mayo Clinic Scottsdale, Ariz)
Neurology 48:1446–1448, 1997   15–15

Introduction.—A 2-year placebo-controlled trial found that interferon-β1b treatment led to a 31% reduction in clinical exacerbations of multiple sclerosis (MS) and a 70% reduction in the formation of new T_2 MRI lesions. Flu-like symptoms occur in most patients after initiation of treatment, and some experience a transient disease worsening. It is suggested that these side effects may result from an increase in interferon-γ–secreting cells. The results of interferon-β treatment were evaluated in a study of 8 patients with MS.

Methods.—The patients were 4 women and 4 men with a mean age of 36.9 years and a mean duration of disease of 5.4 years. Entry criteria included having an average of at least 0.5 contrast-enhancing lesions on head MRI per month during the 6 months before interferon-β treatment and no immunosuppressive treatment in the 3 months before study entry (except IV methylprednisolone for an acute exacerbation). Treatment consisted of 8 million IU of subcutaneous interferon-β1b, administered subcutaneously on alternate days. Neurologic evaluations were performed monthly during the 6 months before and after initiation of therapy. Brain MRIs were performed monthly before treatment, weekly during the first 4 weeks of treatment, then monthly again.

Results.—The mean number of gadolinium-enhancing lesions was reduced from 9.6 in the 3 months before treatment to 0.6 in the first 12 weeks after treatment. Five of the 8 patients reported mild flu-like symptoms and 2 experienced increased fatigue. In 1 patient, there was a clinically documented worsening of disease without concomitant opening of the blood brain barrier on MRI. These problems occurred despite improvement on contrast-enhanced MRI findings.

Discussion.—Treatment with interferon-β1b immediately reduced the number of contrast-enhanced MRI lesions, an indication of clinical disease activity, in patients with MS. The symptoms reported after initiation of treatment appear to be related to pre-existing lesions rather than to new disease activity. Unless there is documented clinical deterioration or MRI activity, these symptoms should be treated with nonsteroidal anti-inflammatory drugs and antipyretics.

▶ Patients with MS may worsen temporarily with the initiation of interferon therapies (e.g., interferon-β1a or -β1b). This may lead either to premature termination of therapy or steroid intervention. In this small serial MRI and clinical study, Calabresi and colleagues demonstrate that blood-brain barrier impairment usually normalizes quickly with the onset of interferon therapy, and the clinical worsening may occur without cranial MRI evidence of new disease activity. Confirmation of this potentially important observation is awaited.

J.H. Noseworthy, M.D.

Peripheral Blood Stem Cell Transplantation in the Treatment of Progressive Multiple Sclerosis: First Results of a Pilot Study
Fassas A, Anagnostopoulos A, Kazis A, et al (George Papanicolaou Hosp, Exokhi/Thessaloniki, Greece)
Bone Marrow Transplant 20:631–638, 1997   15–16

Introduction.—Experimental investigations with animals have indicated that inherited or induced autoimmune disease might be cured by bone marrow transplantation. This may be true for the animal model of multiple sclerosis (MS), which responds to total-body irradiation and chemotherapy, followed by bone marrow transplantation. The feasibility and toxicity of hematopoietic stem cell transplantation in the treatment of MS was assessed in 15 patients.

Methods.—The median age for 15 patients with progressive MS was 37 years (range, 24–54 years). All patients were severely disabled (median Kurtzke Expanded Disability Status Scale [EDSS], 6.0 and Scripps Neurologic Rating Scale [SNRS], 42). All patients had evidence of clinical deterioration of at least 1.0 point on the EDSS during the previous 12 months. Cyclophosphamide (4 g/m²) and G/GM-CSF (5 µg/kg/day) were administered for stem cell mobilization. There was no neurotoxicity. On days +1 and +2, antithymocyte globulin (2.5–5.0 mg/kg/day) was administered for

TABLE 1.—Transplant-Related Toxicity

Toxicity	Grade (WHO)	No. of patients	Cause
Allergy		14/15	
erythema	1	4	BCNU, stem cell inf., ATG
fever and erythema	2; 1	9	ATG
fever and hypotension	4	5	Stem cell inf., ATG
bronchospasm	3	2	Stem cell inf., ATG
anaphylaxis	4	2	ATG
Oral		7/15	
soreness, erythema	1	6	
ulcers	3	1	
GI bleeding	3	1/15	Steroids
Liver enzymes	1	3/15	
Infection		13/15	
bacteremia	3	9	*Staph.* sp., *E. cloacae, Kl. oxytoca*
fungemia	3	1	*C. albicans*
pneumonia	3	3	
UTI	2	2	*E. faecium, S. haemolyticus*
enteritis	2	3	*E. clocae, Citrobacter* sp.
FUO	2	1	
Neurologic		6/15	
aggravation of visual impairment		2	on days +3, +4
headache		2	on day +3
confusion-disorientation		1	on day +5
deterioration of ataxia		1	on day +10
vertigo		1	on day +11

Abbreviations: WHO, World Health Organization; *UTI,* urinary tract infection; *FUO,* fever of unknown origin; *BCNU,* carmustine; *ATG,* antithymocyte globulin.
(Courtesy of Fassas A, Anagnostopoulos A, Kazis A, et al: Peripheral blood stem cell transplantation in the treatment of progressive multiple sclerosis: First results of a pilot study. *Bone Marrow Transplant* 20:631–638, 1997.)

in vivo T-cell depletion. The main toxic reactions were allergy (93%) and infections (87%). Six patients experienced mild, transient neurotoxicity immediately after transplant (Table 1).

Results.—The median follow-up was 5 months. Seven of 15 patients had durable neurologic improvements on the EDSS. On the SNRS, 15 of 15 patients improved. One patient worsened at 3 months and 2 relapsed.

Conclusion.—Autologous hematopoietic stem cell transplantation may be feasible in patients with MS. Disability is not aggravated and patients may have a clinical benefit with this approach.

▶ Bone marrow transplantation is under study at a number of centers worldwide as a possible candidate for treatment of severe MS. This experimental, costly, and potentially risky form of therapy (fatality rate up to 5%) needs to be addressed in well-designed pilot programs. In this first report from the center in Thessaloniki, Greece, Fassas et al. report that peripheral blood stem cell transplantation was relatively well tolerated. They suggest that patients with progressive MS may benefit from this procedure as 6 of 15 progressive patients with MS (8 primary progressive, 7 secondary progressive) had improvement of at least 1 EDSS point at the 6-month evaluation.

This claim of potential efficacy must be carefully considered, however, for a number of reasons. The difficulties in relying on unblinded evaluation by EDSS have been noted by many observers in open-label MS trials. It is uncommon for patients with progressive MS to show marked improvement with any form of immunosuppressive therapy. The finding that 6 of 15 patients had improvement by at least 1 EDSS point is, therefore, of potential interest but must be balanced by the observation that 11 of the enrolled patients had clinical evidence of "very recent deterioration before hematopoietic stem cell transplantation." Hence, some of the posttransplantation improvement may simply have been regression to the EDSS level before their recent pretreatment deterioration.

The authors' claim that this was a well-tolerated treatment must be balanced by several observations: A single patient had an anaphylactic reaction to ATG, 14 of 15 treated patients experienced treatment-related toxicity (see Table 1), there was transient neurotoxicity after stem cell infusion, and the treatment is costly and has uncertain long-term benefit. The MRI data were not presented in this article but will be of considerable interest when published.

J.H. Noseworthy, M.D., F.R.C.P.C.

NEUROSURGERY

SCOTT R. GIBBS, M.A., M.D.

Reservation Card for the Year Book

Yes! I would like my own copy of *Year Book of Neurology and Neurosurgery*® at the price of **$81.00** (**$90.00** outside the U.S.) plus sales tax, postage, and handling. Please begin my subscription with the current edition according to the terms described below.* I understand that I will have 30 days to examine each annual edition.

Name _____

Address _____

City _____ State _____ ZIP_____

Method of Payment

Check (in U.S. dollars, drawn on a U.S. bank, payable to *Year Book of Neurology and Neurosurgery*®)

❑ VISA ❑ MasterCard ❑ Discover ❑ AmEx ❑ Bill me

Card number _____ Exp. date: _____

Signature _____

Prices are subject to change without notice.   PMC-352

Subscribe to the related journal in your field!

Yes! Begin my one-year subscription to *Journal of Vascular Surgery* (12 issues).

Name _____

Institution _____

Address _____

City _____ State_____

ZIP/PC _____ Country _____

Specialty _____
(Students/residents, please list Institution)

Method of payment

Enclose payment (check or credit card number) and we'll send an extra issue FREE!

❑ Check (in U.S. dollars, drawn on a U.S. bank, and payable to *Journal of Vascular Surgery*)

❑ VISA   ❑ MasterCard   ❑ Discover

❑ AmEx   ❑ Bill me   Exp. date_____

Card #_____

Signature _____

*Includes Canadian GST

Individual/student subscriptions must be in the name of, billed to, and paid for by the individual.

Airmail rates available upon request.
Prices subject to change without notice.

Subscription prices (through 9/30/99)

		USA	Canada*	Int'l
Individuals	❑	$161.00	$212.93	$199.00
Institutions	❑	306.00	368.08	344.00
Students, residents	❑	83.00	129.47	121.00

J024991YA

---

*Your Year Book service guarantee:

When you subscribe to the *Year Book*, you will receive advance notice of future annual volumes about two months before publication. To receive the new edition, you need do nothing—we'll send you the new volume as soon as it is available. If you want to discontinue, the advance notice allows you time to notify us of your decision. If you are not completely satisfied, you have 30 days to return any *Year Book*.

||||

BUSINESS REPLY MAIL

FIRST-CLASS MAIL   PERMIT NO 135   ST LOUIS MO

POSTAGE WILL BE PAID BY ADDRESSEE

SUBSCRIPTION SERVICES
MOSBY, INC.
11830 WESTLINE INDUSTRIAL DRIVE
ST. LOUIS   MO 63146-9988

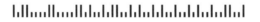

||||

BUSINESS REPLY MAIL

FIRST-CLASS MAIL   PERMIT NO 135   ST LOUIS MO

POSTAGE WILL BE PAID BY ADDRESSEE

SUBSCRIPTION SERVICES
MOSBY, INC.
11830 WESTLINE INDUSTRIAL DRIVE
ST. LOUIS   MO 63146-9988

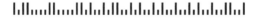

Want to speed up the process?

**To order a *Year Book* or *Advances*,
you also may call 1-800-426-4545**

**To subscribe to a journal today,
call toll-free in the U.S.:
1-800-453-4351
or fax 314-432-1158
Outside the U.S., call: 314-453-4351**

Visit us at: *www.mosby.com/periodicals*

Mosby, Inc.
Subscription Services
11830 Westline Industrial Drive
St. Louis, MO   63146 U.S.A.

 Mosby

The Human Brain: An Enviable Adaptation or Fatal Mutation?

The last 2.8 million years have been good to the hominid and homo lineage—we have come a long way from our distant ancestral neighbors of Sterkfontein.

Our capacious endocranium has burgeoned from the force of an ever-enlarging neocortex. Laid bare, the cerebral lobes induce awe among those brave enough to look. Is it because they embody the individual, or is it simply because they are the latest creation of neurogenesis and evolution? Among other things the pace and manner of our brain evolution will be a matter for future paleoanthropologists to ponder hopefully.

We have accomplished interplanetary travel. We have placed complex communications systems in geosynchronous orbits. We have harnessed nuclear energy! And, *we* have learned to successfully operate upon and repair the organ responsible for all of these achievements—the brain.

But why, while our neighbors are swatting deadly sand flies along the White Nile in a sprawling agglomeration of African huts, do we sit on our fat buttocks—men picking their sideburns and women filing their nails—idly watching the latest lurid reports of our leader's limbic indiscretions. Must we resurrect faradisation to stimulate those afflicted with this variant of cerebral dormancy or is the shear heft of a flaccid mind too much to overcome? Surely our minds were intended for some higher purpose!

Clearly, there has been a decrement in critical thinking, self-control and optimal utilization of our minds. Is industrialization to blame for creating a unique circumstance in our history, wherein we are so relatively comfortable and protected that the demand for intellectual acuity is lessened? Certainly, at some time in our savage past the unbending forces of nature, especially the threat of starvation and death, promoted responsibility, critical thinking, disciplined behavior, concentration, and directed ingenuity. These adaptive traits are essential to our survival.

There is little reason for the complacency that seems to have infected us, because the threat of our extinction looms ever larger as we fail to be forward-thinking about reconciling environmental maintenance with development. Sustainable development in the 21st century will depend upon industrial, governmental, and individual responsibility, combined with scientific literacy.

Our world has fast become scientific and technological, yet despite our many marvelous achievements a vast segment of our society is plagued by scientific illiteracy. The National Science Foundation surveyed adult Americans and revealed that more than half are unaware that the Earth orbits the sun yearly. Less than 1 out of 10 can define a molecule and 80% percent cannot define DNA. Nearly 1 out of 7 American adults could not locate the United States on an unlabeled world map! This problem is not exclusively American. Japan and other countries face a similar paucity of scientific literacy. Overall, our intellectual repository is weakening and this is likely to present grave consequences. A modicum of scientific understanding is necessary for informed public support, and it is public support that influences the political decisions about important, and especially expensive, medical, scientific, and environmental issues. What is the common denominator? Brains—educated brains!

As neurospecialists, rarely does a day pass that we do not speak of the brain, its ventricles, various lobes and sundry parts with second nature familiarity. But, the vast majority of people are entirely unfamiliar with the brain, its functions and overall importance to the individual and to humanity. As neurospecialists, we are about the brain. We know it well and it is our responsibility to teach about its role in behavior choices, critical analysis, emotional modulation, conflict resolution, and how it is harmed by abusive practices. We must teach, not from the vantage point of a detached armchair expert, but as explainers in a learner-centric approach. We must encourage and nurture intelligence thereby advancing our human condition. While we cannot expect lay people to be interested in the arcane details that so excite neuroscientists, we must engage people, especially our young children, in an imaginative and practical understanding of the individual and collective value of our single greatest asset. We must be willing to teach to help ourselves and our children as the vector of our global intellectual capital will likely determine the fate of our species.

Scott R. Gibbs, M.A., M.D.

Reflections on Neurosurgery—A Thread of Continuity

This year I owe a large debt of gratitude to Dr. Glenn Pait for his ready assent to assist me in developing this new section of the YEAR BOOK, "Reflections of Neurosurgery". Our record of achievement in the neurosciences is an astonishingly rich stream of unique events whose artistry of experience is the progenitor of our artistry of creation. The history of our profession is a magnificent adventure that prepares us to better comprehend our present and anticipate our future and it is hardly necessary to dwell on the heuristic value of our past to recognize that our surgery and practice today is inseparable from the experience of all the surgeons who have preceded us. I have deliberately not placed this section at the end of the YEAR BOOK so that it may precede and serve as a historical mooring for our latest developments in neurosurgery.

Scott R. Gibbs, M.A., M.D.

We often assume that what we read and view today is a first. However, in most instances this is certainly not the case. The authors of various papers and chapters will change, but diseases and their consequences will remain for new generations to treat. With the passing of time and the energies of many, we gain a better understanding of diseases and their demands inflicted upon our patients. The following illustrations are just a very few examples of the writings and advancements of those who, like ourselves, sought to help their patients. These early writers are our forefathers, our colleagues.

T. Glenn Pait, M.D., F.A.C.S.

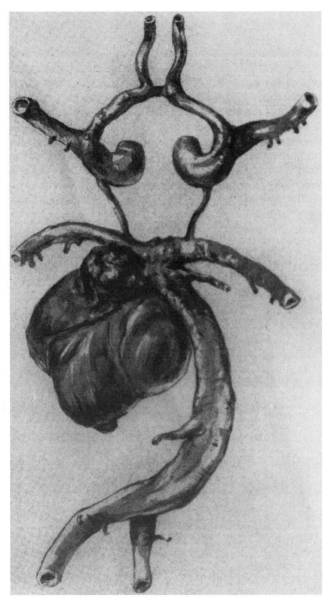

FIGURE 1.—Autopsy of giant aneurysm of the posterior cerebral artery. (Courtesy of Paul B. Hoeber, Inc., Publishers, New York, from Sosman MC, Vogt EC: Aneurysms of the internal carotid artery and the Circle of Willis, from a roentgenological viewpoint. *The American Journal of Roentgenology and Radium Therapy* 15:221, 1926.)

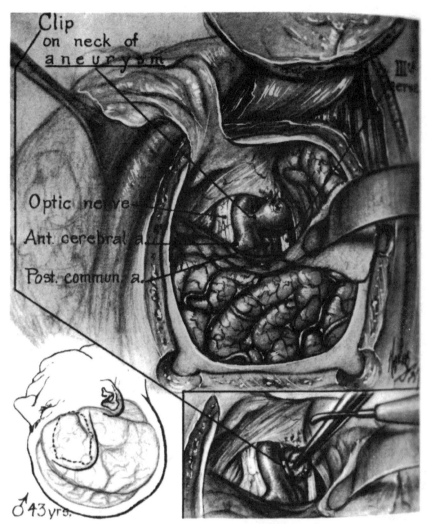

FIGURE 2.—First aneurysm clipping—left posterior communicating artery aneurysm by Walter E. Dandy on March 23, 1937. (Courtesy of Lippincott-Raven Publishers, Philadelphia, from Dandy, WE: Intracranial aneurysms of internal carotid artery. *Ann Surg* 107:654–659, 1938.)

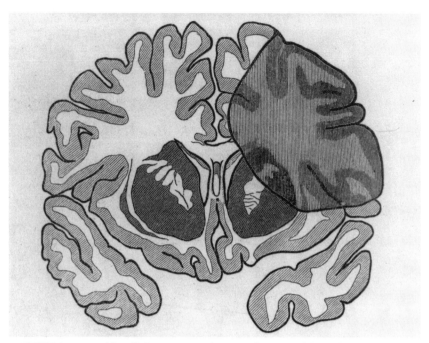

FIGURE 3.—Successful cerebral surgery in October 1888. Illustration of depth of tumor—intracranial fibroma. (Courtesy of Lea Brothers & Co., Philadelphia, from Keen WW: Three successful cases of cerebral surgery. *Am J Med Sci* 96:320–357, 1888.)

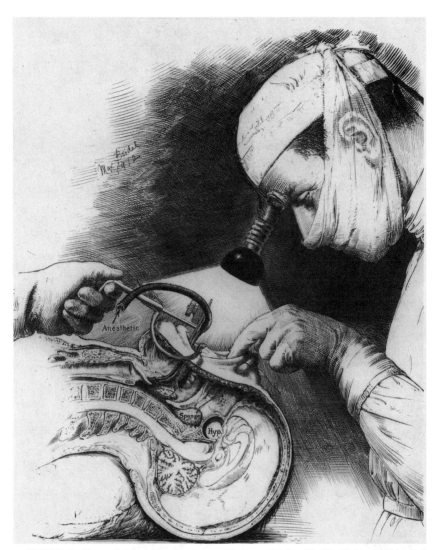

FIGURE 4.—Transsphenoidal hypophysectomy. (Courtesy of Johns Hopkins University School of Medicine, from Cushing H: The Weir Mitchell lecture—Surgical experiences with pituitary disorders. *JAMA* 63:1515–1525, 1914.)

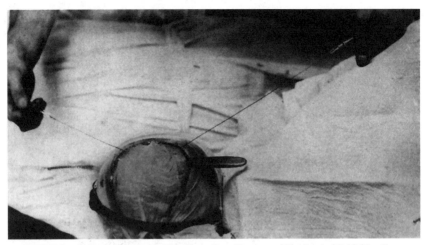

FIGURE 5.—Gigli wire saw for making a bone flap. (Courtesy of The Surgical Publishing Company of Chicago, from Cushing H: Technical methods of performing certain cranial operations. *Surgery, Gynecology, and Obstetrics* 6(3):227–246, 1908.)

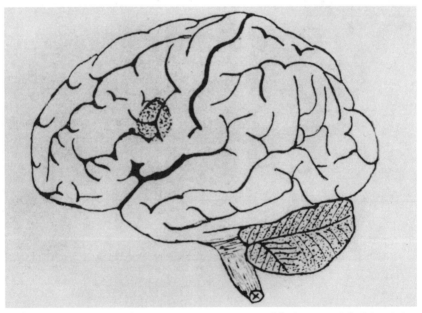

FIGURE 6.—Localization of brain tumor in 1895. (Courtesy of the American Medical Association, Chicago, from Lamphear E: Lectures on intracranial surgery. *JAMA* 24:655–658, 1895.)

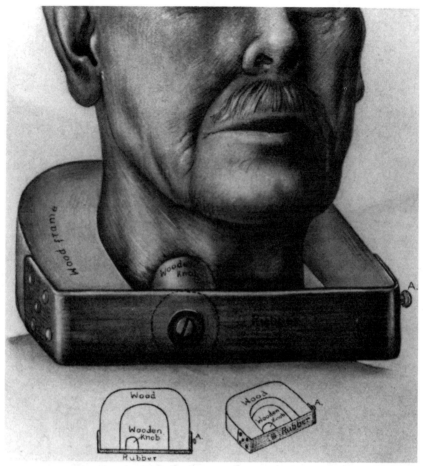

FIGURE 7.—Instrument to compress the common carotid artery in 1924. (Courtesy of J.B. Lippincott Company, Chicago, from Locke, Jr. CE: Intracranial arterio-venous aneurysm or pulsating exophthalmos. *Annals of Surgery* 80:1–24, 1924.)

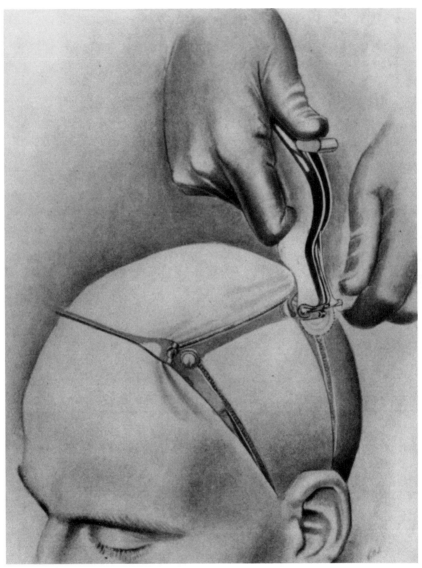

FIGURE 8.—Osteoplastic craniotomy using a "skull plough." (Courtesy of William Wood and Co., New York, from Rogers L: Osteoplastic craniotomy. A new technique for the resection and turning down of bone-flaps from the skull. *The British Journal of Surgery* 18:221, 1930–31.)

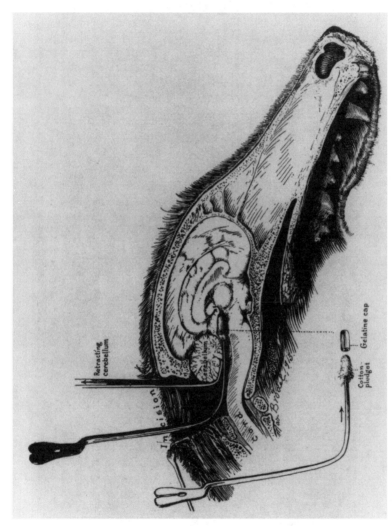

FIGURE 9.—Experimental production of hydrocephalus. (Courtesy of the AMA, Chicago, from Dandy WE, Blackfan KD: Internal hydrocephalus. An experimental, clinical and pathological study. *American Journal of Diseases of Children* 8:406–482, 1914.)

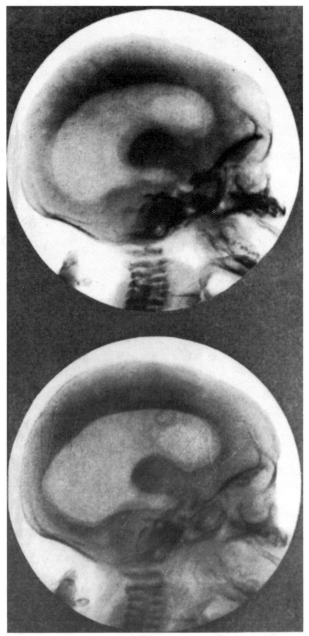

FIGURE 10.—Ventriculography. (Courtesy of Lippincott-Raven Publishers, Philadelphia, from Dandy WE: Ventriculography following the injection of air into the cerebral ventricles. *Annals of Surgery* 68:569–579, 1918.)

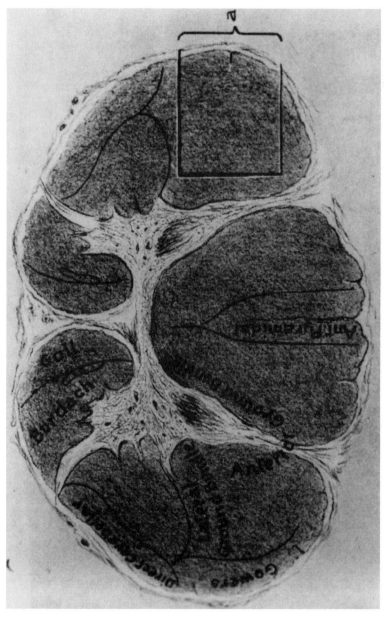

FIGURE 11.—Section of the spinal cord for insufferable pain. (Courtesy of the American Medical Association, Chicago, from Frazier CH: Section of the anterolateral columns of the spinal cord for the relief of pain. *Archives of Neurology and Psychiatry* 4:137–147, 1920.)

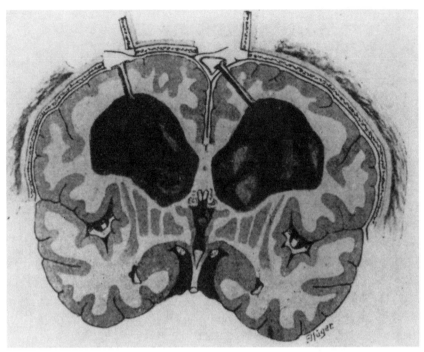

FIGURE 12.—Treatment of hydrocephalus using a vein graft. (Courtesy of the American Medical Association, Chicago, from Davidoff LM: Treatment of Hydrocephalus. *Archives of Surgery* 18:1737–1762, 1929.)

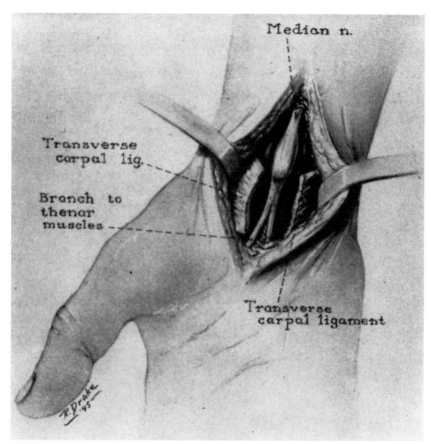

Median n.

Transverse
carpal lig.

Branch to
thenar
muscles

Transverse
carpal ligament

R. Drake
'45

FIGURE 13.—Carpal tunnel syndrome: Tardy median palsy surgical procedure presented by Cannon and Love at the Central Surgical Association, Chicago, IL, Feb. 22–23, 1946. (Courtesy of Mosby, Inc., St. Louis, from Cannon BW, Love JG: Tardy medial palsy; median neuritis; median thenar neuritis amenable to surgery. *Surgery* 20:210, 1946.)

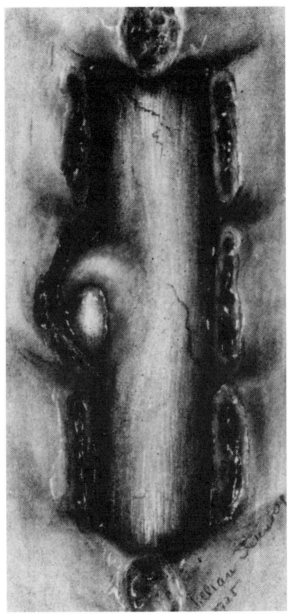

FIGURE 14.—Vertebral disc chondroma. (Courtesy of The Surgical Publishing Company of Chicago, from Elsberg CA: Extradural spinal tumors—primary, secondary, metastatic. *Surgery, Gynecology and Obstetrics* 46:1–, 1928.)

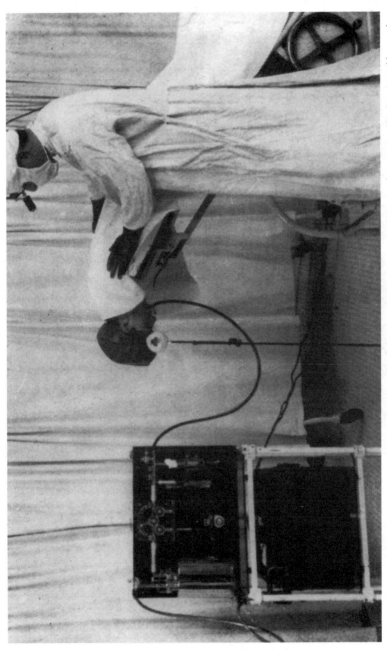

FIGURE 15.—Surgical positioning for thoracic spine surgery. (Courtesy of the Surgical Publishing Company of Chicago, from Frazier CH: Certain problems and procedures in the surgery of the spinal column. *Surgery, Gynecology and Obstetrics* 14:552–560, 1913.)

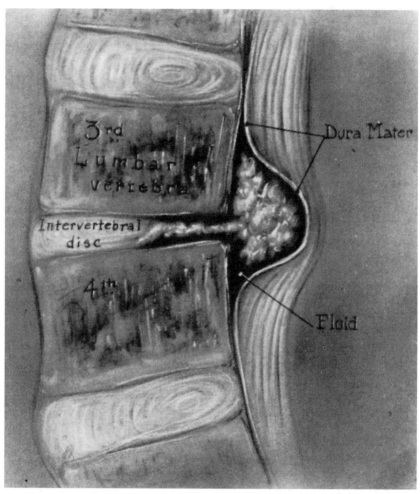

FIGURE 16.—Lumbar disc herniation compressing the cauda equina. (Courtesy of Lippincott-Raven Publishers, Philadelphia, from Dandy WE: Loose cartilage from the intervertebral disc simulating tumor of the spinal cord. *Archives of Surgery* 19:660–672, 1929.)

16 Aneurysms and Intracranial Hemorrhage

Intracranial Aneurysms

Endovascular Occlusion of Experimental Aneurysms With Detachable Coils: Influence of Packing Density and Perioperative Anticoagulation
Reul J, Spetzger U, Weis J, et al (Univ Hosp Rheinisch-Westfälische Technische Hochschule Aachen, Germany)
Neurosurgery 41:1160–1168, 1997   16–1

Background.—With endovascular occlusion of saccular aneurysms of the cerebral arteries, good results have been achieved using detachable coils, even in so-called "surgical aneurysms." However, recent reports have found the rate of recanalization to be higher than expected. This outcome is less likely if the coils are packed very tightly. This study examined the effects of coil packing density on outcome, as well as the influence of perioperative anticoagulation on the rate of permanent occlusion.

Methods.—Thirty arterial bifurcation aneurysms were microsurgically created in rabbits. All were occluded with coils, some with electrically detached platinum coils and others with mechanically detached tungsten coils. In both groups, coil placement continued until no additional coils would fit into the aneurysmal lumen, and the lumen was no longer filled with radiographic contrast material. In each case, "packing density" was assessed by angiography to determine the degree of occlusion. Angiograms had to show no visible neck remnant for the occlusion to be considered complete. Some of the animals received heparin anticoagulation. The rabbits were observed for 3–6 months, after which angiographic and histologic analyses were performed.

Results.—Nine of the 30 aneurysms were completely occluded; 10 were occluded subtotally, with greater than 95% occlusion but residual filling at the aneurysmal neck; and 11 were partially occluded. Follow-up angiograms demonstrated recanalization in 14 aneurysms; the rest showed no change from the initial angiographic findings. The pathologic findings did not always agree with the angiographic results. Recanalization was documented in 5 of 9 aneurysms that appeared completely occluded on angiography. Of the 9 aneurysms with initial complete occlusion, only 4 showed endothelial-like tissue at the aneurysmal orifice.

Conclusions.—When endovascular coil systems are used to treat intracranial aneurysms, the packing density of the coils is positively related to the occlusion rate. However, permanent occlusion may not occur even if the coils are densely packed. Endovascular coils are not an alternative to surgical clipping for every aneurysm; they should be considered only when surgical clipping would be associated with clearly increased risk. Heparin anticoagulation has no adverse effects on the results of this technique.

▶ This is a somewhat unusual article. The controlled experiment, to assess the role of anticoagulation in recanalization of coiled aneurysms, is of less interest than the empiric observations of recanalization rates in both the control and treatment groups. The impact of anticoagulation in this model is easily dismissed: there is none. However, the surprisingly high rate of recanalization of aneurysms that appeared completely occluded on the initial post-coiling angiogram is much more interesting. This startling finding, in both heparin–treated and untreated groups, was independent of the type of coil used. The histological demonstration of persistent vascular channels within aneurysms that appeared tightly packed and completely filled with coils on angiography may explain it. Because of the intrinsic limitations of angiographic resolution, an aneurysm that appears completely occluded may, nonetheless, contain microscopic, active vascular channels. With the passage of time, and under the influence of the hemodynamic stresses that are especially prominent at arterial bifurcation points, these persistent microscopic channels can enlarge and cause the aneurysm to recanalize. It would appear that, contrary to an aneurysm with a completely occluded base, the mechanical stresses to which an aneurysm compacted with coils is submitted are sufficient, at least experimentally, to favor recanalization, presumably until neo-endothelialization occurs at the point where the aneurysm meets the artery. These observations suggest that the long–term, angiographic follow–up of patients whose aneurysms appear completely obliterated is warranted. How long such patients should be followed remains an open question.

R. Leblanc, M.D., M.Sc., F.R.C.S.C.

Technical Aspects and Recent Trends in the Management of Large and Giant Midbasilar Artery Aneurysms

Lawton MT, Daspit CP, Spetzler RF (Mercy Healthcare Arizona, Phoenix)
Neurosurgery 41:513–521, 1997   16–2

Introduction.—For patients with basilar artery aneurysms, the surgical approach to the cranial base often involves removal of the petrous bone. Because radical petrosectomy carries considerable morbidity, interest in alternative approaches to the midbasilar artery has been spurred. Such approaches should diminish the extent of temporal bone removal, thus reducing complications, while maintaining good surgical exposure. The authors present their experience with 2 such approaches to midbasilar artery aneurysms—the extended orbitozygomatic and far-lateral approaches—and compare these with the standard transpetrosal approaches.

Patients and Outcomes.—The 5-year experience included 28 patients undergoing surgery for large or giant aneurysms of the midbasilar artery. A pterional-subtemporal or extended orbitozygomatic approach was used in 10 patients, a presigmoid transpetrosal approach in 5, and a far-lateral approach in 13. Twenty-one patients had good outcomes, with Glasgow Outcome Scale scores of 1 or 2; 3 patients were left with permanent, treatment-related neurologic deficits. There were 4 deaths. The orbitozygomatic approach replaced the pterional-subtemporal approach in the later part of the series. Hypothermic circulatory arrest was used in 18 patients, leading to improved exposure of the midbasilar region with either the orbitozygomatic or far-lateral approach. As the use of these procedures increased, the use of transpetrosal approaches decreased.

Conclusions.—This experience illustrates the use of the modified orbitozygomatic and far-lateral approaches to achieve surgical exposure of the midbasilar region for patients with large and giant aneurysms. In selected patients, these approaches can replace the standard transpetrosal approaches, leading to reduced morbidity. Temporal bone-conserving approaches must be used with hypothermic circulatory arrest.

▶ In recent years, interest in skull base surgery has virtually blossomed. Nowhere have skull base techniques been more fruitfully applied than in the domain of cerebrovascular surgery. Lawton et al. expand on the pioneering work of Drake, Yasargil, and Kempe in extending our reach to the basilar artery. They describe techniques wherein aggressive but selective bony resection allow better illumination, an unobstructed view, and greater access and maneuverability in tight corners of the posterior fossa. Combined with hypothermic cardioplegia, these techniques permit treatment of the most challenging aneurysms of the basilar artery, with a minimal amount of retraction on vital neural structures and with reasonable, if not ideal, surgical results. The authors also provide a sobering discussion of the difficulties and possible complications of hypothermic cardiac arrest, which should give pause to all who may be contemplating these approaches.

R. Leblanc, M.D., M.Sc., F.R.C.S.C.

Screening For Ocular Hemorrhages in Patients With Ruptured Cerebral Aneurysms: A Prospective Study of 99 Patients
Frizzell RT, Kuhn F, Morris R, et al (Univ of Alabama, Birmingham)
Neurosurgery 41:529–534, 1997   16–3

Background.—Terson's syndrome and other ocular hemorrhages can occur in up to 40% of patients with ruptured cerebral aneurysms. Microsurgical vitrectomy can safely restore vision in patients with visual loss because of Terson's syndrome. Prospectively screening a selected group of patients with aneurysms may result in a higher rate of vitrectomy in patients with more extensive subarachnoid bleeding.

Methods.—An ophthalmologist screened 99 patients with ruptured cerebral aneurysms for Terson's syndrome and other types of ocular hemorrhage. Follow-up data were available for 7 of 8 patients with Terson's syndrome. When indicated, vitrectomy was done to restore vision.

Findings.—Seventeen percent of the patients with ruptured cerebral aneurysms had ocular hemorrhages. Eight percent had Terson's syndrome. The sensitivity of the screening of patients with a history of transient or prolonged comas was 100% in patients with Terson's syndrome and 89% in patients with other ocular hemorrhages. Overall, 55% of the patients had a history of transient or prolonged comas. Fifty-three percent had ocular hemorrhages. Vitrectomy improved vision dramatically in 2 of the 8 patients with Terson's syndrome. Other ocular hemorrhages did not require surgical treatment.

Conclusions.—Ophthalmologic screening of patients with a history of transient or prolonged comas after ruptured cerebral aneurysms was very sensitive in detecting ocular hemorrhages. Such bleeding was relatively common in these patients with subarachnoid hemorrhage, who were seen in an academic neurologic practice. In patients with no spontaneous visual improvement, vitrectomy dramatically reverses blindness.

▶ If the eyes are the window to the soul, so, too, do they offer insight into aneurysmal subarachnoid hemorrhage. Sir Charles Symonds, then a Fellow at the Peter Bent Brigham Hospital in Boston, achieved the first antemortem diagnosis of a cerebral aneurysm in a patient who had a third nerve palsy. Cushing, his mentor, believed that the patient harbored a temporal lobe tumor, which he then attempted to remove with the expected result. As his reward, Sir Charles was relegated to the autopsy room and halls of the pathology department to better elucidate, in a retrospective fashion, the signs and symptoms that we now associate with aneurysmal subarachnoid hemorrhage. Since Symonds' original publication in the *Guys Hospital Report*, a pupil sparing third nerve palsy has been recognized as a hallmark of posterior communicating artery aneurysms.[1] To his credit, Cushing commented on the significance of Symonds' paper but nonetheless felt compelled to state that, although we could now diagnose cerebral aneurysms, he could think of no other condition less amenable to surgical intervention. Dandy would, of course, prove him wrong by successfully treating patients with cerebral aneurysms, prominently illustrating his surgical technique in a patient whose aneurysm had produced a third nerve palsy.[2] Following Symonds, Sir Geoffry Jefferson described the visual findings associated with carotid ophthalmic aneurysms.[3] The ophthalmological features described by these outstanding clinicians came to be recognized as helpful in the bedside diagnosis of cerebral aneurysms, just as the presence of subhyloid hemorrhages seen through the ophthalmoscope came to be recognized as a feature of subarachnoid hemorrhage.

Preceding these insights was Terson who observed that subarachnoid hemorrhage could be associated with bleeding into the vitreous chamber of the eye.[4] Although Terson may be faulted for wrongly thinking that vitreous hemorrhage results from the spread of blood from the subarachnoid space at the base of the brain to the subhyloid region of the globe along the optic nerve, later investigators have not been more successful than Terson in discovering the true mechanism accounting for the syndrome that bears his name. The visual loss that occurs in Terson's syndrome can be dramatic and worrisome, but the spontaneous visual recovery that most patients exhibit can be just as striking. In view of this generally benign evolution, when should one perform a vitrectomy? The wise neurosurgeon will, perforce, leave this decision to the ophthalmologist, but he or she will receive no insight from the article by Frizzel et al. as the indications for vitrectomy and its timing are not given, beyond a general statement that surgery was performed in 2 of their cases when spontaneous recovery was felt to be delayed.

R. Leblanc, M.D., M.Sc., F.R.C.S.C.

References

1. Symonds CP: Contributions to the clinical study of intracranial aneurysms. *Guy's Hospital Reports* 73:139–158, 1923.
2. Dandy W: Intracranial anterial aneurysms. Ithaca, New York, Comstock Publishing Company, Inc., 1944.
3. Jefferson G: Compression of the chiasma, optic nerve and optic tracts by intercranial aneurysms. *Brain* 60:444–497, 1937.
4. De l'hemorrhagic dans le corts vitre au cours de l'hemorrhagic cerebrale. *Clin Opthalmol* 6:309–312, 1900.

Ruptured Giant Intracranial Aneurysms: Part I. A Study of Rebleeding
Khurana VG, Piepgras DG, Whisnant JP (Mayo Clinic and Mayo Found, Rochester, Minn)
J Neurosurg 88:425–429, 1998   16–4

Purpose.—Subarachnoid hemorrhage (SAH) is present at diagnosis in about one fourth of giant aneurysms. Little is known about the rate of rebleeding from giant aneurysms compared with the rate of that from smaller lesions. This study evaluated the frequency of rebleeding and associated factors.

Methods.—The retrospective study included 109 patients treated for initial SAH from a giant aneurysm. These patients accounted for one fourth of all patients treated for giant intracranial aneurysm at the Mayo Clinic over a 23-year period. All but 7 patients were referred from other centers. Aneurysmal diameter was 25–60 mm; three fourths of the aneurysms were located in the anterior intracranial circulation. Surviving patients were studied for a mean of 1.7 years.

Results.—Twenty-eight percent of patients had an episode of rebleeding some time during the study. When the date of first rehemorrhage was known, it was within less than 15 days after the initial hemorrhage in 63% of patients. On analysis of 63 patients admitted to the Mayo Clinic within 7 days after their initial hemorrhage, 14% had a first rehemorrhage after admission. For these patients, the cumulative frequency of rebleeding at 14 days after admission was 18%. In some patients, CSF drainage, cerebral angiography, and delayed recurrence played a role in the rebleeding. Patients with intraaneurysmal thrombosis could still have rebleeding. One third of patients having recurrent SAH at the Mayo Clinic died in the hospital.

Conclusions.—The rate of rebleeding from giant aneurysms is similar to that from smaller aneurysms. Rebleeding is fatal in about one third of patients; it can occur in the presence of intra-aneurysmal thrombus, and is not strongly linked to interventions such as CSF drainage or cerebral angiography.

Ruptured Giant Intracranial Aneurysms: Part II. A Retrospective Analysis of Timing and Outcome of Surgical Treatment
Piepgras DG, Khurana VG, Whisnant JP (Mayo Clinic and Mayo Found, Rochester, Minn)
J Neurosurg 88:430–435, 1998   16–5

Background.—The benefits of early surgery for patients with small ruptured aneurysms, as long as the patients are in good neurologic condition, have been well described. It is not as easy to determine the optimal time for surgery in patients with giant aneurysms, largely because the risk of rebleeding is uncertain. Also, some giant aneurysms cannot be easily clipped. The effect of timing of surgery on the outcomes of ruptured giant intracranial aneurysms was analyzed.

Patients.—The 23-year experience included 109 patients with ruptured giant aneurysms, all but 7 of whom were referred from other hospitals. The aneurysms ranged in size from 20 to 60 mm. One hundred and five patients survived to undergo surgery; 84% underwent direct surgery on the aneurysm. For patients initially seen in the study hospital or referred promptly, surgery was performed an average of 4–5 days after admission. Condition was often worse, and surgery performed earlier, for patients admitted earlier. Patients with aneurysms in the posterior circulation tended to be operated on later than patients with aneurysms in the anterior circulation. In two thirds of cases in which direct surgery was possible, the parent vessel had to be temporarily occluded. Occlusion time in this group averaged 16 minutes.

Outcomes.—The rate of favorable outcome among patients undergoing surgery was 72% with aneurysms of the anterior circulation and 78% with aneurysms of the posterior circulation. Mortality was 21% overall and 9% for surgical management. Among patients seen after their first hemorrhage, the rate of favorable outcome was 42% for patients undergoing early surgery and 82% for those undergoing intermediate or delayed surgery.

Conclusions.—Ruptured giant intracranial aneurysms are associated with unique technical problems, and are best managed by prompt referral to centers specializing in the management of such lesions. Though surgery should be performed as soon as possible, it should be planned carefully, because hasty treatment increases the risk of unfavorable outcome. Rebleeding patterns are similar to those encountered in smaller lesions.

▶ The authors reviewed 109 cases of SAH due to rupture of giant aneurysms (25mm or more in diameter) treated between 1973 and 1996, 74% being anterior circulation aneurysms. The cumulative rate of rebleeding at 14 days after admission was 18.4%, which was comparable to the rate of rebleeding of smaller aneurysms. The overall management mortality rate was 21.1% and the surgical mortality was 8.6%. These were also not too different from those of smaller aneurysms. Early surgery (Day 0–3) showed favorable outcome in 42% and unfavorable outcome in 58%, whereas delayed surgery (Day 4 or later) showed favorable outcome in 82% and unfavorable outcome in 18%. This may mean that in ruptured giant aneurysms, delayed surgery with preoperative thorough planning is advisable. More accumulation of data, however, should be necessary to draw any conclusion.

K. Sano, M.D., Ph.D.

Does the Size of Intracranial Aneurysms Change With Intracranial Pressure? Observations Based on Color "Power" Transcranial Doppler Ultrasound
Wardlaw JM, Cannon J, Statham PFX, et al (Western Gen Hosp Natl Health Service Trust, Edinburgh, Scotland)
J Neurosurg 88:846–850, 1998   16–6

Purpose.—Because it is independent of the angle of insonation, color "power" transcranial Doppler (TCD) US is more sensitive to movement than conventional Doppler US. Some authors have claimed that power TCD can demonstrate random motion with a net motion of zero. In a previous study using color power TCD, the authors noted that aneurysms appeared to pulsate more than adjacent normal artery with each cardiac cycle. They also observed greater pulsatility in recently ruptured aneurysms than in unruptured ones. This study investigated whether the increased pulsatility of aneurysms noted on color power TCD represents a true change in aneurysmal size and whether intracranial pressure (ICP) influences the aneurysmal dimensions.

Methods.—The study included 9 patients with recent subarachnoid hemorrhage and hydrocephalus requiring intraventricular CSF drainage. Each patient had angiographic confirmation of aneurysm. The investigators performed color power TCD studies of the intracranial arteries and aneurysm through the temporal bone window. The power TCD studies were performed at various known ICP levels. In 4 patients, power TCD was done before and after the ventricular drain was placed.

Results.—During color power TCD studies performed at high ICPs, the aneurysms appeared highly pulsatile with small maximum cross-sectional areas. In contrast, aneurysms studied at low ICPs showed much less pulsatility and much larger size. Intracranial pressure had no significant effect on either the pulsatility or cross-sectional area of normal arteries. Aneurysm pulsatility decreased significantly after insertion of ventricular drains.

Conclusion.—Color power TCD appears to demonstrate real fluctuations in aneurysm size with changes in ICP. Low ICPs are associated with larger and less pulsatile aneurysms, whereas high ICPs are linked to smaller, more pulsatile lesions. Color power TCD offers a new approach to visualizing intracranial vascular dynamics. With further research, the technique may help in predicting the likelihood that an aneurysm will burst, among other applications.

▶ The results of color power TCD depend on the predetermined (by the investigator) flow velocity threshold-value for creating the color image. Flow within both arteries and aneurysms is divided into (1) threshold-flow which appears as a colored area, and (2) subthreshold flow with velocity lower than the threshold which is not visualised. During systole, the flow acceleration increases the proportion of threshold to subthreshold flow and produces an expansion of the colored area.

Arteries and aneurysms are completely different vascular systems. In systole, the proportion of blood volume that accelerates above the color threshold is likely to be much higher in aneurysms compared with arteries. The artery is a conduit within which laminar flow is maintained constantly. Diastolic flow cannot fall below a certain minimal velocity because this would endanger perfusion. If the Doppler color threshold is set below this minimal velocity, a substantial proportion of arterial blood volume will have a velocity above the color threshold in diastole, and the observed expansion of color in systole will be relatively small.

Conversely, the aneurysm is a "cul de sac" and its "vortex" or "swirl-type" flow serves no physiologic purpose. In diastole, most of the aneurysmal blood may have a very low velocity (below the color threshold) or flow may come to a halt (this is how aneurysms get thrombosed). As a result, in systole, the proportion of aneurysmal blood volume that accelerates above the color threshold is much higher and creates the appearance of the aneurysm's pronounced expansibility.

High ICP accentuates this differential effect of the systole-diastole cycle in the arterial and aneurysmal flow. Aneurysms get smaller because of compression by brain. In diastole, aneurysmal flow velocity becomes even lower because the total intracranial blood volume gets reduced and directed towards arteries and functioning brain. In systole, blood pressure rises above normal to overcome the increased ICP. As a result, during systole the proportional blood volume within aneurysms that accelerates above the color threshold is even higher, and the aneurysm appears even more expansible.

The question thus remains. Is the expansion in color painting a consequence of aneurysm expansion or flow acceleration within the aneurysm in systole bringing the color threshold nearer to the aneurysm wall? It would be interesting if the authors' results could be reproduced by either computer modelling or on artificial tubes imitating the artery-aneurysm structure.

Nevertheless, if the authors are accurate in their suppositions, the technique is a useful contribution with substantial potential clinical applications. Data on arterial and aneurysmal expansibility may be useful in the management of patients with subarachnoid hemorrhage, especially those who are compromised because of high ICP. Such data could also be useful in decision making with regard to the urgency of surgical intervention in patients with multiple, unruptured or incidental aneurysms.

Other patients likely to benefit are those who are seen with sudden, severe headache but whose computer tomography and CSF analysis are negative for subarachnoid hemorrhage. It is currently unclear whether episodes of pronounced aneurysmal expansion can mechanically stimulate the trigeminal perivascular nerve endings and, therefore, cause the headache without rupture. Usually, such patients are not investigated by angiography. Doppler may identify those who harbor an expanding aneurysm and need urgent treatment.

D.E. Sakas, M.D.

Subarachnoid Hemorrhage

Neuroprotective Effect of an Antioxidant, Ebselen, in Patients With Delayed Neurological Deficits After Aneurysmal Subarachnoid Hemorrhage
Saito I, Asano T, Sano K, et al (Kyorin Univ, Tokyo; Saitama Med Ctr School, Kawagoe; Fuji Brain Inst Hosp, Shizuoka; et al)
Neurosurgery 42:269–278, 1998   16–7

Introduction.—Ebselen is a lipid–soluble seleno–organic compound with antioxidant activity through a glutathione peroxidase-like action that has both cytoprotective and anti-inflammatory effects in some disease models. It may be able to protect brain tissue against ischemic insults. The effect of ebselen on the outcome of subarachnoid hemorrhage (SAH) was assessed in a multicenter placebo–controlled double–blind clinical trial.

Methods.—Eighty-four patients with aneurysmal SAH of Hunt and Kosnik grades II through IV at admission were randomized to either

2–week treatment with ebselen (150 mg twice daily) or placebo fine granules dispersed in water within 96 hours of ictus. The Glasgow Outcome Scale score was measured at 2 weeks, 1 month, and 3 months after beginning of treatment. The incidence of delayed ischemic neurological deficits (DINDs) clinically diagnosed as caused by vasospasm and the incidence and extent of low-density areas on postoperative computed tomographic scans were assessed.

Results.—Of 286 patients evaluated, 145 and 141, respectively, were treated with ebselen and placebo. DINDs were observed in 52 patients who received ebselen and 58 patients who received placebo. Patients who received ebselen had a significantly better outcome and a corresponding significant reduction in the incidence and extent of low-density areas on CT scan than patients who received placebo.

Conclusion.—Treatment with ebselen did not significantly prevent clinically diagnosed DINDs, but the severity of resulting brain damage significantly decreased and the overall outcome of patients with DINDs significantly improved. Ebselen may be a useful neuroprotective agent in the treatment of SAH.

▶ The authors present the results of a carefully planned and executed Phase II (multicenter double–blinded placebo–controlled) clinical trial of ebselen, a glutathione peroxidase–like lipid soluble compound, as a protective agent against DINDs in patients after aneurysmal SAH. Ebselen did not affect the incidence of DIND; however, it showed a beneficial effect on outcome and produced a decrease in incidence and extension of the low–density areas on CT. The study suggests that inhibition of oxidative stress improves outcome in a subpopulation of patients after SAH that developed cerebral ischemia. Despite the authors hopes, however, blocking lipid peroxidation does not affect an incidence of vasospasm after clinical studies with SAH-like trilizad, another potent inhibitor of lipid peroxidation, have shown. These findings suggest a clinical usefulness of ebselen for amelioration of deleterious effects of DIND on outcome after SAH.

R.M. Pluta, M.D., Ph.D.

Comparison of the Use of Medical Resources and Outcomes in the Treatment of Aneurysmal Subarachnoid Hemorrhage Between Canada and the United States
Glick HA, Polsky D, Willke RJ, et al (Univ of Pennsylvania, Philadelphia; Pharmacia and Upjohn Inc., Kalamazoo, Mich; Univ of Virginia, Charlottesville; et al)
Stroke 29:351–358, 1998   16–8

Introduction.—Because Canada spends a smaller percentage of gross domestic product on health care and exerts greater government control over expenditure than does the United States, differences between the health care systems of Canada and the United States have received growing attention. To assess differences between Canada and the United States in the use of medical resources and in clinical outcome in the treatment of aneurysmal subarachnoid hemorrhage during the first 90 days after randomization, data from a randomized trial of tirilazad mesylate were used. A better understanding of the size and scope of the differences in treatment between the 2 countries over an extended period was gained by including postdischarge use of medical resources.

Methods.—There was a total of 877 patients; of these, 683 were enrolled in the United States and 194 were enrolled in Canada. Means and confidence intervals around the differences in means were analyzed to compare the countries in patient characteristics, use of medical resources, and outcomes. Multivariable regression analysis was also used to predict these differences.

Results.—In Canada, the average hospital stay was 4.2 days longer, but most of the extra stay was among patients who were admitted in poor neurologic condition. In Canada, however, hospital stays were generally substantially less intensive. Patients in the United States spent 3.7 more days in nursing homes and rehabilitation centers than did patients in Canada. The Glasgow Outcome Scale score, rates of death, and occurrence of vasospasm did not differ between the 2 countries.

Conclusion.—A shift in the sites of formal care rather than the length of this care was the cause of the apparent difference in length of stay between Canada and the United States for patients admitted in good neurologic condition. The length and sites of care, however, differed between the 2 countries for patients admitted in poor neurologic condition. The differences in the use of medical resources could not be justified, as there were no significant differences in outcomes.

▶ This work is 1 of very few cross-national comparison studies that include data on postdischarge medical resource utilization. Despite the self-acknowledged limitations of this study, it offers interesting observations and speculations regarding the forces within the United States hospital payment system that influence medical resource utilization. I am not surprised that the overall clinical outcomes between the 2 countries are not significantly different.

Although the authors do not address this issue, medical resource utilization is surely influenced by patient and family expectations superimposed upon the health care delivery system to which they have become accustomed. And, I suspect, this accounts for a significant portion of the additional use of medical resources in the United States. We have generations of people in the United States who have an entitlement mentality regarding their health care and have learned to expect—and even demand, all of the best of our health care system without the burden of payment or any other barrier to entry. Our system is undergoing a metamorphosis away from health care on demand, which eventually will be reflected in our societal expectations for health care. At that time, we will likely see less of our gross national product expended on health care.

S.R. Gibbs, M.A., M.D.

Intra–aortic Balloon Counterpulsation Augments Cerebral Blood Flow in the Patient With Cerebral Vasospasm: A Xenon–enhanced Computed Tomography Study

Nussbaum ES, Sebring LA, Ganz WF, et al (Univ of Minnesota, Minneapolis)
Neurosurgery 42:206–214, 1998   16–9

Introduction.—The most widely used circulatory assist device and a mainstay of therapy for transient state of severe cardiac dysfunction is the intra–aortic balloon counterpulsation. The balloon catheter is positioned in the descending thoracic aorta distal to the origin of the left subclavian artery and proximal to the renal vessels after percutaneous insertion via the femoral artery. The displacement of blood that would otherwise remain in the aorta during diastole results with inflation at the time of aortic valve closure, which improves flow to the coronary arteries, peripheral circulation, the carotid and vertebral arteries. A previous study showed improvement in cerebral blood flow in a canine model. Experience with a patient is now reported.

Methods.—In a patient who had subarachnoid hemorrhage and concomitant myocardial infarction, the clinical use of intra–aortic balloon counterpulsation to treat cerebral vasospasm was reported. The patient had ineffective treatment with hypertensive, hypervolemic, and hemodilution therapy, and then intra–aortic balloon counterpulsation was recommended. To obtain serial measurements of cerebral blood flow with and without intra–aortic balloon counterpulsation over a 4–day period, xenon–enhanced computed tomography was used.

Results.—In this patient, intra–aortic balloon counterpulsation dramatically improved cardiac function. Significant improvement in cerebral blood flow with intra–aortic balloon counterpulsation was demonstrated with xenon–enhanced computed tomography. Before intra–aortic balloon counterpulsation, the average global cerebral blood flow was 20.5±4.4 mL/100g/min, and after the procedure, it was 34.7±3.8 mL/100g/min. Before intra–aortic balloon counterpulsation, the lower the cerebral blood flow, the greater the improvement with the procedure. Cerebral blood flow improved from 33% to 161% above baseline with an average of 69.3%. There were no complications with this procedure.

Conclusion.—In a patient with vasospasm, this is the first report demonstrating the ability of intra–aortic balloon counterpulsation to improve cerebral blood flow. In select patients with refractory cerebral vasospasm who do not respond to traditional treatment measures, intra–aortic balloon counterpulsation is a rational treatment option.

▶ Despite decades of research, vasospasm after aneurysmal subarachnoid hemorrhage remains an ominous, incurable enigma. Patients with heart insufficiency after a rupture of intracranial aneurysm face a very gruesome perspective even if the aneurysm is clipped. In such cases, the use of the most effective treatment against delayed ischemic neurological deficits, the 3H (hypervolemia, hemodilution, hypertension) therapy is limited and dangerous. Such, luckily rare patients in neurosurgical practice, are candidates for the presented treatment. The idea presented by Nussbaum et al to use intra–aortic balloon counterpulsation for treatment of severe vasospasm opens a new avenue for research to use physical forces to improve cerebral blood flow in patients with vasospasm.

R.M. Pluta, M.D., Ph.D.

The Efficacy and Safety of Angioplasty for Cerebral Vasospasm After Subarachnoid Hemorrhage
Bejjani GK, Bank WO, Olan WJ, et al (George Washington Univ, Washington, DC)
Neurosurgery 42:979–987, 1998   16–10

Purpose.—Cerebral vasospasm is a common and potentially life-threatening or disabling complication of subarachnoid hemorrhage. Patients with symptomatic vasospasm are increasingly treated with cerebral angioplasty. The authors have been performing intraluminal angioplasty since 1983. They have reported their results in terms of efficacy and safety, including the influence of timing on the clinical results.

Methods.—The 3½-year retrospective study included 31 patients with 43 aneurysms and 1 with arteriovenous malformations. The patients were 23 women and 8 men with a mean age of 44 years. Hunt and Hess grade was 1 in 4 patients, 2 in 7 patients, 3 in 15 patients, and 4 in 5 patients. Angioplasty was performed after aneurysm clipping or coiling in all patients but 2. The major indication for angioplasty was neurologic deficit caused by vasospasm that failed to resolve despite hypertensive hypervolemic hemodilution therapy. The data review focused on clinical improvement after angioplasty and how it was affected by the timing of angioplasty.

Results.—The average time to angioplasty was 7 days after subarachnoid hemorrhage. In 21 patients, angioplasty was performed within 24 hours of refractory clinical deterioration. In a total of 81 dilated vessels, there were 3 angioplasty-related complications: 2 cases of femoral hematoma and 1 of retroperitoneal hematoma. Twelve procedures were associated with dramatic clinical improvement, 11 with moderate improvement, and 9 with little or no improvement. Patients undergoing early angioplasty tended to have better clinical improvement. Recovery at discharge was graded as good in 8 patients, with a Glasgow Outcome Scale score of 11. Eleven patients were left with moderate disabilities and 10 with severe disabilities, with Glasgow Outcome Scale scores of 2 and 3, respectively. Two patients died, neither as a result of angioplasty. Follow-up in 27 patients revealed good outcomes in 25, moderate disability in 1, and death in 1.

Conclusion.—For patients with symptomatic cerebral vasospasm that does not respond to hyperdynamic hypervolemic therapy, angioplasty appears to be a safe and effective form of therapy. Substantial clinical improvement is possible with early angioplasty performed within 24 hours of subarachnoid hemorrhage. However, even delayed angioplasty provides good results, probably by keeping cerebral ischemia from getting worse and extending to other territories.

▶ This very nice paper convincingly demonstrates the efficacy of balloon angioplasty for the treatment of vasospasms after subarachnoid hemorrhage. The authors stress several important points. One is that patients have a much better recovery when treated within 24 hours after clinical deterioration. Another important point is that no major complication was observed. Taking these 2 facts into account, we, in our practice, attempt angioplasty of vasospasm as soon as the patient deteriorates, usually within 1 hour. A CT scan is first performed to exclude massive brain infection; then the patient is brought to the angiography suite for an angiogram and, if possible, angioplasty.

We have observed the same dramatic reversal of neurologic deficits as that described by the authors. We do not think it is necessary to wait for the demonstration of the inefficacy of hypertensive hypervolemic hemodilution therapy and nimodipine. These 2 treatment modalities are used routinely in high-risk patients and can be introduced or continued at the same time as angioplasty. I think it would even be useful to treat high-risk patients before neurologic symptoms develop, at the time when Doppler velocities regularly increase and when a decrease in cerebral blood flow can be demonstrated.

Balloon angioplasty should now be considered part of the standard treatment of cerebral vasospasm. It needs to be performed immediately after the onset of symptoms and by a highly qualified interventional neuroradiologist. This necessitates referring patients with subarachnoid hemorrhage to specialized centers.

N. de Tribolet, M.D.

Effect of 5% Albumin Solution on Sodium Balance and Blood Volume After Subarachnoid Hemorrhage

Mayer SA, Solomon RA, Fink ME, et al (Columbia-Presbyterian Med Ctr, New York)

Neurosurgery 42:759–768, 1998   16–11

Background.—Patients with subarachnoid hemorrhage (SAH) are at risk of excessive natriuresis and volume contraction. These could be important risk factors for vasospasm-related delayed cerebral ischemia (DCI). The effects of postoperative administration of 5% albumin solution on sodium balance and blood volume in patients with SAH were studied, as well as factors affecting renal sodium excretion after SAH.

Methods.—The randomized trial included 43 patients with acute SAH. They received either hypervolemic or normovolemic treatment for 7 days after aneurysm clipping. Both groups received a baseline infusion of normal saline, 80 mL/hr. In addition, they received 250 mL of 5% albumin solution every 2 hours for central venous pressure (CVP) values of 8 mm Hg or less in the hypervolemia group and 5 mm Hg or less in the normovolemia group. The hemodynamic parameters, renal function, sodium balance, and blood volume responses to these treatments were compared.

Results.—Baseline measurements showed relative volume expansion in both groups. The amounts of total fluid, sodium, and 5% albumin solution given were significantly greater in the hypervolemia group than in the hypovolemia group. Central venous pressure values and serum albumin levels were also higher in the hypervolemia group. These patients had an even cumulative sodium balance. In contrast, those in the normovolemia group had a persistently negative sodium balance, the result of sodium losses occurring on postoperative days 2 and 3. Twenty-four–hour sodium balance was negatively correlated with glomerular filtration rate and positively associated with serum albumin levels, after correction for sodium intake. Hypervolemia therapy seemed to paradoxically decrease glomerular filtration rate; blood volume decreased by 10% in both groups. One patient receiving hypervolemia treatment had pulmonary edema requiring diuresis.

Conclusions.—For patients with SAH, giving supplemental 5% albumin solution to keep CVP at greater than 8 mm Hg prevents sodium and fluid losses without affecting blood volume. This is so even in patients who are hypervolemic at baseline. Post-SAH natriuresis may be partly mediated by elevations in glomerular filtration rate. Administration of 5% albumin solution not only expands volume, it also reduces glomerular filtration rate while promoting renal sodium retention. By reducing fluid requirements, supplemental albumin may lead to a reduced frequency of pulmonary edema.

▶ Volume depletion produced by the syndrome of inappropriate secretion of antidiuretic hormone in response to aneurysmal SAH can be responsible for vasospasm-related delayed ischemic deficits. Therefore, 3H therapy (hypervolemia, hemodilution, and hypertension) has found proponents all over the world despite its severe complications, i.e., pulmonary edema. It is widely used, but the optimal methods for hemodilution remain to be defined. Mayer and colleagues successfully started to explore this area. In this thorough randomized study of 43 consecutive patients after aneurysmal bleeding, they sought to establish the role of supplemental volume expansion with 5% albumin on the blood volume and sodium levels. They did not find a positive impact of albumin on blood volume, but the supplemental delivery of albumin prevented sodium and fluid losses and limited the amount of total fluid required to maintain CVP at desirable levels. The authors suggested that the use of 5% albumin as a supplemental colloid volume expander significantly lowered the risk of pulmonary edema. However, to finish their excellent work, the authors should consider performing a double-blind, placebo-controlled trial.

R.M. Pluta, M.D., Ph.D.

Cigarette Smoking–induced Increase in the Risk of Symptomatic Vasospasm After Aneurysmal Subarachnoid Hemorrhage

Lasner TM, Weil RJ, Riina HA, et al (Univ of Pennsylvania, Philadelphia; Case Western Reserve Univ, Cleveland, Ohio; Dept of Veterans Affairs, Cleveland, Ohio)

J Neurosurg 87:381–384, 1997   16–12

Objective.—Previous studies have found that in patients with aneurysmal subarachnoid hemorrhage (SAH), the thickness of blood within the basal cistern on CT scan is positively correlated with risk of angiographic vasospasm. Other factors commonly present in patients with aneurysmal SAH—including smoking, hypertension, sentinel hemorrhage, and alcohol abuse—have not been evaluated for associations with symptomatic vasospasm. This prospective study sought to identify additional risk factors for symptomatic vasospasm in patients with SAH.

Methods.—The study included 70 consecutive patients with aneurysmal SAH who did not die before trauma and were not comatose postoperatively. There were 49 women and 26 men (mean age, 50 years; 74% white). All received hypervolemic therapy and nimodipine given as prophylaxis for vasospasm. The occurrence of cerebral vasospasm was suggested by elevation of transcranial Doppler velocities and otherwise unexplained neurologic deterioration 3 to 14 days after SAH. The diagnosis was confirmed by cerebral angiography or clinical improvement after induced hypertension. Potential demographic and clinical risk factors for this complication were evaluated by multivariate logistic regression.

Results.—Sixty-four percent of the patients smoked cigarettes, 46% had hypertension, and 10% were alcohol abusers. Nineteen percent of patients had sentinel bleeding, and 49% had a Fisher grade 3 SAH, i.e., thick subarachnoid clot. Symptomatic vasospasm occurred in 29%. Factors independently associated with this complication included cigarette smoking (odds ratio, 4.7) and Fisher grade 3 SAH (odds ratio, 5.1). The other factors investigated were nonsignificant; they were age, sex, race, hypertension, coronary artery disease, diabetes mellitus, alcohol abuse, illicit drug use, sentinel headache, Hunt and Hess grade, World Federation of Neurological Surgeons grade, and location of the ruptured aneurysm.

Conclusion.—In patients with aneurysmal SAH, cigarette smoking is associated with a more than fourfold increase in the risk of symptomatic vasospasm. This factor is independent of Fisher grade. In contrast to previous reports, young age and clinical grade do not appear to be significant predictors of vasospasm. Knowledge of the risk factors for cerebral vasospasm may help to guide monitoring of individual patients after aneurysmal SAH.

▶ Add this to the long list of deleterious effects of tobacco abuse. This is the first prospective analysis of cigarette smoking as a coexisting risk factor for symptomatic vasospasm. Plaudits to the authors for their diligence on this long-awaited, but not particularly surprising, confirmation.

S.R. Gibbs, M.A., M.D.

Other Intracranial Hemorrhage

Acute Posttraumatic Subdural Hematomas: "Intradural" Computed Tomographic Appearance As a Favorable Prognostic Factor
Domenicucci M, Strzelecki JW, Delfini R (Rome "La Sapienza" Univ)
Neurosurgery 42:51–55, 1998   16–13

Introduction.—The mortality rate for patients having surgical evacuation of acute subdural hematomas is as high as 90%. Early surgery, young patient age, a Glasgow Coma Scale score of more than 5, and the presence of a lucid interval are thought to be factors that are prognostically favorable in the surgical treatment of subdural hematomas.

Methods.—A review was conducted of 31 patients with posttraumatic acute subdural hematoma who submitted to surgery. The interval from their trauma to surgery was less than 4 hours; they had Glasgow Coma Scale scores of less than 8. Preoperative CT images were examined, and patients were divided between those who had preserved subarachnoid spaces and those who did not to determine the immediate and long-term results.

Results.—Intact subarachnoid spaces and the absence of blood in the CSF were seen in the preoperative CT scans of 5 of the 31 patients. A much better postoperative course was found with these patients.

Conclusion.—For patients with acute subdural hematomas, the presence of intact subarachnoid spaces on CT scans may be interpreted as an extremely favorable prognostic factor. The protective effect of the integral visceral membrane of the hematoma—which prevents the diffusion of neurotoxic and vasoactive substances into the subarachnoid spaces—may be part of the reason.

▶ These author's observations and findings are consistent with my personal experience, and they suggest that obliteration of the subarachnoid space in patients who have sustained an acute subdural hematoma portends a poorer neurologic outcome. In trauma, the subarachnoid space may become obliterated by subarachnoid hemorrhage or the direct effect of a massive subdural hematoma. The literature is replete with reports of the neurotoxic and vasoactive effects of extravasated blood; consequently, there is little mystery about poorer neurologic outcomes in patients with subdural hematomas and posttraumatic subarachnoid hemorrhage.

The subarachnoid space allows percolation of a noncompressible but displaceable CSF buffer, and I think of it as the final buffer between the brain and the hemorrhagic insult. I believe that once this buffer has been obliterated, the venous outflow through the subadjacent cortical veins becomes partially or completely obstructed. The arterial inflow remains relatively uncompromised, resulting in severe parenchymal congestion, secondary brain injury, reduced brain compliance, and midline shift that is classically out of proportion to the dimensions of the hematoma.

The classic article by Seelig et al[1] established the "4 hour rule" based upon a series of 82 patients with acute subdural hematoma. The authors found that patients operated upon within 4 hours of injury had a 30% mortality rate, compared with a 90% mortality rate if surgery occurred more than 4 hours after injury. It would be interesting to know what percentage of those operated upon early had a relatively well-preserved subarachnoid space. The radiographic findings of an intact subarachnoid space may be a more accurate prognostic sign than measurements of clot dimensions and/or midline shift because the patient's tolerance of the latter may vary widely, depending upon brain compliance and degree of brain atrophy.

S.R. Gibbs, M.A., M.D.

Reference

1. Seelig JM, Becker DP, Miller JD, et al: Traumatic acute subdural hematoma: Major mortality reduction in comatose patients treated within four hours. *N Engl J Med* 304:1511–1518, 1981.

The Dilemma of Discontinuation of Anticoagulation Therapy for Patients With Intracranial Hemorrhage and Mechanical Heart Valves
Wijdicks EFM, Schievink WI, Brown RD, et al (Mayo Clinic and Found, Rochester, Minn)
Neurosurgery 42:769–773, 1998   16–14

Introduction.—For patients with mechanical heart valves, the risk of anticoagulant–related hemorrhage is approximately 1% per patient per year. When intracranial hemorrhage develops, the decision must be made about whether to continue anticoagulant therapy, which may enlarge the hemorrhagic volume; to restart anticoagulant therapy early, which could cause recurrent hemorrhage; or to reverse anticoagulant therapy, which could place the patient at risk of embolization. Risk factors for embolization may include atrial fibrillation, cage–ball valves in the mitral position, and reduced ventricular function. A large retrospective study evaluated the effects of discontinuing anticoagulation therapy in patients with intracranial hemorrhage and mechanical prosthetic valves.

Patients.—The review included 39 consecutive patients with intracranial hemorrhage and mechanical heart valves. There were 27 men and 12 women, median age 69; 4 patients had a history of transient ischemic attacks or minor stroke. Intracranial hemorrhage developed a median of 6 years after valve replacement. The hemorrhage consisted of acute subdural hematoma in 20 patients, lobar hematoma in 10, subarachnoid hemorrhage in 4, cerebellar hematoma in 3, and basal ganglionic hematoma in 2. There were 13 deaths within 2 days of admission; the remaining 26 patients all received fresh frozen plasma and vitamin K. Acute subdural hematoma was evacuated in 15 patients; clipping of an anterior communicating aneurysm was performed in 1.

Outcomes.—The patients were kept off anticoagulation therapy for a median of 8 days. There were no cases of transient ischemic attack, ischemic stroke, valve thrombosis, or systemic embolization. There were no recurrent intracranial hemorrhages while the patients were in the hospital, after anticoagulation therapy was restarted, or after treatment with antiplatelet agents.

Conclusions.—As long as there is no history of systemic embolization, temporary cessation of anticoagulation therapy appears to be a safe management option for patients with intracranial hemorrhage and mechanical heart valves. Stopping anticoagulants for 1–2 weeks is usually long enough to monitor the evolution of parenchymal hematoma, to perform clipping or coil injection in ruptured aneurysms, or to perform evacuation of an acute subdural hematoma. Afterward, anticoagulation therapy, with or without antiplatelet therapy, can be safely restarted. The authors call for multicenter studies of this issue.

▶ Limited information on treatment of patients who suffer from intracranial hemorrhage and were receiving anticoagulant therapy was available so far. This article dealing with patients with implanted prosthetic heart valves is important, even if the material presented includes a limited number of patients. Weighing the pros and cons in such cases is not an uncommon dilemma and the decisions are quite different. Among 39 surviving patients, there were no thromboembolic complications, despite immediate discontinuation of anticoagulation medication for up to 3 months (median, 8 days). Even in the group of 9 patients, considered by all criteria as a very high risk, none suffered any ill effects. So far, the general attitude in such cases was to suspend the anticoagulant therapy for a rather short time, a few days perhaps. The statement of the authors that temporary reversal of anticoagulant therapy is safe for the group mentioned, brings one to the idea of applying this experience in a much greater number of patients being on anticoagulant therapy for other reasons e.g., atrial fibrillation or venous thrombosis. The limited number of patients is probably insufficient for definite therapeutic guidelines, but suggests the need of further investigations, undertaken perhaps as a multicenter study.

B. Klun, M.D., Ph.D.

17 Brain Tumors

Gliomas

Surgical Treatment of Insular Gliomas
Vanaclocha V, Sáiz–Sapena N, García-Casasola C (Univ of Navarra, Pamplona, Spain)
Acta Neurochir (Wien) 139:1126–1135, 1997   17–1

Introduction.—To prevent tumor progression and to increase the recurrence–free interval, any well–delineated low grade glioma should be removed radically. A higher incidence of recurrences has been associated with the addition of radiotherapy to partial removal compared to radical removal and no radiotherapy. Surgical treatment of gliomas in the insular area are challenging because of the proximity to the internal capsule and the branches of the middle cerebral artery. Intra-operative mapping of the endangered brain areas by electrical stimulation can help avoid induction of neurological sequelae, but the patient must be awake during surgery. A review was conducted of surgical removal of glial tumors of the insular area.

Methods.—There were 23 patients with insular gliomas in a 7–year period. As general anesthesia usually leads to more conservative resections, the surgical procedure was performed under local anesthesia whenever possible to increase the radicality of the resection.

Results.—Complete resection was performed in 20 of 23 patients (86.9%) and subtotal resection in 3 patients (13.1%). There were 2 oligodendrogliomas removed, 5 grade I astrocytomas, 9 grade II, 4 grade III, and 3 grade IV tumors. Five patients had neurological deficits after surgery. Hemiparesis occurred in 4 patients, who recovered about 6 months later, and 1 patient had motor dysphasia that took a week to recover. Malignant change occurred in 2 of the 17 patients operated on for low grade insular gliomas.

Conclusion.—In all patients, complete surgical removal of insular gliomas should be considered and at least attempted. If there is good anatomical knowledge and an experienced team available, Sylvian gliomas can be removed safely. Wider resection is achieved when the procedure is performed under local anesthesia, resulting in good control of the possible neurological deficits that might appear. Long–term survival is better with a wide removal in comparison to subtotal removal and radiotherapy.

▶ Because of its proximity to such eloquent and functional structures as the internal capsule, centrum semiovale and lenticulostriate arteries, the insular region has been a neurosurgical and anatomical taboo—a place out of bounds, untouchable and interdicted for routine interventions even for the more experienced neurosurgeon. For many decades, we have been discouraged from senior teaching staff to not act surgically, giving the green light only to more conservative procedures, such as stereotactic biopsies and lately radiosurgery. The present authors offer a more provocative approach to deep insular gliomas, accomplishing a 86.9% complete resection, thus preventing tumor progression and malignization and obtaining longer recurrence-free intervals. Special importance is given to a functional approach, using intra-operative mapping by electrical stimulation on fully awake and cooperative patients, intra-operative ultrasound, and observation for minimal signs of neurological deficits appearance. This approach has made it possible for more experienced surgical teams to encourage a more aggressive surgical removal of insular gliomas.

R. Marino Jr., M.D.

Preoperative Activation and Intraoperative Stimulation of Language-related Areas in Patients With Glioma
Herholz K, Reulen H-J, von Stockhausen H-M, et al (Max-Planck-Institut and Neurologische Universitätsklinik, Köln, Germany; Ludwig-Maximilians-Universität, München, Germany)
Neurosurgery 41:1253–1262, 1997   17–2

Background.—Operating on gliomas close to language-related regions in dominant inferior frontal or superior temporal cortex is associated with a high risk of postoperative aphasia. Intraoperative stimulation methods for tailoring the extent of resection and decreasing this risk can be performed. The accuracy of preoperative localization of language-related cortex by MRI-guided positron emission tomography (PET) was assessed.

Methods.—Eight patients, aged 25–47 years, were studied. All had gliomas in the left dominant hemisphere. Preoperative MRI-guided PET and intraoperative electric stimulation of the cortex were performed.

Findings.—More intense and better-lateralized local increases in cerebral blood flow in the PET examination were elicited by a verb-generation task than by a naming task. For the verb-generation task, preoperative and intraoperative findings were significantly correlated. Cerebral blood flow increases during preoperative activation were significantly higher in cortical sites with aphasic disturbance during electric stimulation than in sites without intraoperative language impairment. Areas with cerebral blood flow increases exceeding an optimal threshold had a sensitivity and specificity of 73% and 81%, respectively, in predicting aphasic disturbance during intraoperative stimulation.

Conclusion.—With further technical improvements, language function imaging may become a preoperative diagnostic tool in patients with tumors close to language-related brain structures. Further research is needed to determine whether preoperative activation data may be acccurate enough to obviate the need for intraoperative stimulation.

▶ In contrast with other organs, the brain has an exquisite interdependence of physiology and topography, in which successful surgery for a neoplasm provides complete tumoral resection combined with optimal preservation of normal tissue surrounding the tumor. Our times have witnessed an impressive development of brain imaging and sophisticated methods of functional brain localization. The work of Herholz et al. is a good example of high technology used to illuminate the surgical act with precise information to shield, in this case, language-related areas near the tumor.

Rather than setting a new standard of technological intervention, the results of this study provide a wealth of extremely useful data for further research into the complex issue of clear-cut delimitation of tumor boundaries and normal brain tissue. As the effective spatial resolution of PET is about 10 mm, this method is still far from optimal. In the case of nervous tissue, it should be less than 1 mm. Also, the results of neuroimaging are still somewhat at variance with the information obtained by electric stimulation, producing a significative number of false positives and false negatives.

The beauty of this study lies in the confluence of an array of methods designed to circumscribe the language areas by imaging studies, electrophysiologic recording, and ingenious grammatical tasks. Each of these methods has splendid perspectives for improvement. Also, a feasible perspective can be found in the development of computer software for processing all gathered information to give an unambiguous plane of the functional areas in a given patient.

J. Sotelo, M.D.

Meningiomas

Surgical Management of Meningiomas Originating in Meckel's Cave
Samii M, Carvalho GA, Tatagiba M, et al (Nordstadt Hosp, Hannover, Germany)
Neurosurgery 41:767–775, 1997   17–3

Introduction.—Approximately 1% of all intracranial meningiomas are accounted for by primary Meckel's cave meningiomas. At the time of diagnosis, they may be confined to the area of Meckel's cave, but they may grow beyond the area, if left unrecognized, and extend into the middle and posterior fossae, the cavernous sinus, the internal carotid artery, and the basal cranial nerves. There is no general agreement about the approaches of choice for treating these tumors. Primary Meckel's cave meningiomas were reclassified according to tumor location and extension. A retrospective review was conducted to study the characteristics of Meckel's cave meningiomas and to determine the impact of this new classification on the surgical management of these lesions and the outcomes of the patients.

Methods.—There were 21 patients with meningiomas originating in Meckel's cave in this retrospective analysis of all meningiomas involving the cranial base. Tumors were classified according to the tumor extension into 4 different types. Type I tumors were mainly confined to Meckel's cave. Type II tumors were defined as Meckel's cave meningiomas with extension into the middle fossa. Type III tumors extended into the posterior fossa. Type IV tumors extended into both middle and posterior fossae.

Results.—Regardless of tumor type, trigeminal neuralgia resolved in all patients. Only in type III meningiomas did trigeminal hypesthesia show postoperative improvement. Total removal without further morbidity was frequently achieved in types I and III. The extent of tumor extirpation was limited in some patients by cavernous sinus infiltration, especially in types II and IV.

Conclusion.—A good prognosis was seen with types I, II, and III Meckel's cave meningiomas. Very good outcomes were achieved in most cases. Without further morbidity and with postoperative improvement of the preexisting symptoms, radical tumor removal can usually be achieved, particularly in tumor types I and III. Type IV meningiomas, however, are usually only resected subtotally. A high risk of additional morbidity may result from surgery in such instances, particularly to the third, fourth, and fifth cranial nerves. In all tumor types, the postoperative outcome regarding facial pain is usually very good. In most patients, trigeminal hypesthesia may persist after tumor removal.

▶ Vigilance in the evaluation of trigeminal neuralgia and atypical face pain will rarely reveal a lesion in the region of the trigeminal nerve; a minority of these lesions will be meningiomas. This generous series supports 6 relatively intuitive patterns of tumor growth; these patterns dictate various surgical approaches. I have recently grown fond of the zygomatic-subtemporal approach to the Gasserian ganglion, the cavernous sinus for lesions with a middle fossa component with and without cavernous sinus involvement (author's types I, II, III (cavernous sinus), IV, and V (cavernous sinus). I find the exposure wide and shallow and the retraction minimal. This technique, however, is not to the exclusion of the transsylvian approach, as facility with multiple exposures of the same area is important for individualization of the approach to various bodies, tails and tongues of the target lesion.

C.P. Bondurant, M.D.

Factors Associated With Survival in Patients With Meningioma

McCarthy BJ, Davis FG, Freels S, et al (Univ of Illinois, Chicago; Harvard Med School, Boston; Chicago Inst of Neurosurgery and Neuroresearch; et al)
J Neurosurg 88:831–839, 1998   17–4

Introduction.—Recent studies have suggested that survival from meningioma may be better in women than in men. National Cancer Data Base (NCDB) data were analyzed to identify factors affecting survival in patients with meningioma.

Methods.—The tumors were reported by approximately 1,000 hospitals participating in the American College of Surgeons tumor registry program. The investigators analyzed data on more than 9,000 cases of meningioma diagnosed in 2 periods: 1985–1988 and 1990–1992. A proportional hazards model was used to identify factors affecting survival.

Results.—Overall 5-year survival was 69%. Survival was 81% for patients aged 21–64 years, compared with 56% for those aged 65 years or older. Overall 5-year survival was 70% for patients with benign tumors, 75% for patients with atypical meningiomas, and 55% for those with malignant meningiomas. For benign tumors, factors significantly associated with survival included age at diagnosis, tumor size, surgical treatment, hospital type, and radiation therapy. For malignant tumors, the significant factors were age at diagnosis, surgical treatment, and radiation therapy. With all types of treatment, 5-year symptom recurrence rate was 19% for patients with benign tumors vs. 32% for those with malignant tumors. The 5-year tumor recurrence rate after complete removal of a benign tumor was 20.5%.

Conclusion.—This study provides the most complete data to date on survival from meningioma in the United States. The NCDB, though not population based, can provide useful information on patient characteristics and treatments for benign and malignant brain tumors. Age is a significant predictor of mortality in all types of melanomas; however, sex is not significant after adjustment for other factors by multivariate analyses.

▶ In this article, the authors analyzed prognostic factors in patients with meningiomas selected using the International Classification of Diseases for Oncology codes 9530–9537. They thus obtained 8,891 benign meningiomas, 165 atypical meningiomas, and 771 malignant meningiomas. One of the major findings was that younger patients fared better than older ones. However, in the classification used, the youngest age group is from 0–44 years. It would have been much more interesting to separate pediatric cases from adult cases. Indeed, pediatric tumors are, in general, very different from adult ones.

The survival rates were better for patients with benign or atypical meningiomas, as compared with those with malignant meningiomas. For the latter group, it was found that those undergoing surgery, but not receiving radiation therapy, did significantly better than all other groups. This is extremely surprising and in opposition to well-conducted studies showing that adjuvant radiation therapy improves the outcome for malignant meningiomas. The same is true for the finding that in benign meningiomas, no significant differences in survival rates were found for those who underwent partial resections with or without radiation therapy. Indeed, many groups have published the fact that radiation therapy improves the outcome of partially resected benign meningiomas. It is not surprising to find that the 5-year survival rate was better after surgery alone than after radiation therapy alone, but it is extremely surprising to find that the survival rate was worse in those with total compared with partial surgical resection.

In the discussion section, the authors admit that there might have been misclassifications and that they could not validate the completeness and quality of clinical data. In my opinion, this means that this type of study is useless for the clinician who needs clear guidelines for the treatment of meningiomas. These tumors must be completely resected, whenever possible, which means that the resection must include the dural attachment, including a margin of normal dura and any infiltrated bone. Some skull base meningiomas, particularly in the cavernous sinus, cannot be completely removed and must be closely followed and radiation therapy offered when the tumor progresses. Malignant meningiomas should receive adjuvant radiotherapy whatever the extent of resection.

Atypical meningiomas remain a problem and should be immediately radiated if incompletely resected; they should be very closely followed, even if the resection has been complete. For small meningiomas—for example, those in the cavernous sinus—stereotactic radiotherapy offers very promising prospectives.

N. de Tribolet, M.D.

Pituitary Tumors

Transcranial Epidural Approach to Pituitary Tumors Extending Beyond the Sella
Dolenc VV (Univ Med Ctr, Ljubljana, Slovenia)
Neurosurgery 41:542–552, 1997   17–5

Introduction.—Pressure is exerted on to the surrounding structures by pituitary tumors that grow to the extent of the volume of the sella. Traditionally, such tumors were operated on through the transphenoidal and/or transcranial approach, but this resulted in complications, such as pneumatocephalus, cerebrospinal fluid leak, mechanical lesions of the internal carotid artery or visual apparatus, and failure to remove the tumor completely. A new approach through the triangular windows avoided these complications. Results of the classical approach were compared with the new approach in a group of patients with pituitary tumors extending into the parasellar and other regions beyond the sella.

Methods.—In a 15–year period, 210 patients who had pituitary tumors extending into the parasellar and other regions beyond the sella were operated on using the transcranial approach. Using central cranial base specimens, the anatomic relationships of the sellar and parasellar regions were studied. After careful study of the triangles of the lateral wall of the cavernous sinus, including anteromedial, paramedial, and Parkinson's triangle, as well as practical experience dealing with tumors in the region, the use of the triangular windows became the key access to the pituitary tumors in the enlarged sella and in the neighboring areas.

Results.—Using the classical approach in 120 patients, complete removal was achieved in 66.5%. In 8% of these patients, postoperative cerebrospinal fluid leak occurred. In 6%, visual function was impaired. The new approach was used on 90 patients, and a complete excision was achieved in 92.5% of these patients. Only 1 patient had postoperative impairment of the visual function, and only 1 other patient had cerebrospinal fluid leak. For 26% of the patients in the classical approach group, postoperative improvement of the visual function was achieved, whereas 52% of the patients in the new approach had improvement. No mortality was found in either group.

Conclusion.—The previous transcranial approach is inferior to the new approach to pituitary tumors extending beyond the sella (regarding the rate of completeness of the tumor resection). By preserving intact the diaphragm sellae and the dura covering the central cranial base around the sella, the risks of surgical complications can be avoided using the new approach. Endocrinological disorders were not addressed by this approach, nor was the functional efficacy of surgical treatment relating to hormones.

▶ The author describes a novel, original and well-conceived approach to the sella and parasellar regions through the cavernous sinus, creatively using the anatomical corridors and various triangles of the cavernous sinus structures. This technique is a logical extension of Dolenc's concepts and techniques, which have contributed so much to cranial base microsurgery. However, this approach is extremely demanding technically, reserved only for those familiar with the intricate anatomy of the cavernous sinus and with the pterional-orbito-clinoidal craniotomy approach. It was not designed for the general practitioner of neurosurgery, since it should be considered a very aggressive surgical approach, even for resourceful neurosurgeons, who should carefully analyze *when* it is appropriate to use it as an alternative to classical transcranial intradural approach, transphenoidal approach or radiation therapy in dealing with residual and/or recurrent pituitary tumors.

The aim of this transcavernous approach is to provide a better possibility for the removal of invasive tumors located beyond the borders of the sella and to lower the morbidity of these lesions. However, authors with the larger series of pituitary tumors know of the almost impossible task in eliminating or performing a "total" removal of an invasive or "malignant" pituitary adenoma, since they microscopically invade dural structures and the surrounding tissues. Only an extensive study of patients with hyperactive endocrine syndromes along with their pituitary tumors could provide the necessary markers for the assumption of their total removal, since tumors on the lateral aspects of the contralateral internal carotid artery are impossible to remove by this approach, as related by the author in this article. This is an important contribution. Dolenc once again demonstrates that the cavernous sinus is not an off-limit structure as some of us were taught during our training programs.

R. Marino Jr., M.D.

Surgical Technique

The Role of Neuroendoscopy in the Treatment of Pineal Region Tumors
Robinson S, Cohen AR (Rainbow Babies and Childrens Hosp, Cleveland, Ohio; Case Western Reserve Univ, Cleveland, Ohio)
Surg Neurol 48:360–367, 1997   17–6

Introduction.—There is still controversy regarding the optimal treatment for pineal tumors and the often associated noncommunicating hydrocephalus. At the time of presentation, about 90% of patients with pineal region tumors have hydrocephalus. An external ventricular drain or a ventriculoperitoneal shunt has traditionally been used to control hydrocephalus, but the incidence of its malfunction is significant. An alternative surgical strategy allows treatment of the symptomatic hydrocephalus as well as safe tumor biopsy. This technique for the initial management of patients with pineal region neoplasms and symptomatic hydrocephalus was described.

Technique.—Through a single precoronal burr hole, endoscopic third ventriculostomy and, if possible, tumor biopsy is performed. The standard coronal burr hole for a third ventriculostomy is in the midpupillary line. This provides a direct approach to the floor of the third ventricle. The burr hole is moved anteriorly when third ventriculostomy is combined with biopsy (Fig 1). A balloon catheter is inserted through a working channel of the endoscope in the floor of the third ventricle and is repeatedly inflated and deflated to enlarge the fenestration.

Cases.—Four patients with hydrocephalus and tumors of the pineal region were treated by this technique and in all instances, noncommunicating hydrocephalus was controlled by the third ventriculostomy without the need for ventricular shunt placement. There was successful biopsy endoscopically in 3 of the 4 tumors, a mixed malignant germ cell tumor, an epidermoid tumor, and a low-grade astrocytoma of the midbrain. No biopsy was performed on a patient with a posterior third ventricular tumor whose hydrocephalus was controlled by endoscopic third ventriculostomy. His tumor, a germinoma, was removed via an anterior transcallosal craniotomy. No operative complications were found.

Conclusion.—Without the need for ventricular drainage or shunting, formal tumor resection can be performed nonemergently when indicated.

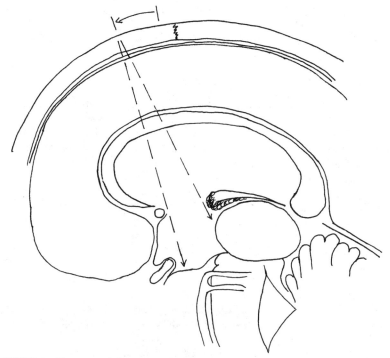

FIGURE 1.—Trajectory: The standard coronal burr hole for a third ventriculostomy is in the midpupillary line, just anterior to the coronal suture. This trajectory provides a direct approach through the foramen of Monro to the floor of the third ventricle, but a poor approach to the posterior third ventricle. When third ventriculostomy is combined with biopsy of a pineal region mass, the burr hole is moved anteriorly, using the preoperative sagittal MRI as a guide. This allows a trajectory to both the floor of the third ventricle and to the posterior third ventricle. (Reprinted by permission of the publisher from Robinson S, Cohen AR: The role of neuroendoscopy in the treatment of pineal region tumors. *Surg Neurol* 48:360–367, copyright 1997 by Elsevier Science Inc.)

Patients with neoplasms of the pineal region and symptomatic hydrocephalus can be safely and minimally managed with neuroendoscopy.

▶ The authors report endoscopic third ventriculostomy surgical techniques and simultaneous performance of endoscopic biopsies of pineal region neoplasms for obstructive hydrocephalus caused by pineal region tumors in 4 patients. For this type of obstructive hydrocephalus, endoscopic third ventriculostomy is the procedure of choice. Attempting the simultaneous biopsy of a pineal tumor is attractive for planning future treatment of a neoplasm. When endoscopic biopsy is not feasible in the setting of a third ventriculostomy, we do a stereotactic needle biopsy of a neoplasm in the same setting or as a second-stage surgery. In addition to the tumor biopsy, the cystic nature of a tumor can be fenestrated into the ventricular system. In selecting a precise burr hole site for this purpose, stereotactic techniques can be beneficial.

H.D. Jho, M.D., Ph.D.

Cranioplasty With Autogenous Autoclaved Calvarial Bone Flap in the Cases of Tumoural Invasion

Vanaclocha V, Sáiz-Sapena N, García-Casasola C, et al (Univ of Navarra, Pamplona, Spain)
Acta Neurochir (Wien) 139:970–976, 1997   17–7

Background.—Ideally, bone flaps raised during craniotomy are replaced at the end of the procedure. However, because of the risk of tumor recurrence, flaps invaded by tumor cells cannot be replaced. Outcomes of bone flap autoclaving to avoid the risk of tumor recurrence were analyzed.

Methods.—Sixty-two patients underwent autoclaving of the bone flap during craniotomy between 1989 and 1995. Thirty-five patients had meningiomas; 16, bone tumors; 5, metastases; and 8, scalp tumors. Infiltrated bone flaps were removed, cleaned, autoclaved for 20 minutes at 134° C and 1 kg/cm^2, and reimplanted. Follow-up ranged from 10 to 58 months. Skull radiographs and photographs were obtained at follow-up visits, and clinical examinations were performed. When needed, a CT scan was done to determine bone flap thickness.

Findings.—Follow-up radiographs showed partial resorption in 19.3% of the patients. Loss of thickness in another 56.4% was noted on CT. The external aspect remained unchanged in all patients. Biopsies obtained at a repeat surgical procedure in 6 patients showed newly formed bone partly repopulated by osteocytes and retaining areas of sequestered bone.

Conclusions.—Autoclaved bone replaced in direct contact with living bone is repopulated gradually with osteocytes. Thus, cranial vault autoclaved autologous bone flap is a good alternative in patients with bone flaps that are invaded by tumor cells but not destroyed.

▶ A number of companies produce a custom cranioplasty product. Some of these products are made of synthetic material and others of biometallic mesh. These are fine products, and, in my experience, "they fit like a glove." However, these implants are relatively expensive and they require a second surgical procedure. To prevent a second procedure, I have made an alginate mold of the involved bone and cast a methylmethacrylate implant that was implanted at the same surgery.

I am certain many neurosurgeons have developed creative solutions to this problem, and some may have thought about the possibility presented in this article, but uncertainty of the outcome may have prevented them from trying it. The authors present their favorable experience with a technique, and outcome that is encouraging. Their technique, based upon the repopulation and remodeling of denatured bone matrix, is not a new concept; in fact, in the orthopedic literature this is a time-tested technique used for limb salvage in resection of skeletal tumors.[1-3]

This appears to be a safe, inexpensive, convenient, and effective solution for cranioplasty in cases with nondestructive tumor involvement of the calvarium. Because some resorption of the flap did occur in some cases, it may be best to reserve this technique for areas other than the forehead.

Also, since the osteogenicity of the flap is lost in autoclaving, it would be interesting to evaluate treatment of the devitalized bone matrix with bone morphogenic protein and/or bone-derived growth factor to expedite the repopulation of osteocytes and prevent resorption.

S.R. Gibbs, M.A., M.D.

References

1. Kriecbergs A, Köhler P: Diaphyseal reconstruction by autoclaved bone. *Acta Orthop Scand* 58:61–67, 1987.
2. Harrington KD, Johnston JO, Kaufer HN, et al: Limb salvage and prosthetic joint reconstruction for low-grade and selected high-grade sarcomas of bone after wide resection and replacement by autoclaved autogenic graft. *Clin Orthop* 211:180–214, 1986.
3. Köhler P, Kriecbergs A: Chondrosarcoma treated by reimplantation of resected bone after autoclaving and supplementation with allogenic bone matrix: A case report. *Clin Orthop* 294:281–284, 1993.

Tumor Devascularization by Intratumoral Ethanol Injection During Surgery: Technical Note
Lonser RR, Heiss JD, Oldfield EH (Natl Inst of Neurological Disorders and Stroke, Bethesda, Md)
J Neurosurg 88:923–924, 1998   17–8

Background.—Selective catheterization of tumor vessels for delivery of occlusive materials has led to preoperative reductions in the vascularity of tumors. The authors' experience with percutaneous infusion of vertebral hemangiomas and other vascular lesions has suggested that direct injection of ethanol could produce rapid tumor devascularization, thus reducing bleeding and facilitating surgical resection. This study assessed the effects of intratumoral ethanol injection on tumor hemostasis and resectability.

Methods.—The study included 4 patients undergoing surgery for CNS neoplasms. There were 3 spinal epidural and 1 cerebellar neoplasm. Partial intra-arterial embolization was performed before surgery in 1 case. The tumors were injected with dehydrated absolute ethanol, 1 mL, using a tuberculin syringe. Cotton patties were used to minimize ethanol leakage and contact with normal tissues. A 28-gauge needle, with injection in increments of 0.1–0.2 mL, was used to promote retention of ethanol in the tumor and to limit retrograde leakage. Tumor blanching was used as the end point for injection at a specific site.

Results.—Ethanol injection produced immediate and complete regional tumor devascularization in all 4 cases. Noninjected parts of the tumor bled actively during excision; when these regions were injected with ethanol, active bleeding stopped and the lesion blanched. After injection, the tissues became soft, even semiliquid, thus making the resection easier and more effective. There were no complications of ethanol injection.

Conclusion.—Directly injecting small amounts of ethanol into CNS tumors produces incremental tumor devascularization. This procedure results in immediate and complete devascularization of injected regions, thus reducing intratumoral bleeding and promoting ease and effectiveness of resection. Precautions must be taken to keep absolute ethanol from coming into contact with normal tissues because it is neurotoxic.

▶ Pesky bleeding is predictable with some types of tumors in the CNS, and, in some cases, these tumors may be amenable to preoperative embolization, although this rarely completely devascularizes a tumor. Of course, there are surgical strategies for devascularizing, but some still require an "attack and pack" approach to resection to minimize blood loss. Punctilious ethanol has been used as a devascularizing and sclerosing agent for intra-abdominal tumors and endocrine tissues; however, until this report, I am not aware of any description of its direct intraoperative use in neurosurgery. I have used this technique recently on several occasions, and I have found that it works quite well. Because dehydrated absolute ethyl alcohol is inexpensive and easily accessible, this technique should become part of the neurosurgeon's hemostasis armamentarium for highly vascular tumors that are incompletely embolized and for patients with circumstances that preclude preoperative embolization. As the authors have cautioned, absolute ethanol is neurotoxic. They have described several techniques for preventing its contact with normal tissue.

S.R. Gibbs, M.A., M.D.

Miscellaneous Tumors

Brainstem Tolerance to Conformal Radiotherapy of Skull Base Tumors
Debus J, Hug EB, Liebsch NJ, et al (Harvard Cyclotron Lab, Cambridge, Mass; Univ of Heidelberg, Germany)
Int J Radiat Oncol Biol Phys 39:967–975, 1997   17–9

Background.—With new conformal radiation techniques, it is possible to escalate the radiation dose to the target while reducing the dose to critical structures nearby. For patients with tumors of the head and neck and skull base, significant radiation may be delivered to the brainstem during radiation therapy. Though several studies have looked at the ability of the cervical spinal cord to tolerate radiation, none has examined tolerance by the brainstem. Patients receiving high-dose conformal radiation therapy for tumors of the skull base were studied to determine long-term incidence of brainstem toxicity.

Methods.—The analysis included 367 patients with skull base tumors— 195 chordomas and 172 chondrosarcomas—treated over a 21-year period. All patients received combined megavoltage photon and 160 meV proton radiotherapy. Three-dimensional treatment planning was done, target volumes were delineated, and dose distributions to critical nontarget structures and dose-volume histograms were calculated. The average radiation dose per fraction was 1.8 Gy or Cobalt Gray Equivalent (CGE). Mean prescribed dose to the target was 68 CGE. No patient received a radiation dose to the brainstem surface of greater than 64 CGE, or 53 CGE to the brainstem center. The patients were followed for an average of 42.5 months.

Results.—The rate of brainstem toxicity attributable to treatment was 4.6%, with 3 patients dying of these brainstem effects. The actuarial rate of freedom from high-grade toxicity was 94% at 5 years and 88% at 10 years. The maximum radiation dose to the brainstem was significantly associated with the risk of brainstem toxicity. Other factors increasing toxicity risk were volume of brainstem receiving 50 CGE or more, 55 CGE or more, and 60 CGE or more; the number of surgical procedures performed; and the presence of diabetes or high blood pressure. Independent prognostic factors on multivariate analysis were number of surgical procedures performed, brainstem volume receiving 60 CGE, and prevalence of diabetes.

Conclusions.—In patients receiving conformal radiation therapy for tumors of the skull base, the brainstem's ability to tolerate radiation depends more on the tissue volume included in high-dose regions than on the maximum dose to the brainstem alone. Certain predisposing factors and a history of multiple surgical procedures also affect brainstem tolerance of radiation. Future trials of high-dose conformal radiation therapy should consider volume constraints to the brainstem and other normal structures. More research is needed to identify factors associated with increased risk of radiation toxicity.

▶ Very few studies have addressed the problem of brainstem tolerance to radiotherapy. Debus et al. report a very large experience (367 patients) of conformal radiotherapy for skull base tumors (chordomas, chondrosarcomas). Unfortunately, these series include patients with very short follow–up (6 months) compared to the mean delay of onset for radiation–induced brainstem toxicity (17 months, range, 4.5–92 months).

Nevertheless, the occurrence of severe brainstem injury (5.5%) is not rare with 1% of death. One can suspect this rate to be higher in this population with a minimum follow–up of more than 92 months (actuarial rate of survival free of high–grade toxicity is 88% at 10 years).

The authors have identified risk factors for brainstem toxicity, including maximum dose to the brainstem, volume of brainstem receiving more than 50 CGE, number of surgical procedures, prevalence of diabetes or high blood pressure.

This unique article offers 2 very important conclusions. The identification of risk factors must be allowed, to avoid a part of these complications, and to help predict the individual risk of such complications. The second conclusion is that the radiosurgery with gamma knife allowing a dramatic reduction in the risk of brainstem injury (no death reported) when treating skull base tumors must be considered the first intention.

If the toxicity of radiotherapy is acceptable for malignant lesions such as chondrosarcomas, then the aim is to treat small, benign, well demarcated tumors of the skull base like brainstem injury (lethal or not) and carcinogenesis must be kept in mind.

We believe that conformal radiotherapy (and or stereotactic radiotherapy) must not be considered for benign, skull base lesions out of very special cases, contradicting radiosurgery and microsurgery with demonstrated evolution.

J. Regis, M.D.

Brain Tumor and Pregnancy

Isla A, Alvarez F, Gonzalez A, et al (Hosp "La Paz," Madrid)
Obstet Gynecol 89:19–23, 1997   17–10

Background.—Previous reports have described women in whom brain tumors were diagnosed during pregnancy. Such cases have been considered uncommon. Seven women with neurologic symptoms related to brain tumors during pregnancy were reported.

Patients.—The 7 patients were identified from a 12-year series of 126,413 pregnancies. The presenting symptoms consisted of focal seizures in 3 patients, neurologic signs in 2, symptoms of intracranial hypertension in 1, and sudden hemorrhage in 1. The patients' mean age was 32. Computed tomography, MRI, or both were performed in every case.

Outcomes.—Six patients were delivered of a viable fetus without complications; one had a miscarriage. Surgery was performed in 6 patients. The seventh, who had neuroradiologic evidence of a fast-growing brainstem glioma, was managed with radiotherapy. This patient died 3 months after delivery of a healthy infant. The histologic diagnoses in the 6 surgical patients were meningioma in 2, ependymoma in 2, and low-grade astrocytoma in 2, with one of the latter having multiple ependymomas. One patient with meningioma and 1 with astrocytoma underwent estrogen and progesterone receptor studies, which were positive in both cases.

Conclusions.—Brain tumors during pregnancy are rare but may be related to pregnancy hormones. The rate of tumor growth may be mediated through specific intracellular receptors. Treatment should be individualized. Surgery may be deferred if the tumor is diagnosed during the first half of gestation and if the tumor is a small one without neurologic signs. If the tumor is diagnosed during the second half of gestation, corticosteroids can be used to accelerate fetal maturation, and the patient can undergo early cesarean section followed by brain surgery.

▶ A variety of host factors have been associated with the development and progression of tumors in the CNS. Cushing and Eisenhardt,[1] in their famous treatise on meningiomas, were the first to describe a provocative relationship between pregnancy and the rapid progression of neurologic symptoms in women with meningiomas. Since the recognition of this intercurrent relationship, the hormonal milieu during pregnancy and during the menstrual cycle has been implicated and, not surprisingly, investigations have revealed hormonal receptors for a variety of CNS tumors. Although brain tumors in pregnancy are rare, several practical points may be gleaned from this work.

Neurodiagnostic imaging may proceed as usual with MRI or CT (with shielding of the fetus). Iodinated contrast agents are physiologically inert and reportedly pose little risk to the fetus; although good material and fetal hydration are essential.[2] The timing of craniotomy must be individualized; it depends upon the size of the tumor and gestational duration at presentation, the severity of neurologic symptoms, and the response to corticosteroid therapy. Corticosteroid therapy may reduce maternal tumorigenic cerebral edema, and it may also precociously stimulate the fetal lecithin-sphingomyelin index (a marker for lung maturation),[3] but long-term use—especially in the third trimester—may cause fetal adrenal suppression and resultant neonatal hypoadrenalism.[3] Anticonvulsants may be administered to gravid patients who are at high risk for seizures and at a relatively low risk for deleterious effects; however, blood levels should be monitored closely throughout the pregnancy and puerperium as the changes in serum-binding proteins will change the unbound fraction of an anticonvulsant.[4]

Although the occurrence of CNS tumors during pregnancy has been well reviewed by Roelvink et al.,[5] our best understanding of the epidemiology and intercurrent effects of pregnancy, by tumor type, will only be revealed through a large, collective, multi-institutional data set. Internet collaboration holds this potential.

S.R. Gibbs, M.A., M.D.

References

1. Cushing H, Eisenhardt L: *Meningiomas: Their Classification, Regional Behavior, Life History, and Surgical End Result.* Springfield, Ill, Charles C. Thomas, 1938.
2. Dalessio DJ: Neurologic diseases, in Burrow CN, Ferris TF (eds): *Medical Complications During Pregnancy.* Philadelphia, WB Saunders, 1982, pp 435–447.
3. Biggs JSG, Allan JA: Medication and pregnancy. *Drugs* 21:69–75, 1981.
4. Kochenour N, Emery MG, Sawehuk RJ: Phenytoin metabolism in pregnancy. *Obstet Gynecol* 56:577–582, 1980.
5. Roelvink NC, Kamphorst W, van Alphen HAM, et al: Pregnancy-related primary brain and spinal tumors. *Arch Neurol* 44(2):209–215, 1987.

Ependymoma: Results, Prognostic Factors and Treatment Recommendations
McLaughlin MP, Marcus RB Jr, Buatti JM, et al (Univ of Florida, Gainesville)
Int J Radiat Oncol Biol Phys 40:845–850, 1998   17–11

Purpose.—Postoperative radiotherapy improves survival in patients with ependymomas. However, there is disagreement about whether treatment should include craniospinal, whole brain, or partial brain irradiation. The prognostic factors are also unclear. A 23-year experience with postoperative radiotherapy for the treatment of ependymomas was reviewed.

Methods.—The experience included 41 patients with ependymomas who were receiving postoperative radiotherapy with curative intent. The patients were 23 children and 18 adults; most of the younger children but relatively few of the adult patients had high-grade tumors. All patients were free of metastases outside the CNS. The ependymomas were supratentorial in 10 patients, infratentorial in 22, and in the spinal cord in 9. Surgery, consisting of stereotactic biopsy, subtotal resection, or gross total resection, was performed in all patients. Craniospinal radiotherapy was administered to most patients with high-grade lesions, with less-extensive irradiation for those patients with low-grade lesions. For patients with spinal cord ependymomas, partial spine or whole spine irradiation was given.

Results.—Twenty-one of the 32 intracranial tumors recurred at the primary tumor site. There were no recurrent spinal cord tumors. Ten-year overall survival was 51%, with relapse-free survival of 46%. Survival was 100% for patients with spinal cord tumors, 45% for those with infratentorial tumors, and 20% for those with supratentorial tumors. Tumor site was the only factor significantly related to survival on multivariate analysis. None of the other factors evaluated—including grade, sex, age, duration of symptoms, extent of resection, primary tumor dose, extent of treatment field, interval between surgery and radiotherapy, and days of radiotherapy—was significant.

Conclusions.—The primary tumor site is the main site of treatment failure in patients with ependymomas, the results suggest. The authors recommend partial brain fields for the treatment of all supratentorial and low-grade infratentorial tumors. Spinal cord ependymomas can be treated with limited fields, resulting in excellent tumor control and low complication rates. The only patients who need craniospinal irradiation are those with radiologic or pathologic evidence of craniospinal seeding.

▶ The term *ependymoma* raises prognostic uncertainty regardless of histological grade. The most important factor seems to be the location of the primary tumor, with a clearly-defined gradient in which supratentorial tumors carry the worst prediction, followed by those located in the infratentorial area and spinal cord; the latter are curable in almost all cases. The article by McLaughlin et al. helps to delineate the profiles and clinical outcome of ependymomas. From this long-term follow up a clear image of the course of ependymomas after optimal treatment can be drawn: for supratentorial tumors, recurrence at the primary site after surgery and radiotherapy is the rule; long-term survival, in spite of surgical salvage, is only around 20%; more than half of recurrences take place within the first 2 years after treatment. Infratentorial lesions present a somewhat less depressing perspective: half of patients recover. In contrast, all patients with spinal cord ependymoma survive, with splendid functional recovery in those cases in which the tumor was located in the cauda equina. Along the neuraxis, the lower location of ependymoma has the better prognosis, and the upper location has the less favorable. The site of the tumor seems to be far more influential than the histological characteristics of neoplastic grade, mainly because of surgical accessibility for radical excision. As with other neoplasms of the nervous system, tumor infiltration of brain parenchyma and recurrence after surgery and radiotherapy continue to represent the principal problems of ependymomas.

J. Sotelo, M.D.

Benign Skull Lesions
Tucker WS, Nasser-Sharif FJ (Univ of Toronto)
Can J Surg 40:449–455, 1997   17–12

Background.—Little information is available on the demographics and characteristics of patients with benign skull lesions. The 10–year experience of 4 neurosurgeons was reviewed to provide this information.

Methods and Findings.—Thirty-one patients were included. Twenty-five were women. A total of 32 lesions were excised. Mean patient age was 41.9 years. Sixty-three percent of the tumors were osteomas. The parietal bone was the most common location. Most patients with calvarial tumors had no neurologic symptoms. Plain skull radiography and computed tomography were useful diagnostic studies. Seven patients underwent nuclear bone scanning, and all had craniectomy, most with cranioplasty. Three patients had new neurologic symptoms after surgery. Symptom resolution was incomplete in 1 patient.

Conclusions.—Benign skull lesions require neurosurgical intervention. Surgical excision can confirm the diagnosis, improve cosmesis, and slow the progression of neurologic dysfunction. Primary care physicians need to be able to recognize such lesions and refer patients to the surgeon for appropriate treatment.

▶ Benign lesions are rare in the neurosurgical practice. This valuable study of 31 patients with benign skull lesions brings to our attention those rare but usually rewarding lesions. Craniotomy proved safe and curative (very low morbidity, no mortality and only 1 recurrence) for treatment of those tumors. Analysis of the clinical data from one center collected for 10 years by 4 neurosurgeons confirmed the known incidence and distribution of the lesions. The most common diagnosis was a parieto-frontal osteoma in women about 40 years old. Other rare lesions, such as intraostial meningiomas, hemangiomas, osteoid osteoma, eosinophilic granuloma, sinus mucocoele and hyperthrophic bone, were also treated successfully with excision and acrylic cranioplasty. As expected, neurological deficits were rare, and normal X-rays and computed tomography with bone and tissue density scanning were the most useful for establishing the diagnosis. A very thorough discussion summarizes the findings and natural history of the disease. However, general descriptive statistics are heavily biased toward the group of patients with osteomas, which skewed distribution of the lesions, and negatively affects the summary. One needs to be very careful in summarizing the data in such studies to avoid statistically-driven errors leading to statements of lesser value.

R.M. Pluta, M.D., Ph.D.

Demographics, Prognosis, and Therapy in 702 Patients With Brain Metastases From Malignant Melanoma
Sampson JH, Carter JH Jr, Friedman AH, et al (Duke Univ, Durham, NC)
J Neurosurg 88:11–20, 1998   17–13

Background.—Brain metastases commonly develop in patients with malignant melanoma. These patients have limited treatment options and, in most cases, a poor prognosis. The current retrospective review identified demographic factors associated with the development of clinically significant brain metastases, as well as factors affecting prognosis.

Methods and Findings.—Of 6,953 patients with melanoma treated at 1 center, 702 had clinically significant brain metastases. Development of brain metastases was associated with male sex; primary lesions on mucosal surfaces or on the skin of the trunk, head, or neck; thick or ulcerated primary lesions; and histologic findings of acral lentiginous or nodular lesions. Patients with brain metastases had a median survival of 113.2 days. Metastases contributed to the deaths of 94.5% of these patients. Survival time was significantly shorter in patients with primary lesions in the head or neck region than in patients with other brain metastases. Patients with a single brain metastasis, patients without lung or multiple other visceral metastases, and patients whose initial presentation included a brain metastasis had a significantly better prognosis. The small number of patients surviving for more than 3 years had a surgically treated, single brain metastasis in the absence of other visceral metastatic disease.

Conclusions.—Though the prognosis is dismal in most patients with brain metastases resulting from melanoma, a subgroup of patients likely to survive for longer periods can be identified. In such patients, surgical resection can significantly extend meaningful survival. The recommendation of surgery should be based mostly on the resectability of the brain metastases and on the status and number of other organs with metastatic lesions.

▶ The authors describe a retrospective review of 702 patients with clinical or radiological evidence of brain metastases who were treated at Duke University Medical Center over the past 20 years.

This is a useful review of a tumor that, in general, has a dismal prognosis. The authors identify factors associated with the development of brain metastases: male gender; primary lesions located on mucosal surfaces or on the skin of the trunk, head, and neck; thick or ulcerated primary lesions; and histological findings of acral lentiginous or nodular lesions.

The overall median survival time of all patients with brain metastases was less than 4 months, and patients with primary lesions located on the head or neck region had significantly shorter survival time than other patients with brain metastases.

As in other series, there was a very small group of patients who survived for more than 3 years, and these patients were characterized by the presence of surgically-treated single brain metastases in the absence of other visceral metastatic disease.

Although this series suffers from the drawbacks of a retrospective study, it is particularly useful because it is a large series from a single institution, and does provide an important overview of the disease. The authors also give useful guidelines for recommending surgical resection of brain metastases. The authors quite reasonably conclude that craniotomy with excision of brain metastasis is most useful in patients with metastatic disease limited to the brain or to the brain and 1 other organ only, and that aggressive surgical therapy in such patients is associated with a neurological improvement in 50% of cases, and can extend the period of meaningful survival. There is a brief discussion of the usefulness of stereotactic radiosurgery in patients with multiple metastases, but, clearly, a prospective study of this treatment modality is required to provide more information.

A.H. Kaye, M.D., M.B.B.S., F.R.A.C.S.

Survival Rates in Patients With Primary Malignant Brain Tumors Stratified by Patient Age and Tumor Histological Type: An Analysis Based on Surveillance, Epidemiology, and End Results (SEER) Data, 1973–1991
Davis FG, Freels S, Grutsch J, et al (Univ of Illinois, Chicago; Chicago Inst of Neurosurgery and Neuroscience; H Lee Mofitt Cancer Ctr, Tampa, Fla)
J Neurosurg 88:1–10, 1998   17–14

Introduction.—Although annual reports of population–based survival rates for all patients with malignant primary brain tumors are available, survival data for patients according to histological tumor types is more limited. Using the most recent data from the Surveillance, Epidemiology, and End Results program from 1973 to 1991, researchers stratified population–based survival rate estimates by patient age and histological tumor type.

Methods.—The study sample included 22,526 patients who were diagnosed with primary malignant brain tumors between 1973 and 1991; patients with a previous or subsequent cancer diagnosis were excluded. Tumors were classified by histological type based on the International Classification of Diseases for Oncology morphology codes. Three histological groups with a high proportion of benign tumors were excluded, leaving 21,947 malignant cases among 12 tumor types. Three age groups were defined: children ($\leq$20 years at diagnosis), younger adults (21 to 64 years), and older adults ($\geq$65 years). The year of diagnosis was used to define 3 time periods: 1973 to 1980, 1981 to 1985, and 1986 to 1991. Survival rates were compared for histological type, age, and year of diagnosis.

Results.—The distribution of tumor type varied across patient age, with astrocytoma predominating in younger patients and glioblastoma multiforme (GBM) in older patients. For most histological groups, there was a pattern of declining survival rates with increasing patient age and overall improvements in survival across the 3 time periods, adjusting for age at diagnosis. Two– and 5–year survival rates improved over time for children and adults with medulloblastoma and for adults with astrocytoma and oligodendroglioma. Gender differences in survival existed for patients with medulloblastoma in the 1970s, but have since disappeared. Patients with GBM consistently exhibited the poorest survival rates across all 3 age groups.

Conclusion.—Overall survival of patients with brain tumors has improved over the last 2 decades, particularly for patients with medulloblastoma. Adults with astrocytoma or oligodendroglioma also experienced improved survival rates. These gains appear to have resulted from therapeutic advances rather than from a shift in patient age at diagnosis. Among adults, there was a pattern of declining survival rates with increasing patient age at diagnosis. The most intractable brain tumor continues to be GBM.

▶ This report provides population–based survival rate of 22,526 malignant brain tumors diagnosed between 1973 and 1991. A similar study conducted by the Committee of Brain Tumor Registry of Japan published the data of 31,211 cases of brain tumors treated between 1969 and 1983.[1] This occupied the whole issue of the Journal and included 3,006 cases of astrocytoma; 1,551 cases of malignant astrocytoma and 2,846 cases of glioblastoma. The 5–year survival rates of astrocytoma, malignant astrocytoma and glioblastoma were 48.6%, 14.5%, and 10.1%, respectively in cases treated between 1969 and 1973, whereas those in cases treated between 1974 and 1978 were 55.3%, 22.1%, and 10.3%, respectively. This means that glioblastoma continues to be the most intractable tumor and awaits further developments of tumor treatments.

K. Sano, M.D., Ph.D., Dr.h.c., F.A.C.S.

Reference

1. Neurologia medico-chirurgica (Tokyo) 32:385–547, 1992.

18 Carotid Occlusive Vascular Disease

Carotid Artery Stents: Early and Intermediate Follow-up With Doppler US
Robbin ML, Lockhart ME, Weber TM, et al (Univ of Alabama, Birmingham; Atlanta Cardiology Group, Ga)
Radiology 205:749–756, 1997   18–1

Introduction.—Carotid artery stent placement is being studied as a treatment for extracranial carotid artery stenosis. The authors' study protocol includes both angiographic and US follow-up. Although angiography is the standard, color Doppler US is quick, noninvasive, and less expensive. Ultrasound was evaluated for use as a follow-up study after placement of carotid artery stents.

Methods.—The analysis included Doppler US scans performed after stent placement in 170 carotid arteries of 119 patients. Angiographic correlation was available in each case. One hundred sixty-seven cases involved stents placed in the internal carotid artery (ICA), and 80% involved stents extending across the bifurcation into the common carotid artery (CCA). The US scans were evaluated for their ability to detect stenosis, occlusions, and other complications. Prospective criteria for stenosis included a peak systolic velocity of greater than 1.25 m/sec, an ICA to CCA peak systolic velocity ratio of 3:1 or greater, and intrastent doubling of peak systolic velocity. Retrospective criteria included a peak systolic velocity of greater than 1.7 m/sec, an ICA end diastolic velocity of greater than 0.4 m/sec, an ICA-CCA peak systolic velocity ratio greater than 2.0, and an ICA-CCA end diastolic velocity ratio greater than 2.4.

Results.—Eighty-seven scans were performed immediately after stent placement and 83 were performed intermediately at an average follow-up of 7 months. There were 2 cases of stent occlusion. Twenty-six stented arteries showed at least 1 abnormality among the prospective US criteria, and 47 had 1 or more positive retrospective criteria. The angiographic findings corresponded with the US findings, with only 1 significant stenosis in an ICA stent. Ultrasound showed moderate collapse of a CCA stent in 1 case.

Conclusion.—This study shows the ability of follow-up US to detect significant stenosis, occlusion, or collapse of carotid artery stents. Ultrasound may prove to be a sensitive technique for the detection of intrastent stenosis. The authors call for more study with longer follow-up to clarify the US criteria for recurrent stenosis.

▶ This article relates the experience of the University of Alabama–Birmingham group in comparing Doppler US with angiography for determination of stenosis or occlusion in patients after the carotid angioplasty and stenting. This group has the largest experience with this procedure, evidenced in part by the excellent technical results of this study. However, the near-complete absence of poststenting occlusion or high-grade stenosis (4/171 patients) preludes meaningful analysis of the sensitivity of US in detecting these lesions. The mere fact that US can detect Doppler flow through the stent is of interest and suggests that this technique may be useful for routine follow-up in patients undergoing carotid angioplasty and stenting.

M.R. Mayberg, M.D.

Superficial and Deep Cervical Plexus Block for Carotid Artery Surgery: A Prospective Study of 1000 Blocks
Davies MJ, Silbert BS, Scott DA, et al (St Vincent's Hosp, Melbourne, Australia)
Reg Anesth 22:442–446, 1997   18–2

Introduction.—The advantages of cervical plexus block over general anesthesia include identification of a high-risk group for postoperative stroke, faster recovery, lower cost, easier monitoring, and avoidance of the complications of general anesthesia. The success rate, complication rate, and patient acceptance were assessed in 924 patients undergoing combined superficial and deep cervical plexus blocks.

Methods.—Nine-hundred twenty-four patients underwent 1,000 carotid artery surgeries using superficial and deep cervical plexus blocks. Data were recorded prospectively. Patients were interviewed by telephone on or about the third postoperative day by an independent anesthesiologist regarding any problems with anesthesia and whether the patients would be willing to have the same form of anesthesia if they needed similar surgery in the future.

Results.—Lidocaine was used in 88% of the surgeries. Surgical supplementation of the blocks was required in 53% of the surgeries. Clinical evidence of intravascular injection of local anesthetic was observed in 6 blocks (0.6%). Sedation was needed in 66% of the surgeries. Conversion to general anesthetic was required in 25 surgeries (2.5%). Ninety-one percent of the patients reported no problems with the block, and 93% indicated they would undergo the same anesthetic for any future similar surgery.

Conclusion.—Superficial and deep cervical plexus block has a high success rate and patient acceptance rate. The complication rate was low. Intravascular injection of local anesthetic should be prevented as it is the most serious complication of this block.

▶ This article probably represents the largest single institutional experience with regional anesthesia for carotid endarterectomy. In the hands of these authors, the technique of combined deep plus superficial cervical block was effective and safe. It should be noted, however, that some sequelae, such as phrenic nerve dysfunction and Horner's syndrome, were not monitored in this study. Of importance is the fact that 4.1% of patients could not be neurologically monitored because of conversion to general anesthetic or oversedation. Thus, although regional anesthesia is a reasonable alternative for carotid endarterectomy, the surgeon must be prepared to operate without neurologic monitoring in a small percentage of cases.

M.R. Mayberg, M.D.

Hemodynamic Instability After Carotid Endarterectomy: Risk Factors and Associations With Operative Complications

Wong JH, Findlay JM, Suarez-Almazor ME (Univ of Alberta, Edmonton, Canada)
Neurosurgery 41:35–43, 1997   18–3

Introduction.—Some degree of hemodynamic instability frequently develops after carotid endarterectomy. The postoperative hemodynamic fluctuations are usually transient, and their clinical significance is unknown. The incidence of hypertension, hypotension, and bradycardia after carotid endarterectomy (CEA) was noted and hemodynamic variables predictive of postoperative stroke, death, or cardiac complications were assessed in 291 CEAs performed in 265 patients.

Methods.—Medical charts were retrospectively analyzed from hemodynamic data collected from patients' time of arrival in the recovery room until the end of the first postoperative day. Primary outcome events were stroke or death within 30 days of surgery. Secondary outcome events were postoperative cardiac complications.

Results.—Of 290 CEAs (hospital documentation was missing for 1 patient) 26 (9%), 36 (12%), and 159 (55%) resulted in postoperative hypertension, hypotension, and bradycardia, respectively. Fifteen (5%) of CEAs resulted in postoperative stroke or death. There was a significant correlation between postoperative hypertension and stroke and a statistical trend with cardiac complications. Independent preoperative risk factors for postoperative hypertension were angiographic intracranial carotid stenosis greater than 50%, cardiac dysrhythmia, preoperative systolic blood pressure higher than 160 mm Hg, neurologic instability, and renal insufficiency. There were no primary or secondary correlations between preoperative hypotension and bradycardia.

Conclusion.—Hemodynamic instability was frequently seen after CEA. Only postoperative hypertension was positively correlated with stroke or death or possible cardiac complications. Patients undergoing CEA, and particularly those at increased risk for postoperative hypertension, should be monitored in a setting that can respond appropriately to neurologic and cardiovascular emergencies.

▶ Increasing pressures to reduce cost have led to various patient management protocols for CEA, including the reduction or elimination of postoperative ICU monitoring. This retrospective community study does not directly address any change in outcome related to this practice, but it does provide some data regarding the incidence of hypotension, hypertension, and bradycardia after CEA. The association noted in this study between postoperative hypertension and stroke or cardiac complication may not be causal; i.e., hypertension may have been the result of these conditions. It is not clear why patients with hypertension (systolic blood pressure greater than 220) were not treated before this level was reached. I believe that postoperative hemodynamic monitoring after CEA is important, although a prospective trial would be needed to validate that belief.

M.R. Mayberg, M.D.

Epidemiology of Carotid Endarterectomy Among Medicare Beneficiaries: 1985–1996 Update
Hsia DC, Moscoe LM, Krushat WM (US Department of Health and Human Services; Rockville, Md; US Department of Health and Human Services, Baltimore, Md)
Stroke 29:346–350, 1998   18–4

Introduction.—The annual trend for carotid endarterectomies (CEAs) in the United States has twice changed direction, according to projections from the National Hospital Discharge Survey. The use of the procedure peaked in 1985, had gone out of favor by 1991, and had subsequently recovered by 1996. The medical developments pertaining to CEAs paralleled these trends. The decline was caused by concerns about the effectiveness of the procedure and proper indications for surgical interventions, but, since 1991, controlled trials have affirmed its use in selected patients. Changes in the rate and outcome of CEAs among Medicare beneficiaries were reviewed.

Methods.—To calculate CEA frequency, rate, and perioperative mortality by patient demography and hospital characteristics, codes from the *International Classification of Diseases, 9th Revision, Clinical Modification* were analyzed.

Results.—In 1985, there was an initial peak of 61,273 CEAs (20.6 per 10,000 Medicare beneficiaries. In 1989, the number of procedures declined to 46,571 (14.3 per 10,000). In 1996, the number of procedures rose to 108,275 (28.6 per 10,000). The patients were predominantly male, white, and aged 65–74. Surgery occurred predominantly in nonprofit, urban, large, and teaching hospitals. There was a decline in the perioperative mortality rate from 3% in 1985 to 1.6% in 1996.

Conclusion.—Prompt response to reports from clinical trials were shown by the frequency and rate of CEA. Over time, perioperative mortality rates improved and converged but did not attain the rates reported by the trials. There was twice the average perioperative mortality rate in patients 85 years of age and older.

▶ The Medicare Medical Provider Analysis and Review data provide an opportunity to study a variety of issues related to health care delivery including demographics, utilization, and certain crude measures of outcome. This analysis of Medicare data for CEA documents previously reported trends in the frequency of CEA in the Medicare population. It appears that several well-designed, randomized, prospective clinical trials for CEA have influenced clinical decision making in this population.

Of interest, this report also documents some small but potentially important trends, such as increased frequency of CEA among elderly men and whites, with more cases being performed at large, urban and teaching hospitals. The data also show a correlation between CEA volume per hospital and perioperative death. Although the perioperative mortality rate for CEA appears to be decreasing, the authors caution that the observed incidence of perioperative death for the overall Medicare population is greater than that observed in the clinical trials.

I would disagree with their contention that the data from this analysis infer less efficacy for CEA, because no information is available regarding indications for surgery, co-morbidity, etc. Clearly, the decision to recommend CEA should be based upon a number of scientifically validated factors related to the patient, the lesion, and the experience of the surgeon, but not upon aggregate national Medicare statistics.

M.R. Mayberg, M.D.

A Cost Comparison of Balloon Angioplasty and Stenting Versus Endarterectomy for the Treatment of Carotid Artery Stenosis
Jordan WD Jr, Roye GD, Fisher WS III, et al (Univ of Alabama, Birmingham)
J Vasc Surg 27:16–24, 1998   18–5

Introduction.—The standard treatment for high-grade stenosis of the extracranial carotid arteries is carotid endarterectomy (CEA). New methods of revascularization have been explored recently, such as percutaneous transluminal angioplasty (PTA), which hypothetically includes less morbidity, shorter recovery, and lower cost. Patients who had elective treatment for carotid artery stenosis were studied, and the hospital charges for PTA and carotid endarterectomy were compared.

Methods.—During a 14-month period, 218 patients had 234 procedures for the treatment of 239 carotid bifurcation stenoses. Treatment consisted of PTA in 109 cases and CEA in 130 cases. For each hospitalization, hospital charges were reviewed and categorized according to operating room, radiology, cardiac catheterization laboratory, and other hospital charges.

Results.—Among the patients who had PTA, there were 8 strokes (7.7%) and 1 death (0.9%). Among the patients who had CEA, there were 2 strokes (1.5%) and 2 deaths (1.5%). For PTAs, total hospital charges per admission were $30,140, and for CEAs they were $21,670. For PTAs, the average postprocedure length of stay was 2.9 days, and for CEAs it was 3.1 days. For the PTA group, cardiac catheterization laboratory charges were $12,968. The operating room charges for the CEA group were $4,263. When hospitalizations that were prolonged by complications were excluded, the average total charges for the patients who had PTA decreased to $24,848 (mean length of stay, 1.9 days), and the average total charges for patients who had CEA dropped to $19,247 (mean length of stay, 2.6 days).

Conclusions.—PTA for the treatment of carotid artery stenosis cannot be currently justified on the basis of reduced hospital charges alone. Total hospital charges can be reduced in both groups with future cost-containing measures.

▶ CEA is now the established treatment for stenosed extracranial carotid arteries. More recently, PTA with stenting has been advocated as an alternative treatment because it allegedly decreases morbidity, and is associated with a shorter recovery and lower costs.

The authors compared these points. The results are interesting: CEA seems preferable to PTA with stenting. However, coronary artery disease and hypertension were significantly less prevalent in the CEA group, which might influence the results to some extent.

K. Sano, M.D., Ph.D., Dr.h.c., F.A.C.S.

Treatment of Blunt Injury to the Carotid Artery by Using Endovascular Stents: An Early Experience

Duke BJ, Ryu RK, Coldwell DM, et al (Univ of Colorado, Denver)
J Neurosurg 87:825–829, 1997   18–6

Background.—Identifying blunt carotid injury (BCI) before the development of ischemic symptoms necessitates aggressive screening of at–risk patients. Long–term anticoagulation therapy has been the mainstay of treatment. However, many lesions and the risk of distal embolization persist despite medical treatment. Successful treatment with endovascular stent placement for nonpenetrating carotid injuries was reported in the current study.

Patients and Outcomes.—Six patients with BCI were treated. At the time of diagnosis, all were given IV heparin. Angiography was performed within 1 week of injury. Stents were placed in patients with dissections that enlarged despite anticoagulation therapy and with pseudoaneurysms. The stents were self-expanding and did not require in situ balloon dilation, which minimized the amount of manipulation needed. Patients were maintained on heparin therapy after stent placement, but heparin was subsequently discontinued in 3 patients. The other 5 were eventually switched from heparin to coumadin. After 8 weeks, they were switched to 1 aspirin per day for another month.

Conclusions.—Endovascular stents may be a safe, effective alternative to surgery and medical treatment in patients with BCI. Stent placement may be suitable for vessels with progressive dissection being managed medically and for posttraumatic pseudoaneurysms. Further research is warranted.

▶ Duke et al. describe a simple, apparently safe and effective technique to restore patency to an injured carotid artery and to obliterate pseudoaneurysms without the complications associated with long–term anticoagulation, the difficulties of carotid reconstruction, or the unpalatable choice of Hunterian ligation and carotid occlusion.

Their indications for treatment—progressive stenosis or the onset of new symptoms when the patient is adequately anticoagulated, the enlargement of a known pseudoaneurysm or the appearance of a new one—seem reasonable. Their proposal of long–term follow–up by annual computed tomographic angiography for 5 years appears prudent.

R. Leblanc, M.D., M.Sc., F.R.C.S.C.

Carotid Endarterectomy in the U.K. and Ireland: Audit of 30-Day Outcome

McCollum PT, for the Vascular Surgical Society (Ninewells Hosp, Dundee, Scotland)
Eur J Vasc Endovasc Surg 14:386–391, 1997   18–7

Introduction.—Carotid endarterectomy confers a definite advantage of reduced stroke risk to patients who are otherwise medically fit in the presence of ipsilateral symptoms and a carotid artery stenosis of more than 70%. With an expected increase in the number of operations performed, the Vascular Surgery Society of Great Britain and Ireland was concerned about the outcomes. A prospective study with a randomly sampled group of members of the Vascular Surgery Society of Great Britain known to be performing carotid surgery was conducted to establish the current patient stroke and mortality rate and to examine the currently favored operative practices.

Methods.—Fifty-nine consultant surgeons with 709 patients having carotid endarterectomy were examined for their demographic data and 30-day outcomes in a 6-month period. The surgeons completed a 28-question questionnaire for each patient who had the surgery; the main end points were death and postoperative stroke at 30 days. Indications for surgery were ipsilateral transient ischemic attack, amaurosis fugaz/retinal artery occlusion, ipsilateral cardiovascular accident, asymptomatic stenosis, contralateral symptoms, and vertebrobasilar symptoms.

Results.—There was an 82% mean ipsilateral stenosis with a range of 30% to 99%. Preoperative neurologic consults were necessary for 31% of patients. Patches were placed in 54.4% of patients, drains in 71.9%, tacking sutures in 40.1%, and shunts in 67.5%. There were 9 deaths (1.3%) at 30 days with 4 cardiac deaths and 3 neurologic deaths. There were 15 ipsilateral postoperative cardiovascular accidents (2.1%). One or more complications, usually minor, were found in 19% of patients. No independent risk factor for cardiovascular accident, other than seniority of the surgeon, was found, according to statistical analysis.

Conclusion.—For all patients, there was a combined stroke/death rate of 3% at 30 days. These surgeons had a very low morbidity/mortality rate for performing carotid surgery. To ensure that this quality of service does not deteriorate, continued audit is required.

▶ This prospective audit is an example of self-imposed quality assurance and establishment of a local "performance benchmark." The combined stroke and death rate of 3% compares quite favorably with the European and North American Trials.[1-3] Subanalysis of the data revealed that age, use of a shunt, patch grafting, length of the surgery, and district general hospital vs. university hospital did not correlate with a significant increase or decrease in operative risk. The presence of a trainee surgeon did correlate with increased risk of stroke, but the number of unsupervised surgeries was not noted. Also, the number of carotid operations performed by each surgeon did not correlate with increased risk of stroke.

Interestingly, shunts and patch grafts were used in a larger proportion of patients than I see indications for in my practice, and nearly 1 of every 5 patients had some type of minor complication (hematoma, neuropraxia, etc.). A small number of surgeons had disproportionately long delays to surgery, and it was noted that "these were mostly surgeons who had the largest practices." The authors suggested that "there may be a trade-off of high volume caseload against time to surgery."

Quality assurance studies or programs are, of course, designed to detect deficiencies, and the authors readily acknowledge those detected among the surgeons in the United Kingdom and Ireland who voluntarily participated in this study. Perhaps a prospective international audit of neurosurgeons' carotid endarterectomy practices and outcomes would be equally revealing and reassuring. If our collective results are as favorable as we believe, these data would surely bolster our position in reclaiming a larger proportion of carotid vascular surgery.

S.R. Gibbs, M.A., M.D.

References

1. European Carotid Surgery Trialists' Collaborative Group. MRC European Carotid Surgery Trial: Interim results for symptomatic patients with severe (70%–90%) or with mild (0%–29%) carotid stenosis. *Lancet* 337:1235–1243, 1991.
2. European Carotid Surgery Trialists' Collaborative Group. Endarterectomy for moderate symptomatic carotid stenosis: Interim results from the MRC European Carotid Surgery Trial. *Lancet* 347:1591–1593, 1996.
3. North American Symptomatic Carotid Endarterectomy Trial Collaborators. Beneficial effect of carotid endarterectomy in symptomatic patients with high grade stenosis. *N Engl J Med* 325:335–351, 1991.

Prevention of Postoperative Thrombotic Stroke After Carotid Endarterectomy: The Role of Transcranial Doppler Ultrasound

Lennard N, Smith J, Dumville J, et al (Leicester Royal Infirmary, England)
J Vasc Surg 26:579–584, 1997   18–8

Background.—The risk of ipsilateral stroke after carotid endarterectomy (CEA) has been reported to be 5% to 7%. Previous research has shown that postoperative internal carotid artery thrombosis was preceded by a phase of asymptomatic microparticulate embolization. A determination was made of the incidence of particulate embolization after CEA, the effect of Dextran-40 infusion in patients with sustained postoperative embolization, and the value of transcranial Doppler (TCD) monitoring plus adjuvant Dextran treatment on the rate of postoperative carotid thrombosis.

Methods.—One hundred patients undergoing CEA were studied prospectively. Six-hour postoperative monitoring was conducted using a TCD modified to allow automatic, intermittent recordings from the ipsilateral middle cerebral artery waveform. When 25 or more emboli were detected in any 10-minute period, an incremental Dextran-40 infusion was begun.

Findings.—Overall, 1 or more emboli were detected in 48% of the patients postoperatively (Table 1), especially in the first 2 hours (Fig 1). However, only 5 patients had sustained embolization requiring Dextran

TABLE 1.—Incidence of Postoperative Embolization in 100 Patients

No. of emboli	No. of patients	%
0	52	52
1 to 10	23	23
11 to 25	10	23
26 to 50	7	7
51 to 75	2	2
76 to 100	1	1
>100	5	5

(Courtesy of Lennard N, Smith J, Dumville J, et al: Prevention of postoperative thrombotic stroke after carotid endarterectomy: The role of transcranial Doppler ultrasound. *J Vasc Surg* 26:579–584, 1997.)

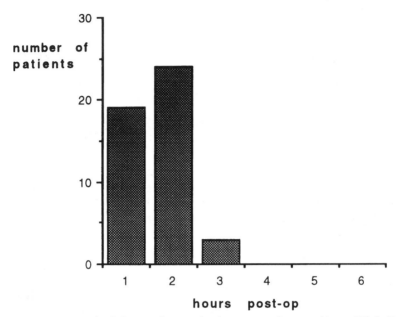

FIGURE 1.—Onset of embolization after carotid endarterectomy. (Courtesy of Lennard N, Smith J, Dumville J, et al: Prevention of postoperative thrombotic stroke after carotid endarterectomy: The role of transcranial Doppler ultrasound. *J Vasc Surg* 26:579–584, 1997.)

treatment. The embolization rate dropped quickly in each of these 5 patients (Fig 2).

Conclusions.—In this series, a small percentage of patients sustained embolization after CEA. Dextran therapy reduced and subsequently stopped all the emboli in patients needing such treatment, contributing to a 0% perioperative morbidity and mortality rate.

▶ TCD ultrasound allows detection of emboli traveling through the cerebral circulation. Usually, the major intracranial arteries, especially the middle cerebral artery, are used for embolus detection. This technology applied to patients undergoing CEA, intraoperatively and postoperatively, has revealed that patients experience a showering of microemboli intraoperatively and postoperatively.[1] Study of embolic patterns by TCD revealed a conspicuous asymptomatic microembolic pattern that is highly predictive for postoperative thrombotic stroke. Early detection of this pattern permits early preventative therapeutic or surgical intervention. In this study, dextran-40 appeared to effectively quell the escalating pattern of microparticulate embolization, thereby preventing thrombotic postoperative stroke.

Currently, TCD is expensive and time consuming as it requires a dedicated technician throughout the monitoring period. Perhaps investigators at centers with this technological luxury will use it to determine an effective, safe

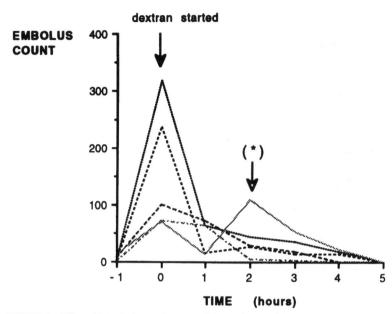

FIGURE 2.—Effect of introducing an incremental-dose infusion of dextran therapy on the rate of embolization (5 patients). Dextran was started at time 0. Rate of embolization in the hour preceding starting of the dextran infusion is also given for comparison. *Asterisk* indicates 1 patient in whom the rate of embolization increased after start of the dextran infusion, necessitating further increase in dose. Thereafter, rate of embolization diminished. (Courtesy of Lennard N, Smith J, Dumville J, et al: Prevention of postoperative thrombotic stroke after carotid endarterectomy: The role of transcranial Doppler ultrasound. *J Vasc Surg* 26:579–584, 1997.)

inhibitor of platelet aggregation that will obviate the need for embolic monitoring.

S.R. Gibbs, M.A., M.D.

Reference

1. Gaunt ME, Ratliff DA, Martin PJ, Smith J, Bell PRF, Naylor AR. On-table diagnosis of incipient carotid artery thrombosis during carotid endarterectomy by transcranial Doppler scanning. *J Vasc Surg* 20:104–107, 1994.

Randomised Trial of Endarterectomy for Recently Symptomatic Carotid Stenosis: Final Results of the MRC European Carotid Surgery Trial (ECST)
Farrell B, for the ECST Organization (Western Gen Hosp, Edinburgh, Scotland)
Lancet 351:1379–1387, 1998   18–9

Objective.—The European Carotid Surgery Trial was designed to compare 2 approaches to patients with episodes of ischemia in the carotid artery territory and stenosis near the origin of the symptomatic internal carotid artery. The 2 approaches were performing carotid endarterectomy (CEA) as soon as possible, and avoiding surgery as long as possible. The benefits of both approaches were expected to vary by patient characteristics, in particular with severity of stenosis. The final trial results are reported.

Methods.—The randomized trial included 3,024 patients at 98 centers. All patients had some degree of carotid stenosis and had experienced 1 or more episodes of transient or mild symptomatic ischemia in the distribution of 1 or both carotid arteries in the previous 6 months. Sixty percent of patients were assigned to undergo CEA as soon as possible; 40% of patients were assigned to the control condition, in which surgery was avoided as long as possible. The patients were followed up for a mean of 6 years, with the results analyzed by intention to treat.

Results.—Major stroke or death occurred in 37.0% of patients assigned to surgery and 36.5% of those assigned to the control group. There was a 7% risk of major stroke or death complicating surgery; this figure did not vary with severity of stenosis. Severity of stenosis did affect the risk of major ischemic stroke ipsilateral to the unoperated, symptomatic carotid artery. This risk was noted especially in patients with greater than 70% to 80% stenosis of the original luminal diameter and for 2–3 years after randomization. For patients with stenosis of greater than 80%, the immediate risk of surgery was counterbalanced by the long-term risk of stroke without surgery. For such patients, the Kaplan-Meier estimate of the 3-year risk of major stroke or death was 26.5% for the control group vs. 14.9% for the surgery group. However, this balance varied considerably with age and sex.

Conclusions.—For most patients with recent, nondisabling ischemic events in the carotid artery territory and stenosis of greater than approximately 80%, CEA is usually indicated. Age and sex also influence the balance of surgical risk and benefit. This article includes a chart to help in estimating the benefits of surgery according to sex, age, and severity of stenosis.

▶ This elegant and thoughtful study confirms and further defines much of what we already knew from the results of the North American Symptomatic Carotid Endarterectomy Trial.[1] Of note, notwithstanding differences in measurement of angiographic stenosis between this and the NASCET study, a clear benefit with surgery was again emphatically demonstrated for high grade stenosis. Additionally, the conclusion that there is less stroke risk reduction after carotid surgery in female patients, as previously suggested in the Asymptomatic Carotid Atherosclerosis Study,[2] represents a further useful refinement for identifying cohorts most likely to benefit from CEA. A caveat with this and other endarterectomy trials is that the results are largely derived from experienced groups of surgeons and hence may not be universally applicable.

J.M. Duff, M.D., M.B., B.Ch.

References

1. North American Symptomatic Carotid Endarterectomy Trial Collaborators: Beneficial effect of carotid endarterectomy in symptomatic patients with high-grade stenosis. *N Engl J Med* 325:445–453, 1991.
2. Asymptomatic Carotid Atherosclerosis Study Executive Committee: Endarterectomy for asymptomatic carotid artery stenosis. *JAMA* 273:1421–1428, 1995.

19 Cranial Operative Techniques

Superimposed Holographic Image-guided Neurosurgery: Technical Note
Ko K (Univ of Medicine and Dentistry of New Jersey, New Brunswick)
J Neurosurg 88:777–781, 1998   19–1

Introduction.—Three-dimensional (3–D) holograms can now be used to record and display radiologic data for clinical purposes, improving the physician's understanding of 3–D form or volume. If the holographic image could be superimposed onto the surgical field, it could allow the surgeon to operate while looking through the holographic image, comparing the real and radiologic views without having to look away from the patient. The author is interested in the possibility of using a superimposed holographic image as an interactive visual map during craniofacial neurosurgical procedures. An initial experience with the use of CT scan-derived reflection holograms superimposed on the operative field during craniofacial surgery is presented.

Methods and Results.—The author created CT-derived narrow band reflection holograms of patients undergoing surgery involving the calvaria. The holograms were then sterilized and placed over the surgical site. Bone sutures served as registration points between the skull and 3-D image. The holographic image, illuminated by the surgeon's halogen headlamp, served as a visual template for the operation. The accuracy of the holograms was within 2 mm, as judged by the titanium constructs fashioned preoperatively to fit the bone defect. The presence of the holograms eliminated the need for freehand contouring of the calvaria. The surgeon had sufficient space to work beneath the holograms, which could be easily rotated out of the surgical field if necessary. There were no patient complaints resulting from use of the holograms, and no complications. The holograms allowed the surgeon to rehearse the procedure in the laboratory and office.

Discussion.—This is the first reported use of holograms superimposed over the surgical field for use in neurosurgery. The detail provided is useful for both planning and performing operations on the calvaria. In this experience, the holograms were valuable in providing a visual reference and in guiding calvarial reconstruction. With further technical development, holography could play a useful role in craniofacial surgery.

▶ A novel application of holographic imaging to superimpose a 3-D image directly onto the operative field during neurological surgery is described. The specific implementation described, craniofacial reconstructive surgery, appears ideally suited to the technical characteristics and specific limitations of the monochromatic holographic technique demonstrated, because the technique allows the surgeon to visualize either existing, pre-operative bone structure or a computer-reconstructed "road map" of the desired postoperative result. With currently available technology, a similar holographic approach would be less suitable for more dynamic or interactive situations, such as intracranial vascular or tumor surgery, where endmarks are less distinct and change over time. As the author concludes, the technology is at present labor intensive and costly, requiring 12–24 hours of bench work per hologram, and specialized laser equipment to generate the hologram. Some of the investment in time is recovered in the operating room from improved operative planning, and the holograms are helpful in patient education. The author has demonstrated the feasibility of this rather elegant application of the physics of holography to 3-D imaging in the operating room.

G. Pjura, M.D.

The First Decade of Continuous Monitoring of Jugular Bulb Oxyhemoglobin Saturation: Management Strategies and Clinical Outcome

Cruz J (Allegheny Univ, Philadelphia; Comprehensive Internatl Ctr for Neuroemergencies, São Paulo, Brazil)
Crit Care Med 26:344–351, 1998   19–2

Introduction.—A broad spectrum of newly derived physiologic variables and concepts from continuous fiberoptic monitoring of jugular bulb oxyhemoglobin saturation includes cerebral extraction of oxygen, cerebral consumption of oxygen, systemic-cerebral oxygenation index, and systemic-cerebral ventilatory index. The outcome of severely brain-injured patients undergoing monitoring and management of cerebral extraction oxygen in conjunction with cerebral perfusion pressure was prospectively compared with the outcome of patients subjected to monitoring and management of cerebral perfusion pressure alone.

Methods.—Of 353 adults with severe acute brain trauma, 178 underwent continuous monitoring and management of cerebral extraction of oxygen and cerebral perfusion (CEO group). The remaining group (controls) of 175 patients underwent monitoring and management of cerebral perfusion pressure only (CPP group). Patients were matched according to age, postresuscitation Glasgow Coma Scale scores, rates of acute surgical intracranial hematomas and brain swelling, pupillary abnormalities, early hypotensive events (before intensive care monitoring), initial levels of intracranial pressure, and cerebral perfusion pressure.

Results.—Sixteen CEO group and 53 CPP group patients died (9% vs. 30%, respectively). The length of cerebral perfusion pressure monitoring was significantly longer in CPP group than CEO group patients (6.5 days vs. 10.5 days).

Conclusion.—Outcome from severe acute brain trauma with associated intracranial hypertension and compromise cerebrospinal fluid spaces is superior in patients undergoing optimal hyperventilation, based on monitoring and management of CEO and perfusion pressure, to the outcome in patients monitored and managed using cerebral perfusion pressure alone.

▶ Perfusion pressure has traditionally been used as an essential parameter to monitor brain functioning in patients with acute brain trauma. However, it is clear that the complex physiopathological events interacting in the first hours after trauma produce tissular changes whose proper exploration requires more than the figures obtained from measuring perfusion pressure.[1] For a decade, J. Cruz has supported the value of monitoring changes in oxygen consumption by the brain to guide initial therapeutic measures after severe brain trauma. Differences in diatomic oxygen content between arteries and veins reflect brain oxygen extraction, a logical and ingenious idea that provides useful information on neuronal vitality, and which could be reinforced perhaps with similar measurements of glucose extraction by the brain. In the hands of Cruz, using this method as the gold standard for optimized downward or upward hyperventilation has resulted in significant decreases in mortality and monitoring time. In these patients, adjustment of $Paco_2$ values, achieved by manipulation of ventilatory frequency according to an algorithm developed by Cruz, leads to improvement of intracranial pressure, cerebral perfusion pressure, and cerebral extraction of oxygen. Based on such valuable experience, with a considerable number of patients reported in various publications, it should be quite important to see articles about the experience of other workers from other institutions with the potential value of measurements of oxygen consumption in the initial therapeutic intervention of acute brain trauma.

J. Sotelo, M.D.

Reference

1. Young A, Willatts S: Controversies in management of acute brain trauma. *Lancet* 352:164–166, 1998.

Endoscope-assisted Brain Surgery: Part 1—Evolution, Basic Concept, and Current Technique

Perneczky A, Fries G (Johannes Gutenberg-Univ, Mainz, Germany)
Neurosurgery 42:219–225, 1998   19–3

Introduction.—Neurosurgical techniques have improved so much that large craniotomies are no longer required. The basic concepts and current techniques used in endoscope-assisted brain surgery are reviewed.

Advances in Operative Techniques.—Improved diagnostic imaging techniques have facilitated exact localization of lesions and precise determination of topographical relations of definite lesions to individual anatomic variations of intracranial structures. This precision may be used to perform individual surgical procedures through keyhole approaches. Keyhole craniotomies, however, have problems caused by the narrow viewing angles and the decrease in light intensity in the depth of the operating field.

Endoscope-assisted Microsurgery.—Objects located directly opposite keyhole craniotomies may be offset with the intraoperative use of rigid rod lens endoscopes. The shaft of these instruments can be easily controlled through the surgical microscope. Both hands are used in endoscope-assisted microsurgery. The endoscope is fixed in its desired position using a mechanical arm affixed to the headholder. Their superior optical quality and maneuverability make rigid lens scopes the best choice in these surgeries. Endoscopic and microscopic images may be viewed at the same time by (1) observation of the microscopic image through the oculars of the microscope and observation of the endoscopic image on a video screen positioned in front of the surgeon; (2) observation of the microscopic image through the oculars of the microscope and display of the endoscopic image on a head-mounted liquid crystal diode screen; (3) projection of both microscopic and endoscopic images on 1 screen in a picture-in-picture mode; (4) projection of both microscopic and endoscopic images into specially designed microscope oculars; and (5) transmission of both microscopic and endoscopic images into a head-mounted liquid crystal diode screen.

Conclusion.—With the ability to determine nearly all individual anatomic and pathoanatomic details of a specific patient, individual lesions may be targeted through a keyhole approach using the particular anatomic windows. With improvements in light intensity and depiction of important anatomic details by intraoperative use of lens scopes the keyhole approach with endoscope-assisted microsurgery may produce maximum efficiency for lesion removal, maximum patient safety, and minimum invasiveness.

▶ The first of a 2-part series by Perneczky and Fries presents a superb and comprehensive view of the evolution and development of the concepts behind the use of endoscopes to assist in microsurgical techniques. Endoscopes have been extensively used in the ventricular system, but these authors have coupled the endoscope with the microscope to serve as an invaluable adjunct to performing surgery through small craniotomies. The authors state that the advantages provided by endoscopes include increased light intensity while approaching an object, clear depiction of details in close-up positions, and extended views and angles. These advantages allow the surgeon to obtain better visualization, decrease the amount of traction on superficial neural vascular structures, and improve the surgical approach to deep-seated lesions through narrow corridors.

D.F. Jimenez, M.D.

Endoscope-assisted Brain Surgery: Part 2—Analysis of 380 Procedures
Fries G, Perneczky A (Johannes Gutenberg-Univ, Mainz, Germany)
Neurosurgery 42:226–232, 1998   19–4

Introduction.—Intraoperative retraction of brain tissue can lead to cerebral infarction through increased local cerebral tissue pressure and diminished cerebral blood flow. Microsurgical techniques and instruments that help to decrease intraoperative retraction of normal intracranial neuronal and vascular structures improve postoperative outcomes. Although it increases operating time and operation-related trauma, resection of the dura and bone edges must be performed to achieve sufficient control of the operative field without retraction of neurovascular components. A retrospective review of 380 endoscope-assisted microneurosurgical operations was conducted to describe the principles upon which the technique of endoscopic-assisted brain surgery is based, give an impression of possible indications for endoscope-assisted microsurgical procedures, and delineate the advantages of endoscopes when used as surgical instruments during microsurgical approaches to intracranial lesions (Fig 3).

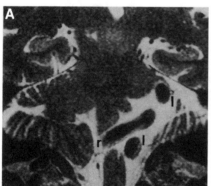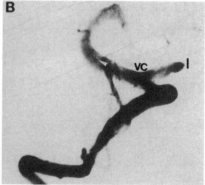

FIGURE 3.—A, T2-weighted magnetic resonance image in the coronal plane, demonstrating the right megadolichovertebral artery transversing and compressing the medulla oblongata (**r**). Note the 2 sections through the left megavertebral artery (**l**). B, angiogram, left oblique view, after contrast injection into the right megadolichovertebral artery. Note the contrast filling of the vertebral conjunction (**vc**), some retrograde flow in the distal portion of the left vertebral artery (**l**), and contrast filling of the megadolichobasilar artery (*white arrowhead*), which is crossing over the pons back to the left side. (Courtesy of Fries G, Perneczky A: Endoscope-assisted brain surgery: Part 2—analysis of 380 procedures. *Neurosurgery* 42:226–232, 1998.)

Methods.—Surgeries were analyzed for time of surgery, usefulness of intraoperative endoscopy, and complication rates. Lens scopes were used that had viewing angles of 0° to 110° with diameters of 2.0–5.0 mm, and newly designed "viewing dissectors" (curved, rigid fiberscopes) with diameters of 1.0–1.5 mm connected to a video unit. Retractor arms fixed to the Mayfield headholder were used to position endoscopes so that the surgeon could use both hands under simultaneous endoscopic and microscopic control.

Results.—Of 380 lesions treated, 205 were tumors, 53 were aneurysms, 86 were cysts, and 36 were neurovascular compression syndromes. Lesion locations were 89 in the ventricular system, 242 in the subarachnoid or intracerebral spaces, and 48 in the sella. Advantages of endoscope-assisted microsurgery approach included reduced size of the craniotomy and less operation-related tissue trauma of approaches to lesions located in the ventricular system and the subarachnoid space at the base of the brain; decreased amount of retraction during tumor removal; and improved visual control of the retrosellar, endosellar, retroclival, and infratentorial structures. This approach was helpful during procedures in the posterior cranial fossa and at the craniocervical junction. Without retraction of dura and bone edges, it allowed for inspection of channels and hidden structures (internal auditory meatus, ventral surface of the brain stem, ventral aspect of root entry zones of cranial nerves, content of the foramen magnum, and upper cervical canal). Endoscopic instrumentation during surgery for large or giant aneurysms was beneficial in dissecting perforators on the back side of the aneurysms and in controlling the completeness of clipping.

Conclusion.—Video–endoscope–assisted microsurgery can be accomplished without retraction of neuronal or vascular structures or resection of dura and bone edges. This approach is easy to learn, time-saving, and trauma reducing. It is likely to improve postoperative outcomes.

▶ This article presents the authors' experience with 380 endoscope-assisted neurosurgical procedures using rigid lens endoscopes which vary in angles between 0° and 120° and in diameters between 2 and 5 mm. The majority of these cases (205) were tumors. Eighty-nine of these procedures were localized to the ventricular system. Based on their experience, the authors conclude that endoscope-assisted neurosurgery is of significant benefit because it allows improved visualization of deep-seated lesions, minimal brain retraction, and smaller craniotomies. There were no intraoperative complications related to the use of the endoscope, and no increase in infection rate. The authors present an elegant and innovative way of approaching neurosurgical pathology and introduce important surgical concepts.

D.F. Jimenez, M.D.

Detailed Evaluation of 2959 Allogeneic and Xenogeneic Dense Connective Tissue Grafts (Fascia Lata, Pericardium, and Dura Mater) Used in the Course of 20 Years For Duraplasty in Neurosurgery
Pařízek J, Měřička P, Hušk Z, et al (Charles Univ, Hradec Králové, Czech Republic)
Acta Neurochir (Wien) 139:827–838, 1997   19–5

Background.—Allogeneic and xenogeneic dense connective tissue grafts have long been used in neurosurgery. A detailed assessment of 2,959 dense connective tissue grafts used for duraplasty was reported.

Methods and Findings.—The grafts, used in 2,665 neurosurgical procedures between 1976 and 1995, were fascia lata (1,767), pericardium (909), and dura mater (283). Similar and favorable clinical outcomes were achieved by duraplasty using either allogeneic or xenogeneic grafts. However, the pliable deep-frozen fascia lata grafts, which could be used anywhere, were reserved for sella turcica plugging, anterior cranial base plasty, aneurysmal wrapping, and lipomyelomeningocele surgery. In most patients, pericardium and dura mater grafts were used over the brain convexity and posterior cranial fossa. Because of its workability, flexibility, decreased thickness, and better transparency, ovine pericardium was better than bovine and allogeneic pericardia. Postoperative complications occurred in 7.3% of the patients. Cerebrospinal fluid fistulas occurred in 2.8%, meningitis in 2.3%, pseudomeningoceles in 2.2%, wound infections in 0.6%, malresorptive hydrocephalus in 0.5%, and adhesions to nerve tissue in 0.5%. Most of these complications healed without the need for surgery. Forty-eight grafts (1.6%) were considered failures, 46 of which were reoperated. Another 39 healed successfully but required 39 shunt procedures for malresorptive hydrocephalus and/or a large pseudomeningocele. Thus, the overall pure complication rate was 3.1%.

Conclusion.—In this detailed investigation of allogeneic and xenogeneic grafts used for duraplasty in neurosurgery, the success rate was 96.9%. Xenogeneic pericardium and allogeneic dura mater grafts were especially suitable over the brain convexity and for posterior fossa duraplasty. Ovine pericardium grafts are superior to bovine and allogeneic pericardia. Deep frozen allogeneic fascia lata grafts are suitable for duraplasty at any location but must be reserved for specific purposes because of their limited supply.

▶ Dense connective tissue grafts are convenient alternatives for closure of traumatic, spontaneous, and iatrogenic dural defects. Newer, thinner, and more pliable grafts (locally, bovine pericardium) have improved the elegance and facility with which structurally sound and water-tight closure can be completed. These materials are, however, foreign bodies; meticulous techniques and vigilance regarding potential infectious sources, such as paranasal sinuses, must be maintained. I have evaluated 2 cases of aseptic meningitis resolving with steroids and 1 case of bacterial graft infection responding only to removal of the graft and replacement with pericranium. These 3 cases, of course, are a tiny minority of the otherwise successful closures. Nonetheless, I continue to enjoy the pliability, resilience, elasticity, and closure integrity of pericranium when available—especially if it has a vascularized pedicle.

C.P. Bondurant, M.D.

Patient Tolerance of Craniotomy Performed With the Patient Under Local Anesthesia and Monitored Conscious Sedation

Danks RA, Rogers M, Aglio LS, et al (Brigham and Women's Hosp, Boston)
Neurosurgery 42:28–36, 1998   19–6

Introduction.—To maximize tumor excision and minimize neurologic deficit for tumors involving eloquent cortex, intraoperative mapping of eloquent cortex during craniotomy performed with the patient under local anesthesia and monitored conscious sedation is a well-established technique. Patients may experience difficulty during this operation, and little is known about patient satisfaction with this procedure. The operative procedure and the patients' subjective responses to it were assessed prospectively.

Methods.—The subjective experiences of 21 consecutive patients having craniotomy and brain mapping under local anesthesia and monitored sedation were formally, intensively, and prospectively assessed. Sixteen patients had midazolam, fentanyl, and sufentanil and 5 had propofol in addition to the other medications. Structured interviews at 2 to 3 days after surgery were conducted by a member of the surgical team. At 1 month after surgery, a psychiatrist conducted a structured interview that was supplemented by preoperative and postoperative assessments of the patients' moods by means of the brief Profile of Mood States questionnaire.

Results.—There were no indications of adverse psychological sequelae of the event at the 1-month follow-up interview, and all patients were entirely comfortable with the experience. The experience was reported as entirely satisfactory, without any intraoperative discomfort or pain, by one half of the patients in the early postoperative interview. Minor difficulties at some stage of the experience was recalled by one third of the patients, and moderate difficulties were reported by one fifth of the patients. To quantify the data, an operating room score with a possible range of 0 to 30 was used. To improve the patients' subjective experience, minor technical changes have been suggested. Patients managed without propofol had a lower incidence of intraoperative problems, but the results did not achieve statistical significance.

Conclusion.—For resection of lesions involving eloquent cortex that might otherwise be considered inoperative, this technique is useful and safe. A level of stress that remains within the tolerance level of the average adult is involved in this procedure.

▶ Brain lesions within eloquent cortex, formerly deemed "inoperable," have been successfully extirpated in patients who have undergone "awake" craniotomy under local anesthesia and light sedation. This has permitted intraoperative brain mapping and optimal resection. As with many "awake" procedures, little has been done to formally study the subjective experience of the patients. This is the first prospective study assessing the patients' impression of the experience. Although some may argue that many of these patients had no good alternative, patient satisfaction is still pivotal. Be mindful that: "Most of our future lies ahead" (Denny Crum, Louisville basketball coach) and, as these authors seem to know, it largely depends upon attention to the details of patient satisfaction.

S.R. Gibbs, M.A., M.D.

Laser-assisted Neuroendoscopy Using a Neodymium-Yttrium Aluminum Garnet or Diode Contact Laser With Pretreated Fiber Tips
Vandertop WP, Verdaasdonk RM, van Swol CFP (Univ Hosp, Utrecht, The Netherlands; Wilhelmina Children's Hosp, Utrecht, The Netherlands)
J Neurosurg 88:82–92, 1998   19–7

Background.—Lasers have proved useful in neuroendoscopy. However, many surgeons are still uncomfortable using high-energy laser endoscopic probes near vital structures, such as the basilar artery in third ventriculostomy. A newly developed laser catheter for use in neuroendoscopy was described.

Methods and Findings.—The new laser is fitted with an atraumatic ball-shaped fiber tip pretreated with a layer of carbon particles, which absorb about 90% of the energy emitted and convert it into heat. As the heat is generated, the temperature at the surface of the tip instantly reaches ablative temperatures at powers of only a few watts per second. Thus, the amount of laser light used and the length of exposure can be limited substantially. The fibertips were used with a neodymium-yttrium aluminum garnet contact laser or a diode contact laser in 49 patients undergoing ventriculocisternostomy, cyst fenetration, colloid cyst resection, or fenestration of the septum pellucidum. The success rate of the procedure, to date, is 100%. The overall outcome success rate is 86%. There has been no increase in morbidity and there have been no deaths.

Conclusion.—Pretreated atraumatic ball-shaped fiber tips make laser application safe and effective in a variety of neuroendoscopic procedures. Because only several watts are needed, compact diode lasers will be the energy source of choice.

▶ The application of neuroendoscopy has been expanding rapidly in recent years. Neuroendoscopy was started with intraventricular procedures for hydrocephalus almost a century ago. Intraventricular endoscopy has advanced to tumor surgery, as well as being used for third ventriculostomies for hydrocephalus. Now, the technique has been implemented in stereotactic intra-axial surgery, extra-axial surgery, skull base surgery, endoscope-assisted microsurgery, pituitary surgery, and spinal surgery. The potential for further development and refinement of neuroendoscopy is enormous, in conjunction with improved surgical equipment, advances in computer technology, video imaging, stereotaxis, and telecommunications.

The miniature carbon tip attached to the diode contact laser reported in this paper by Vandertop et al. is an example of this technology that neuroendoscopic surgeons have been working on. Commercial instrument companies have already entered the race for neuroendoscopic business. As finite cutting tools for intraventricular surgery through an endoscopic working channel, mechanical tools, electric current tools (either of the monopolar or bipolar type), and laser energy tools have been used with various advantages and disadvantages. Laser-powered instruments are attractive in neuroendoscopy because of the ease and precision of their application.

However, uncontrollable penetration into the adjacent tissue has been problematic. A pretreated carbon tip laser seems to overcome this problem. The problem of risk of local heat generation has yet to be answered, and the friable nature of the carbon tip requires improvement. Because it has to be submerged in fluid to prevent burning, the instrument can only be used in a CSF-containing cavity.

H.D. Jho, M.D., Ph.D.

Computed Tomography–guided Transsphenoidal Closure of Postsurgical Cerebrospinal Fluid Fistula: A Transmucosal Needle Technique
Fraioli B, Pastore FS, Floris R, et al (Univ of Rome)
Surg Neurol 48:409–413, 1997   19–8

Background.—Cerebrospinal fluid (CSF) fistula is a serious complication of transphenoidal surgery. Despite careful intraoperative repair and prolonged postoperative lumbar CSF drainage, a new surgical intrasphenoidal plasty can be necessary. A new technique for postoperative transsphenoidal CSF leakage was reported.

Patients and Outcomes.—Five patients with rhinoliquorrhea after a transsphenoidal approach for excising pituitary adenomas and craniopharyngiomas required treatment. Treatment consisted of a computed tomography (CT–guided intrasphenoidal injection of fibrin glue through a 12–gauge spinal needle—a simple, minimally invasive method. In 2 patients, the first attempt was only partially successful; thus, the procedure was repeated. In the last 2 patients treated, 2 cc of fresh autologous blood was given before fibrin glue injection to enhance the mechanisms of healing, possibly inducing adhesions and fibrosis. To date, none of the patients had a recurrence of SCF leakage.

Conclusions.—CT-guided intrasphenoidal injection of fibrin glue through a 12–gauge spinal needle—a simple, safe, mildly invasive technique that can be repeated if necessary—is proposed for the treatment of postoperative transsphenoidal CSF leakage. This may be useful treatment for other types of rhinoliquorrea in selected patients.

▶ CSF leak after transsphenoidal surgery is quite often a complication. Fat graft, flat position, and/or lumbar drainage usually cures the problem, however, some patients face the necessity of surgical repair. The presented innovative method of sealing a defect with CT–guided local autologous blood and fibrin glue injection seems to be safe, simple, only mildly invasive and successful. Another important advantage of this method is its repeatability and the fact that the local injection of the glue may enhance the existing plug (like fat graft) without its removal. The value of the method; however, needs to be confirmed on a larger series of patients.

R.M. Pluta, M.D., Ph.D.

Endoscopic Craniectomy for Early Surgical Correction of Sagittal Craniosynostosis
Jimenez DF, Barone CM (Univ of Missouri, Columbia)
J Neurosurg 88:77–81, 1998   19–9

Objective.—Premature closure of the sagittal suture results in scaphocephaly and other deformations. Conventional open craniectomy can lead to significant blood loss. A technique using endoscopes to minimize scalp incisions, blood loss, and operative times in patients undergoing midline strip craniotomies was described.

Methods.—Four patients (1 girl), aged 2–12 weeks, with scaphocephaly, bifrontal and occipital bosselation, and a midline bony ridge between the anterior fontanelle and the lambda, were treated with endoscopic midline strip craniectomy.

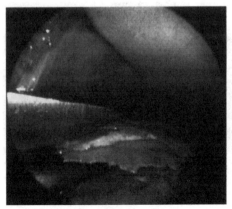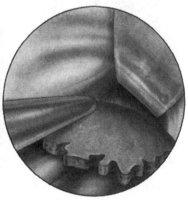

FIGURE 4.—**Left,** endoscopic view of bone-cutting scissors being used to create a paramedian osteotomy. **Right,** artist's rendition of the figure shown at left. The tips of the scissors are seen in the left lower quadrant. Cutting through the posterior edge of the anterior fontanelle, a retractor, elevating the scalp, is seen in the right upper corner. (Courtesy of Jimenez DF, Barone CM: Endoscopic craniectomy for early surgical correction of sagittal craniosynostosis. *J Neurosurg* 88:77–81, 1998.)

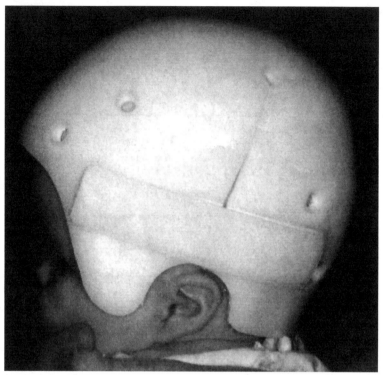

FIGURE 7.—Postoperative photograph of a patient in a polypropylene molding helmet. Anteroposterior growth is partially restricted while allowing increased bitemporal and biparietal expansion to achieve rapid normocephaly. (Courtesy of Jimenez DF, Barone CM: Endoscopic craniectomy for early surgical correction of sagittal craniosynostosis. *J Neurosurg* 88:77–81, 1998.)

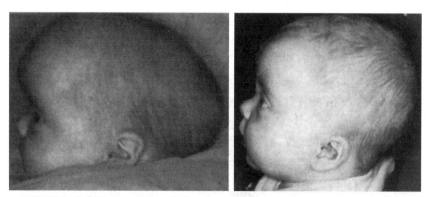

FIGURE 8.—**Left:** preoperative lateral view of a 4-week-old girl who was born with a prominent, palpable midline osseous ridge, marked bifrontal bosselation, occipital cupping, and significant scaphocephaly. **Right:** lateral view of the same infant 7 months postoperatively. (Courtesy of Jimenez DF, Barone CM: Endoscopic craniectomy for early surgical correction of sagittal craniosynostosis. *J Neurosurg* 88:77–81, 1998).

Technique.—A 2-cm incision was made over the anterior fontanelle and another over the lambda. The fontanelle and calvarium were exposed with electrocautery, and the dura was separated from the fontanelle by blunt dissection. Subgaleal dissection was performed to the superior temporal line bilaterally. The dura was dissected free, and a thin strip of bone was removed to the lambdoid sutures. After epidural exposure, lateral paramedian osteotomies, 3- to 4-cm wide and 6- to 9-cm long, were performed. Gelfoam was used to minimize bleeding (Fig 4), and 3 bone wedges were removed. Lambdoid sutures were similarly removed. The scalp was closed, and the patient was fitted with a custom-made cranial remodeling helmet (Fig 7).

Results.—Patients were followed up for 8 to 15 months. No complications or postoperative infections were noted. Duration of surgery ranged from 1.15 to 2.8 hours with an estimated blood volume loss of 2.3% to 26.4%. One child required a transfusion. Children tolerated the helmets well and achieved normocephaly at between 5 and 12 months (Fig 8). All children achieved and maintained a normal cephalic index measurement.

Conclusion.—Endoscopic craniectomy is safe, reduces blood loss during surgery, does not result in an increased complication rate, and achieves excellent results.

▶ Clearly, there has been a trend toward minimally invasive surgery in recent years, and there has been no exception in neurosurgery. The authors have creatively and thoughtfully developed a safe and effective endoscopic technique to correct this developmental deformity. I have personally witnessed this procedure combined with a postoperative cranial molding helmet, and the result is excellent. The authors propose that strip craniectomy produces the best results when the child is less than 2 months old as compensatory deformational skull changes are less well developed. This technique renders bicoronal and midline longitudinal scalp incisions and their attendant blood loss unnecessary.

S.R. Gibbs, M.A., M.D.

A New Technique of Dural Closure: Experience With a Vicryl Mesh
Verheggen R, Schulte-Baumann WJ, Hahm G, et al (School of Medicine, Göttingen, Germany)
Acta Neurochir (Wien) 139:1074–1079, 1997   19–10

Introduction.—Numerous materials have been used to achieve reliable dural closure and avoid postoperative CSF leakages after intracranial surgery. Treatment of dural CSF leaks after posterior fossa surgery is a particularly difficult problem. The technique of dural closure described here uses a composite mesh consisting of polyglactin 910 (vicryl) and poly-p-dioxanone (PDS).

Methods.—During a period of 4 years, 222 patients underwent either a midline or a paramedian suboccipital craniectomy (161 patients) or craniotomy (61 patients) at the study institution. The most common indications for surgery were benign or malignant tumors of the CNS (133 patients) and metastasis (39 patients). Gaping dural defects were covered by autologous dural substitutes in combination with fibrin sealant or hemostyptics in 159 patients and with a vicryl-PDS mesh in 63 patients. In the latter group, a well-cut sheet of the mesh (Ethisorb) was used to cover the entire defect of the craniectomy. Perioperative antibiotic prophylaxis was given to 39.7% of patients receiving the vicryl mesh and 32.7% of those whose dural closure was achieved with muscle patches.

Results.—The 63 patients who received the vicryl-PDS mesh for dural closure after posterior fossa surgery had no infections. In contrast, a deep wound infection occurred in 3 patients in the muscle patch and/or fibrin glue group; 3 additional patients required major surgical debridement and fistulectomy and 2 patients needed broad-spectrum antibiotic therapy after acute meningitis developed. Cerebrospinal fluid collections or leaks arose in 10.41% of the muscle patch group and 6.78% of the mesh closure group.

Conclusion.—The development of CSF leaks after neurosurgical procedures is a serious complication. Leaks are difficult to manage conservatively and may lead to additional morbidity and even a risk of death. A well-fitting piece of Ethisorb vicryl mesh provides a rapid and effective dural closure.

▶ Cranial surgeons have experimented with a variety of dural substitutes. Lyophilized allograft and xenograft,[1, 2] metallic foils,[3, 4] and synthetic materials[5] have been used in cerebral surgery, sometimes to prevent meningocerebral adhesions and in cases in which the dura must be sacrificed or in which a water-tight closure cannot be achieved. The authors report particular satisfaction with vicryl mesh as a dural substitute, although they were unable to statistically demonstrate a reduced rate of cerebrospinal fluid leak.

S.R. Gibbs, M.A., M.D.

References

1. Campbell JB, Bassett CAL, Robertson JW: Clinical use of freeze-dried human dura mater. *J Neurosurg* 15:207–214, 1958.
2. O'Neill P, Booth AE: Use of porcine dermis as a dural substitute in 72 patients. *J Neurosurg* 61:351–354, 1984.
3. Banerjee T, Meagher JN, Hunt We: Unusual complications with use of Silastic dura substitute. *Am Surg* 40:434–437, 1983.
4. Robertson RCL, Peacher WG: The use of tantalum foil in the subdural space. *J Neurosurg* 2:281–284, 1948.
5. Beach HHA: Gold foil in cerebral surgery. *Boston Med Surg J* 136:281–282, 1897.

20 Gene Therapy

Cellular and Molecular Neurosurgery: Pathways From Concept to Reality—Part II: Vector Systems and Delivery Methodologies for Gene Therapy of the Central Nervous System
Zlokovic BV, Apuzzo MLJ (Univ of Southern Calif, Los Angeles)
Neurosurgery 40:805–813, 1997   20–1

Background.—In previous articles, the authors reviewed the possibilities of gene therapy for CNS disorders, including inherited global neurodegenerative disorders, loss of a particular subset of cells to neurodegenerative processes, brain tumors, and stroke. Once candidates for gene therapy have been identified, the issues of delivering genetic material to the brain and regulating gene transcription and expression of the final gene product must be addressed. Vector systems for use in gene therapy for CNS disorders are reviewed, including their potential advantages and disadvantages for clinical application.

Vector Systems for CNS Gene Transfer Therapy.—A number of different vector systems have been studied for use in CNS gene transfer, including retroviruses, recombinant herpes simplex virus, adenoviruses, adeno–associated viruses, plasmid deoxyribonucleic acid encapsulated into cationic liposomes, and neural and oligodendroglia stem cells. Any vector used must address the problem of the blood–brain barrier and/or the blood–brain–tumor barrier. Considered approaches have included local stereotactic CNS injection or infusion of viral vectors; administration of vector producer cells, or cell replacement; administration of genetic material into the local cerebrospinal fluid ventriculocisternal system; osmotic opening of the blood–brain barrier; local intra-arterial infusion; and administration of agents, such as the bradykinin B2 agonist RMP-7, to render the blood-brain-tumor barrier permeable. In vitro studies and a few animal experiments have shown very promising results with gene therapy for various brain disorders. However, key problems remain in areas, such as inefficient transfection of host cells by viral vectors, restricted delivery of genetic material across the vascular barriers of the CNS and brain tumors, nonselective expression of the transgene, and therapeutic control over CNS regulation of transgene expression, as influenced by the specific CNS disease.

Summary.—With advances in cellular and molecular biology, gene therapy for CNS disorders has become a realistic goal. Several different gene therapy approaches to global and localized CNS neurodegenerative disorders and stroke have been identified. This article reviews the vector systems that have been studied for use in CNS gene transfer and identifies the key obstacles that must be overcome to make this form of therapy a clinical reality.

▶ This is Part II of a 2-part series in which the authors review various approaches for gene therapy of the CNS. This second part describes the vector systems and delivery methods for gene therapy.

The authors identify the 2 major problems relating to delivery systems: overcoming the problem of the blood-brain barrier and/or blood-brain-tumor barrier, and ensuring that once the recombinant genetic material is successfully delivered to the target cells within the CNS, the regulation of gene transcription and the expression of its final product can be achieved in a biologically controlled way. The techniques are described simply and lucidly with the pros and cons of each method discussed in an informative manner.

This is an excellent article and is certainly required reading for any neuroscientist interested in gene therapy of CNS disorders.

A.H. Kaye, M.D., M.B.B.S., F.R.A.C.S.

Cellular and Molecular Neurosurgery: Pathways From Concept to Reality—Part I: Target Disorders and Concept Approaches to Gene Therapy of the Central Nervous System
Zlokovic BV, Apuzzo MLJ (Univ of Southern California, Los Angeles)
Neurosurgery 40:789–804, 1997   20–2

Introduction.—Cellular and molecular neurosurgery is an emerging discipline that seeks to develop the potential of gene therapy for disorders of the CNS. Possible applications include gene replacement with a single normal allele to correct enzyme deficiencies and other inherited global degenerative disorders, localized restorative CNS gene therapy to restore a particular subset of cells lost to neurodegenerative processes, and gene therapy for brain tumors or stroke. Studied approaches to gene therapy of CNS disorders are reviewed.

Approaches to CNS Gene Therapy.—The review includes approaches to global CNS gene replacement therapy, cell replacement and restorative gene therapy, gene therapy approaches to brain tumors, gene therapy approaches to stroke, and others. In global gene replacement therapy, viral vector-mediated approaches seek to produce stable expression of normal proteins in deficient brain cells to effect cure of inherited enzyme deficiencies and metabolic diseases, such as the lysosomal storage disorders. Another strategy is the use of neural progenitor cells as vectors for gene therapy; this approach has been used to treat a mouse model of MPS VII, for example. Cellular-genetic strategies have been investigated for use in the repair of particular cell types lost because of neurodegenerative processes. These approaches include cell replacement therapy, viral vector-mediated gene transfer, plasmid/DNA/lipofectin therapy for Parkinson's disease, and experimental approaches for gene therapy for Alzheimer's disease.

A number of different approaches to gene therapy of brain tumors have been investigated, including drug susceptibility genes for selection tumor destruction (so-called suicide genes), herpes simplex virus mutants, antisense strategies addressed against the genes involved in malignant progression and stimulation of tumor growth, and adoptive immunotherapy, which has the potential for highly specific tumor toxicity. Therapeutic genes for use in stroke treatment have been investigated, including administration of an adenoviral vector carrying the human IL-1 receptor agonist protein, and use of the bcl-2 gene to rescue neurons from programmed cell death. Transgenic approaches to manipulate the expression of various hemostasis-related proteins, including the fibrinolytic t-PA/PAI-1 system, have been investigated. Other concepts including transfer of drug-resistant genes to lessen the toxic effects of chemotherapy drugs, and monoclonal antibody gene transfer techniques, such as an antibody against the ErbB-2 receptor, have been studied for use in gene therapy of more accessible non-CNS tissues.

Summary.—Recent years have seen major advances in our understanding of the genetic and biochemical bases of CNS disorders, and in gene therapy approaches to various types of CNS disorders. Though promising, these techniques face major obstacles, including efficacy, selectivity, delivery of genetic material, and regulation of cellular expression of the transgene. Other areas of concern include transient gene expression, viral protein toxicity, drawbacks of antisense therapy, and problems associated with immune responses to transfected proteins.

▶ This is the first part of a 2-part series describing cellular and molecular neurosurgery. The authors review the concept of gene therapy of the CNS, with particular reference to gene replacement therapy and techniques for neurodegenerative disorders, gene therapy for brain tumors, and gene therapy for stroke. Techniques discussed include viral vector mediated CNS transfer of a therapeutic gene, transplantation of genetically modified cells, foetal cell implantation or the use of genetically engineered neural progenitor cells, and production of specific enzyme, neurotransmitter, and/or growth factors. The authors have also described other potentially important techniques, such as adoptive immunotherapy and transfection of CNS tumor cells with drug susceptibility genes, or transduction with "toxic" genes.

The authors have provided an excellent overview of the possibilities for gene therapy of various CNS disorders, and have described each of the techniques lucidly, in a way that can be understood by the practicing neurosurgeon with very little specialist knowledge of molecular biology.

It remains to be seen which of the techniques described will eventually be useful in the treatment of CNS disorders, but the article provides an excellent introduction for both neurosurgeons in training and practical neurosurgeons with an interest in the topic.

A.H. Kaye, M.D., M.B.B.S., F.R.A.C.S.

21 Head Trauma

Use of Hypertonic (3%) Saline/Acetate Infusion in the Treatment of Cerebral Edema: Effect on Intracranial Pressure and Lateral Displacement of the Brain
Qureshi AI, Suarez JI, Bhardwaj A, et al (Johns Hopkins Med Institution, Baltimore, Md)
Crit Care Med 26:440–446, 1998   21–1

Purpose.—Recent reports have described the use of hypertonic saline as a hyperosmolar treatment for intracranial hypertension and cerebral edema. The authors' neurocritical care unit has been giving continuous infusion of hypertonic saline to their patients with acute cerebral injury. This form of hyperosmolar therapy has some important advantages over mannitol in that it is an effective volume expander and does not cause problems with hyperkalemia and impaired renal function. The effects of continuous hypertonic saline/acetate infusion in the treatment of acute cerebral edema were evaluated in a retrospective study.

Methods.—The analysis included 30 episodes of cerebral edema occurring in 27 consecutive patients. Eight patients had head trauma, 5 had postoperative edema, 8 had nontraumatic intracranial hemorrhage, and 6 had cerebral infarction. All were managed with IV infusion of 3% saline/acetate to increase serum sodium concentration to the target range of 145 to 155 mmol/L. The effects of hypertonic saline infusion on intracranial pressure (ICP) and lateral brain displacement were analyzed.

Results.—The head trauma and postoperative edema groups showed reductions in mean ICP within the first 12 hours, in correlation with the rise in serum sodium. However, this effect was not seen in the patients with nontraumatic intracranial hemorrhage or those with cerebral infarction. By 72 hours after the start of hypertonic saline infusion, 4 of 8 patients in the head trauma group had poor ICP control, necessitating treatment with IV pentobarbital. Twenty-one patients underwent repeat CT scanning within 72 hours after the start of hypertonic saline infusion. Lateral brain displacement decreased from 2.8 to 1.1 in the head trauma group and from 3.1 to 1.1 in the postoperative edema group. Again, the benefit was not apparent in the patients with nontraumatic intracranial hemorrhage or cerebral infarction. Six patients had complications necessitating the termination of hypertonic saline infusion; there was pulmonary edema in 3 patients and diabetes insipidus in 3.

Conclusion.—For patients with head trauma or postoperative edema, infusion of 3% saline/acetate appears to give good results in the treatment of cerebral edema. It is an inexpensive treatment with manageable side effects; it does not appear to be effective in patients with nontraumatic intracranial hemorrhage or cerebral infarction, however. The authors call for more research to identify the optimal duration of benefit and the patient population most likely to benefit.

▶ In head trauma, *vasogenic* edema develops primarily in the acute phase (first 24–48 hours) when vasoparalysis, extravasation of complex molecules, and ionic and water shifts may complicate the primary mechanical brain injury. Later on, multiple pathophysiologic and metabolic processes occur and may be associated with astrocytic swelling and cellular ischemia; these result in complex brain swelling (cytotoxic, vasogenic, and interstitial) and hypertonic saline could be detrimental.

In addition, the proportion of edema that is vasogenic in each individual patient varies, depending on the type of trauma, i.e., diffuse axonal injury, focal contusion, or extracerebral hematoma. The improvement in postoperative patients who have undergone resection of focal lesions perhaps suggests that trauma patients with "focal contusions" and pericontusional edema are most likely to benefit.

In postoperative patients, one should make the distinction between 2 types of vasogenic edema. The first is related to excessive tissue retraction (iatrogenic trauma). The second is related to ischemia-reperfusion.[1] Before surgery, brain tissue, adjacent or distal to operable lesions, may become chronically hypoperfused and ischemic. After resection of the lesion, marked increase in blood flow may occur in this tissue (perilesional area) and lead to vasogenic edema, described as *breakthrough* edema after resection of arteriovenous malformations and *reperfusion* (*hyperperfusion*) edema after resection of tumors, carotid endarterectomy or prolonged temporary cerebral arterial clipping.[1]

Further research should clarify the response to treatment of vasogenic edema associated with the aforementioned common types of trauma or postoperative conditions and whether hypertonic saline has an effort on other types of extracellular edema; this could be tested in patients with hydrocephalus and "interstitial" edema that is visualized as periventricular "lucency" on CT or high signal on T2 MRI. Before commencing treatment with hypertonic saline, it is essential that clinicians adopt the correct working hypothesis as to the type, cause, mechanism, and timing of edema on each patient.

D.E. Sakas, M.D.

Reference

1. Macfarlane R, Moskowitz MA, Sakas DE, et al: The role of neuro-effector mechanisms in cerebral hyperperfusion syndromes. *J Neurosurg* 75:845–855, 1991.

Growing Skull Fractures: A Clinical Study of 41 Patients
Gupta SK, Reddy NM, Khosla VK, et al (Postgraduate Inst of Med Education and Research, Chandigarh, India)
Acta Neurochir (Wien) 139:928–932, 1997   21–2

Background.—Growing skull fractures are uncommon complications of head trauma in children. Typically, a skull fracture occurs with an underlying dural tear. The fracture enlarges progressively, producing a cranial defect. Local brain injury, porencephalic formation, and changes in cerebrospinal fluid circulation have been associated with the dural tear. One experience with growing skull fractures was reviewed.

Methods and Findings.—Forty-one patients treated between 1975 and 1995 were included. Patient ages ranged from 1–61 years, with 80.5% of patients younger than 5 years. Injuries were caused by a fall from a height in 93% of cases and by a traffic accident in 7%. In 56% of the patients, the growing skull fracture was parietal or frontoparietal. In 1 patient, it was in the posterior fossa. Nineteen patients underwent CT, which showed an underlying porencephalic cyst, hydrocephalus, or a cyst communicating with the ventricle. A ventriculo-peritoneal shunt only was performed in 5 children. A duroplasty and cranioplasty were done in 24 patients, and a duroplasty alone was done in 8. Acrylic, wire mesh, steel plates, or autologous bone were used for cranioplasty. Three patients died: 2 from postoperative meningitis and 1 from an anesthetic complication. Three patients had CSF leaks after surgery; these were managed by a lumbar drain. Local wound infection occurred in 6 patients.

Conclusion.—Clinicians should examine children with linear skull fractures 2 to 3 months after injury to look for evidence of a growing skull fracture. Underlying brain damage is often progressive in such patients, and neurologic defects can worsen. Surgical repair is indicated for growing skull fractures.

▶ Growing skull fractures are rare complications of head trauma. This rather generous series allows valid evaluation of means as well as extremes. The age range at injury and the age range at presentation are quite broad. Infratentorial as well as supratentorial skull is at risk. Options for treatment and/or repair have evolved through several paradigms; and complications can be significant. Such experience will benefit those now better primed to recognize and handle a complication that may be seen only a few times in ones career.

C.P. Bondurant, M.D.

Effect of Methylphenidate on Attentional Function After Traumatic Brain Injury: A Randomized, Placebo-controlled Trial

Whyte J, Hart T, Schuster K, et al (Temple Univ, Philadelphia; Allegheny Univ of the Health Sciences, Philadelphia)
Am J Phys Med Rehabil 76:440–450, 1997   21–3

Introduction.—After traumatic brain injury, disorders of attention are commonly reported. For most attentional disturbances that follow traumatic brain injury, psychostimulants are among the most commonly used pharmacologic agents. In children and adolescents with attention deficit hyperactivity disorder, methylphenidate has long been used to improve attention and behavioral control. The drug has been shown to enhance vigilance performance, ability to stay on task, complex verbal learning, and the speed with which stimuli are processed for decision-making. In depression, apathy, and arousal deficits in neurologic conditions such as stroke and demention in adults, methylphenidate has also been used. The effects of methylphenidate on attentional function in patients with traumatic brain injury referred specifically for attentional assessment and treatment were evaluated.

Methods.—Using 5 different tasks designed to measure various facets of attentional function, 19 patients were reviewed in a study with a double-blind, placebo-controlled, repeated crossover design. The patients had a median age of 27 years; 15 were men and 4 were women. There were 16 whites, 2 African-Americans, and 1 Hispanic. The 5 tasks were concerned with sustained arousal, phasic arousal, distraction, choice reaction time, and behavioral inattention.

Results.—In the speed of mental processing, methylphenidate produced a significant improvement. The increases in speed did not generally occur at the expense of accuracy. It is still unknown whether improvements in speed could be associated with reductions in accuracy. Orienting to distractions, most aspects of sustained attention and measures of motor speed were not affected. Although the drug may reduce the disruptive impact of distraction on performance by speeding the accomplishment of work before and after a distracting event, there does not seem to be an effect of methylphenidate on distractibility.

Conclusion.—In traumatic brain injury, methylphenidate may be a useful treatment, but primarily for symptoms that can be attributed to slowed mental processing. It is still unknown whether different doses might produce larger effects.

▶ It is widely accepted as fact that important variables affecting intellectual outcome after traumatic brain injury include acute medical management, physical-behavioral rehabilitation, and the brain's repair mechanisms and plasticity. This article suggests that psychopharmacologic treatment may potentially become an additional variable in this process.

The timing of such treatment may be important. In this study, the response of patients treated much later than 18 months after the injury did not differ from that of others treated much earlier. I am inclined to think that the first 18 months offer the best opportunity for maximum psychopharmacologic benefit because of likely positive "interaction" of this treatment with spontaneous biological cellular repair processes.

The duration of the benefit is also an important issue. If the cognitive improvement lasts for only as long as the drug is taken, the patient must depend on it for many years; this may have long-term implications as it is not known whether stimulating increased activity of the "dopaminergic system" by methylphenidate could simultaneously suppress the gradual natural recovery of this system's endogenous stimulatory or regulatory mechanisms.

Future research should correlate closely the response to treatment with findings from advanced neuroimaging such as positron emission tomography, functional MRI, or magnetoencephalography modalities that may make it possible to pinpoint brain lesions and disrupted neurochemical anatomical pathways. I also believe that benefits will be maximized if psychopharmacologic drugs are used as adjuncts to the pharmacologic modulation of the brain's biological cellular repair mechanisms.

D.E. Sakas, M.D.

Cerebral Arteriovenous Oxygen Difference: A Predictor of Cerebral Infarction and Outcome in Patients With Severe Head Injury
Le Roux PD, Newell DW, Lam AM, et al (Univ of Washington, Seattle)
J Neurosurg 87:1–8, 1997   21–4

Introduction.—Several techniques are available to estimate the adequacy of cerebral perfusion pressure (CPP) after severe head injury. Jugular bulb oxygen monitoring, while not measuring absolute cerebral blood flow (CBF) values, provides an estimate of the adequacy of CBF to support cerebral metabolism by measuring the balance between oxygen delivery and consumption. Previous studies have shown an inverse relationship between CBF and arteriovenous oxygen difference ($AVDO_2$) in the absence of infarction or necrosis. A study of 32 head–injured patients examined the $AVDO_2$ response to craniotomy or mannitol administration, the relationships among $AVDO_2$, intracranial pressure (ICP), and CPP, and the associations between $AVDO_2$ and delayed cerebral infarction and outcome.

Methods.—Patients were 21 men and 11 women with a mean age of 34.5. All had an isolated non–penetrating head injury, a Glasgow Coma Scale score of ≤ 8, normal blood pressure, normothermia, hematocrit >30%, and had survived >24 hours after admission. Fifteen patients (group A) underwent craniotomy for evaluation of a traumatic mass lesion and 17 (group B) had no mass lesions but received a mannitol infusion for sustained intracranial hypertension. Outcome was assessed 6 months after head injury.

Results.—Seventeen patients died or were severely disabled. The mean AVDO for all patients before treatment was 8.6 vol%. After craniotomy or mannitol administration, $AVDO_2$ decreased in 27 patients and increased in 5. The mean ICP after craniotomy or mannitol administration was 17.8 mm Hg. Mean CPP was greater in group A than in group B patients; overall, the mean CPP after treatment was 75 mm Hg. No relationship between CPP and $AVDO_2$ was demonstrated. There was a significant association between limited improvement in elevated $AVDO_2$ after craniotomy or mannitol administration and a delayed cerebral infarction. Limited posttreatment improvement in elevated $AVDO_2$ was also significantly associated with an unfavorable outcome.

Conclusion.—Measurement of $AVDO_2$ before craniotomy or mannitol administration was not predictive of delayed cerebral infarction or outcome after severe head injury, but limited improvement in AVDO after treatment was significantly associated with both delayed cerebral infarction and unfavorable outcome. No relationship between CPP and $AVDO_2$ was observed. Results of jugular bulb monitoring can predict outcome after traumatic brain injury.

▶ These clinical investigators determined that in 32 head–injured patients who were treated either with a craniotomy for intracranial hematoma or mannitol for increased intracranial pressure, the failure to see a significant increase in $AVDO_2$ was associated with delayed cerebral infarction and poor outcome after traumatic brain injury. On the basis of these findings, the investigators recommend continuous measurement of $AVDO_2$ by use of a catheter in the jugular bulb. Interestingly, while observing a relationship between ICP and $AVDO_2$ they were unable to demonstrate a correlation between $AVDO_2$ and CPP, once again raising a question regarding the relationship between CPP and ICP. It should be noted that while these investigators recommend continuous jugular bulb catheterization for monitoring $AVDO_2$, they did observe the need for frequent recalibration and a high percentage of erroneous readings because of catheter movement, displacement, intimal impaction, or clot formation. Although this is a well–documented complex study, the case has not been made that measurement of $AVDO_2$ with the aid of continuous jugular bulb catheterization is of sufficient clinical utility at the bedside to warrant adoption for routine use.

C. Watts, M.D., J.D.

Terson's Syndrome in Subarachnoid Hemorrhage and Severe Brain Injury Accompanied by Acutely Raised Intracranial Pressure
Medele RJ, Stummer W, Mueller AJ, et al (Ludwig-Maximilians Univ, Munich)
J Neurosurg 88:851–854, 1998   21–5

Background.—Terson's syndrome refers to retinal or vitreous hemorrhage associated with subarachnoid hemorrhage (SAH). Vitreous hypertension and retinal or vitreous hemorrhage may result from rapid increases in intracranial pressure (ICP), leading to decreased venous drainage of the posterior compartments of the eyes. This study evaluated the incidence of intraocular hemorrhage in patients with severe brain injury vs. SAH and acutely increased ICP.

Methods.—The prospective study included 22 consecutive patients with acute intracranial hypertension—defined as ICP initially exceeding 20 mm Hg—associated with either SAH or severe brain injury. Subarachnoid hemorrhage of World Federation of Neurological Surgeons grades II to IV was present in 13 patients; the other 9 patients had severe brain injury with Glasgow Coma Scale scores of 3 to 10. At the time of admission, a ventricular catheter was placed for ongoing measurement of ICP. Within 1 week after SAH or brain injury, all patients underwent indirect ophthalmoscopy without induced mydriasis. The incidence of Terson's syndrome in patients with SAH and brain injury was compared.

Results.—Retinal or vitreous hemorrhage was found in 46% of patients with SAH and 44% of those with severe brain injury. All of these patients had initial coma, and 7 of 10 had ICP of greater than 30 mm Hg during ventricular catheter placement. Three patients in the SAH group and 1 in the brain injury group had bilateral ocular bleeding. The mortality rate from SAH or brain injury among the patients with Terson's syndrome was 60%.

Conclusion.—Terson's syndrome can occur as a complication of acutely increased ICP, regardless of the cause. This study found a similar incidence of intraocular bleeding in patients with severe brain injury and with SAH. Clinicians should be alert for Terson's syndrome in all patients with acutely increased ICP, as prompt recognition may prevent visual impairment and secondary ocular damage. Patients with Terson's syndrome appear to have a poor prognosis.

▶ It is always preferable to interpret a clinical phenomenon by a single mechanism. In head injuries, however, mechanisms other than a sudden rise of ICP could also lead to Terson's syndrome. The eyeball has several vulnerable sites and vitreoretinal hemorrhages are found within various spaces, i.e., intravitreal, retrovitreal (subhyaloid), superficial, and deeper retina, and under photoreceptors or retinal pigment. Head trauma may be associated with optic nerve injury at the lamina cribosa (perforated sclera) and small tears of the central artery or vein, ciliary vessels or pial plexus followed by diffusion of blood through the retina into the retrovitreal space or vitreous.

Another mechanism may be related to the fact that the sclera and choroid are "fixed" in position but the vitreous and retina are much more mobile. During injury, the orbital contents undergo abrupt differential deceleration because of differences in specific gravity and the firmness of adherence to adjacent tissues. A "sliding" vitreous within the eyeball may exert vitreoretinal traction and precipitate a posterior vitreous detachment, a retinal tear, and hemorrhage from bridging vessels. An embryonic hyaloid artery that persisted in later life within the vitreous could also be torn during such injuries.

Terson's syndrome may accompany traumatic SAH, and either of these conditions is an indicator of a poor prognosis. It would be interesting to find out whether there is a common traumatic mechanism leading to SAH and/or Terson's syndrome. Vitreoretinal hemorrhage is a feature of nonaccidental head injuries that may be caused by the violent shaking of small children.[1] Insights into the mechanisms of Terson's syndrome may improve the pathogenetic classification and management of head injuries. Clinicians should insist on examining the fundi, particularly in children, despite the obstacle of periorbital swelling.

D.E. Sakas, M.D.

Reference

1. Eagling EM, Roper-Hall MJ: *Eye Injuries*. Butterworths, London, 1986.

22 Hydrocephalus

Dutch Normal-pressure Hydrocephalus Study: Randomized Comparison of Low- and Medium-pressure Shunts
Boon AJW, Tans JTJ, Delwel EJ, et al (Westeinde Hosp, The Hague, The Netherlands; Univ Hosp, Rotterdam, The Netherlands; Free Univ Hosp, Amsterdam; et al)
J Neurosurg 88:490–495, 1998   22–1

Introduction.—There is ongoing debate over the appropriate shunt pressure to use for patients with normal-pressure hydrocephalus (NPH). Different studies have used different approaches, but there have been no randomized trials. As part of the Dutch Normal-pressure Hydrocephalus Study, outcomes were compared after placement of a low- vs. medium-pressure shunt in patients with NPH.

Methods.—The randomized, multicenter trial included 96 patients with NPH. They were managed with either a low-pressure ventriculoperitoneal shunt (LPV), 40 mm water, or a medium-pressure shunt (MPV), 100 mm water. Gait disturbance and dementia were graded using an NPH scale. The modified Rankin scale was used to grade disability. The patients were assessed before surgery and 1, 3, 6, 9, and 12 months after surgery. The differences between the preoperative and last follow-up results on the NPH scale and modified Rankin scale were used as the main outcome measures. The 2 treatment groups were compared for mean improvement and proportions of patients showing improvement.

Results.—On intention-to-treat analysis, mRS grade improved by a mean of 1.27 in the LPV group and 0.68 in the MPV group. Seventy-four percent of patients in the LPV group showed improvement, compared with 53% of those in the MPV group. The rates of marked-to-excellent improvement were 45% and 28%, respectively. Patients in the LPV group had a significantly better outcome on the dementia scale; all other outcomes tended to be better with the LPV. The difference was not as great after exclusion of serious events and non–NPH-related deaths. Patients in the LPV group has significantly greater reductions in ventricular size. The rate of subdural effusion was 71% in the LPV group vs. 34% in the MPV group, but this had little impact on patient outcome.

Conclusions.—In patients with NPH, an LPV shunt provides a better outcome than an MPV shunt. However, the differences were not statistically significant. The authors recommend treatment with a low-pressure shunt for patients with NPH.

▶ Shunting for hydrocephalus is the neurological procedure most frequently associated with secondary complications. The most tantalizing complication is over- or under-drainage of CFS. The equilibrium of intracranial pressure in which the hydrodynamics of CFS production, circulation, and absorption occur is so complex that it is difficult to accomplish satisfactory results with a shunt whose performance depends on the intraventricular pressure, which is so variable. When the patient stands in an upright position, the normal ventricular pressure is close to zero; when he is lying down, the mean normal pressure is around 100 mm water. These values could mean that a shunt with an opening pressure of 100 mm water would open only while the patient is lying down and remain closed while he is standing. Moreover, the gravity effect acting upon the shunt might open the valve and produce overdrainage when the patient is standing, even in the case of negative values of ventricular pressure. Thus, while the ventricular pressure varies greatly under normal circumstances, the opening and closing values of a given valve mechanism remain constant. Based on this premise, it can be anticipated that a shunt functioning in relation to intraventricular pressure will not fit properly within the spectrum of hydrodynamic forces taking place inside the ventricular cavities. This article shows large differences in the outcome of shunting for normal-pressure hydrocephalus according to the selection of the valve's opening pressure. With the low-pressure shunt, clinical results are slightly better, but complications caused by subdural effusions are more frequent; with the medium-pressure shunt, clinical results are slightly worse but fewer complications arise. Paradoxically, to achieve maximum clinical improvement, the shunt must function near the limits of excessive drainage, but, to prevent this complication, the shunt must function near the limits of insufficient drainage, therefore losing efficiency. This carefully-designed study also shows that even in the best cases the relief of clinical disturbances caused by normal-pressure hydrocephalus is modest, around 20% in the dementia scale and around 30% in the gait scale. With low-pressure shunts 3 out of 4 patients improve, whereas with medium-pressure shunts the number goes down to 2; however, subdural effusions double in patients with low-pressure shunts (71%) when compared with those in patients with medium-pressure shunts (34%). Treatment for hydrocephalus continues to be a challenge for neurosurgery. In the case of normal-pressure hydrocephalus, whose etiology is still elusive, the optimal treatment seems to go beyond CSF drainage.

J. Sotelo, M.D.

Ventricular Shunt Removal: The Ultimate Treatment of the Slit Ventricle Syndrome

Baskin JJ, Manwaring KH, Rekate HL (Mercy Healthcare Arizona, Phoenix; Phoenix Children's Hosp, Ariz)
J Neurosurg 88:478–484, 1998   22–2

Background.—Slit ventricle syndrome (SVS) can occur as a complication of extracranial ventricular shunt placement in patients with hydrocephalus. Headache results from variable combinations of intracranial hypotension and hypertension. The clinical course of SVS involves recurrent symptomatic exacerbations, leading to repeated and expensive interventions. The use of an algorithm for the evaluation and treatment of SVS was reported (Fig 1).

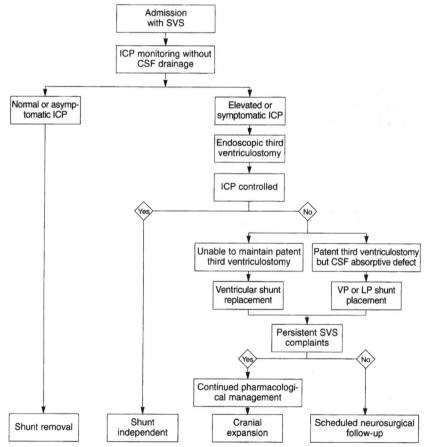

FIGURE 1.—Chart shows management algorithm for patients with slit ventricle syndrome. *Abbreviations: ICP*, intracranial pressure; *SVS*, slit ventricle syndrome; *VP*, ventriculoperitoneal; *LP*, lumboperitoneal. (Courtesy of Baskin JJ, Manwaring KH, Rekate HL: Ventricular shunt removal: The ultimate treatment of the slit ventricle syndrome. *J Neurosurg* 88:478–484, 1998.)

Methods.—The study included 22 patients treated for SVS over a 3-year period. There were 14 females and 8 males with a mean age of 17 years. After admission to the neurosurgical ICU, the patients underwent a trial of iatrogenically maintained "shunt failure." Patients with symptomatic intracranial pressure (ICP) underwent endoscopic third ventriculostomy for treatment of hydrocephalus. Patients who could not maintain a patent third ventriculostomy underwent replacement of the ventriculoperitoneal shunt system for management of persistent hydrocephalus. Those with an additional, more distal defect in CSF absorption underwent either ventriculoperitoneal shunt replacement or insertion of a lumboperitoneal shunt.

Results.—Five of 22 patients had normal ICP measurements despite the lack of CSF drainage. These patients were discharged from the hospital without shunt systems. Endoscopic third ventriculostomy was performed in 16 patients, 10 of whom maintained asymptomatic ICP. This procedure failed to manage ICP in 6 patients; in 4 cases, the failure was apparent before the patient was discharged from the ICU. Five of these patients were managed with reinsertion of a ventriculoperitoneal shunt system, including a high-pressure valve with an antisiphon device or a flow-controlled valve. Overall, 73% of patients had resolution or significant improvement in the SVS symptoms after protocol treatment. At a mean follow-up of 21 months, 64% of patients were no longer shunt dependent.

Conclusion.—Some patients with SVS syndrome need no further intervention after shunt removal. For those with persistent hydrocephalus, endoscopic third ventriculostomy can address the SVS symptoms while avoiding the need for shunt hardware. The study protocol can improve quality of life and simplify medical follow-up for patients with SVS.

▶ Asymptomatic coaptation of the ventricular walls occurs in 20% to 30% of patients with CSF shunts. Consequently, the descriptive semantics ("slit" ventricles) associated with this phenomenon are controversial as "slit ventricle syndrome" is a complete triad of chronic intermittent headache, a slowly refilling shunt reservoir, and the radiographic finding of "slit" ventricles. These patients often have exceptionally low ventricular compliance, or an abnormally elastic brain, that results in ICP spikes correlating with headache. It is essential to differentiate these patients from those with very small ventricles and an incidental headache.

Slit ventricle syndrome can be a vexing problem for the patient, the family, and the neurosurgeon. The authors have developed a straightforward algorithm that may expedite the evaluation and treatment of patients suspected of having SVS. However, as these authors have stated, neurosurgeons choosing to treat this entity must be well-experienced in endoscopic third ventriculostomy, as these patients have anatomical constraints that challenge the most facile endoscopists.

S.R. Gibbs, M.A., M.D.

Posture-related Overdrainage: Comparison of the Performance of 10 Hydrocephalus Shunts in Vitro

Czosnyka Z, Czosnyka M, Richards HK, et al (Addenbrooke's Hosp, Cambridge, England)
Neurosurgery 42:327–334, 1998   22–3

Introduction.—Posture-related overdrainage is the cause of approximately 10% to 30% of shunt revisions in patients treated for hydrocephalus. There are few data on the performance and properties of the variety of different shunts available. Ten models of hydrocephalus shunts were tested to determine their susceptibility to overdrainage of CSF.

Methods.—Five manufacturers were represented in the 10 shunt models. Functional types were siphon-preventing (3), programmable (2), classic differential (4), and flow-regulating (1). The shunts were tested in vitro, using precise computer-controlled equipment designed to evaluate pressure-flow performance curves under various conditions. Following the International Standard Organization/Draft International Standard 7197, hydrodynamic resistance and opening, closing, and operational pressures were evaluated for at least 28 days with normal (atmospheric), and decreased (-23 mm Hg) outlet pressures.

Results.—Most of the 10 tested models of valves produced significantly negative (less than -10 mm Hg) average intracranial pressures in vertical body positions. With the exception of 3 models (the Orbis-Sigma valve, Medtronic PS Medical lumboperitoneal shunt, and Heyer Schulte in-line valve), such pressures may result in overdrainage related to body posture in conjunction with nonphysiologically low hydrodynamic resistance. Shunts with siphon-preventing devices all prevented overdrainage when siphoning occurred. Siphoning could be demonstrated with both programmable shunts and classic differential valves, whereas the design of the Orbis-Sigma flow-regulating valve and its very high dynamic resistance makes it less susceptible to siphoning. Although siphoning, by definition, does not affect lumboperitoneal shunts (the Medtronic PS Medical shunt in these tests), posture-related overdrainage cannot be excluded because the lumbar CSF pressure is increased in vertical body positions. Use of the long distal catheter is likely to reduce the clinically reported rate of complications related to overdrainage. All valves with siphon-preventing devices can be blocked by increased subcutaneous pressure.

Conclusion.—Patients in whom complications related to CSF overdrainage are likely to develop should not receive shunts without mechanisms that prevent very low intracranial pressure in vertical body positions. The presence of negative outlet pressure may not be adequately described in the manufacturers' product literature.

▶ This in vitro study tested the functional performance of 10 commercially available shunting systems. It showed that 3 valves with an antisiphon device and a flow-regulating valve prevented negative proximal pressure from being generated. This type of study is of importance because it allows the potential user of these shunting devices to rely on unbiased independent laboratory tests rather than on the information distributed by the selling company.

From the conclusions of this in vitro testing, the neurosurgeon would be inclined to select certain valve systems for patients at risk for overdrainage. Unfortunately, the results of these studies cannot be directly translated to clinical situations. This opinion is supported by a recent random clinical study comparing a standard pressure differential valve, a valve with an antisiphon device, and a flow-regulating valve.[1] The study did not demonstrate any difference in the rates of patient complications. Thus, it is still unknown why valves with an antisiphon device are not superior in clinical practice to valves that do not have this feature. Further clinical investigations are needed. These include the variations in intracranial pressure after shunting, the variation in CSF flow through the valve during the daytime, and the proportion of CSF secretion that is shunted.

O. Vernet, M.D.
N. de Tribolet, M.D.

Reference

1. Drake JM, Kestle J: Rationale and methodology of the multicenter pediatric cerebrospinal fluid shunt design trial. *Childs Nerv Syst* 12:434–447, 1996.

23 Neurodegenerative Disorders

A Study of Medial Pallidotomy for Parkinson's Disease: Clinical Outcome, MRI Location and Complications

Samuel M, Caputo E, Brooks DJ, et al (Hammersmith Hosp, London; Inst of Neurology, London)

Brain 121:59–75, 1998   23–1

Introduction.—Surgical therapy has recently resurfaced for Parkinson's disease, and pallidotomy has demonstrated significant improvement of the cardinal features of the disease, such as tremor, bradykinesia, rigidity, and gait disturbance, as well as a reduction of levodopa-induced dyskinesias. In patients with medically intractable Parkinson's disease and with marked drug-induced dyskinesias, the effects of unilateral ventral medial pallidotomy were evaluated.

Methods.—Twenty-six patients had motor performance assessed. Under stereotaxic computed tomography guidance, pallidotomy was performed. After 3 months, all patients were followed up, and 9 were followed up after 1 year. To determine which categories of performance improved postoperative, pre- and postoperative performance scores were compared. Medication was compared among patients.

Results.—The diminution of "on" dyskinesias contralateral was the most significant improvement postoperative, found in 67% of patients; 45% had ipsilateral dyskinesia improvement and 50% had axial dyskinesia improvement. There was a 27% improvement of the median "off" motor score and a 25% improvement of contralateral rigidity. Contralateral tremor scores improved by 33% and bradykinesia scores improved by 24%. There was a 22% improvement of ipsilateral rigidity. No significant improvements were seen with medication. Responses were generally maintained after 1 year. Fatal complications occurred in 2 patients, major complications in 4 patients, and minor complications in 10 patients. With increasing operative experience, the complication rate declined.

Conclusion.—Following ventral medial pallidotomy, levodopa-induced dyskinesias are dramatically reduced. Some patients may not be offered an opportunity to increase anti-Parkinsonian medication with pallidotomy, but patient selection should be based on anticipated improvement in levodopa-induced dyskinesias.

▶ The chronic administration of levodopa in Parkinson's disease is well known. (It is now the standard treatment of the diseases associated with the development of fluctuations in motor response and with dystonic-choreic involuntary movements dyskinesias.) The effects of posteroventral medial pallidotomy on main features of Parkinson's disease (bradykinesia, tremor, rigidity, gait disturbance) have been reported by several authors. This meticulous study of the effects of unilateral ventral medial pallidotomy under stereotaxic CT guidance and intraoperative microelectrode recording again showed a significant improvement in contralateral rigidity. The most significant postoperative improvement was the diminution of contralateral dyskinesias. Ipsilateral and axial dyskinesias also improved postoperatively, although to a lesser degree. This study confirms that levodopa-induced dyskinesias are markedly reduced by posteroventral medial pallidotomy, which may offer some patients an opportunity to increase anti-parkinsonian medication.

K. Sano, M.D., Ph.D., Dr.h.c., F.A.C.S.

Diagnostic Yield of Brain Biopsy in Neurodegenerative Disorders
Javedan SP, Tamargo RJ (Johns Hopkins Univ, Baltimore, Md)
Neurosurgery 41:823–830, 1997   23–2

Background.—Although the role of brain biopsy is well established in the diagnosis of patients with suspected neoplastic lesions, few authors have analyzed its diagnostic yield for idiopathic neurodegenerative disorders (meningoencephalitis, CNS vasculitis, and dementia syndromes). The current study determined the diagnostic yield of brain biopsy in these disorders.

Methods.—The analysis included 48 patients undergoing 50 consecutive brain biopsies between 1990 and 1995. Extensive laboratory and radiologic assessments were performed before surgery. Because diagnoses could not be established, brain biopsies were performed.

Findings.—Only 10 biopsies resulted in diagnosis, for a diagnostic yield of 20%. Another 6% of the biopsies were suggestive of diagnoses. Findings on 66% of the biopsies were abnormal but not specific. Eight percent of the biopsies yielded normal findings. Minor complications associated with biopsy occurred in 10% of the patients. Only 4 of the 10 patients with diagnostic biopsies had a meaningful intervention as a result of the procedure. Thus, the overall therapeutic benefit was only 8%. A subgroup analysis showed that patients with focal MRI findings had the greatest likelihood of a diagnostic biopsy. Electroencephalography and laboratory abnormalities did not predict a diagnostic biopsy.

Conclusions.—The current diagnostic yield of brain biopsy for progressive neurodegenerative disorders was only 20% in this study, which is lower than previously reported. The therapeutic benefits of brain biopsy in this population are limited.

▶ The authors demonstrate that only 8% of their open (44 cases) or stereotactic biopsies (6 cases) resulted in clinically relevant changes in the management of their 50 biopsied patients presenting with unexplained neurodegenerative putative diagnosis of herpes encephalitis, chronic meningoencephalitis, dementia syndromes or cerebral vasculitis. In their effort to reevaluate the role of brain biopsy in the management of these disorders, the authors concur on the more limited role for brain biopsy in the present era of advanced non–invasive testing, including neuroimaging and serological testing. Creutzfeldt-Jakob disease was found in 4 patients, thus suggesting an important risk subjected to the operating-room team in this type of diseases.

R. Marino, Jr., M.D.

Deep Brain Stimulation Is Preferable to Thalamotomy for Tremor Suppression
Tasker RR (Toronto Hosp)
Surg Neurol 49:145–154, 1998   23–3

Introduction.—Thalamotomy is an effective procedure to alleviate tremor. Experience with this procedure has shown that deep brain stimulation (DBS) performed at the same site as thalamotomy achieves the same result. This study retrospectively compares the results of DBS and thalamotomy for patients with tremor.

Methods.—The 6–year study included 19 DBS implants, 16 performed for Parkinson's disease (PD) and 3 for essential tremor (ET); and 26 thalamotomies, 23 for PD and 3 for ET. The patients made an informed decision between thalamotomy and DBS. All patients were followed for at least 3 months.

Results.—Tremors were abolished completely in 42% of both groups. Near abolition was achieved in 79% of patients undergoing DBS and 69% of those undergoing thalamotomy. The recurrence rates were 5% and 15%, respectively. Thalamotomy had to be repeated in 15% of cases. No patient required repeat DBS, because tremor recurrence could be controlled by adjustment of stimulation parameters. Fifty-three percent of DBS patients showed a "microthalamotomy" effect resulting from electrode implantation—this effect lasted longer than 1 year in 5 patients. This finding was associated with a good prognosis and underscored the need for precise target selection. Forty-two percent of patients had ataxia, dysarthria, or gait disturbance after thalamotomy, compared with 26% after DBS. When these complications followed DBS, they could usually be controlled by adjusting the stimulation parameters.

Conclusions.—DBS and thalamotomy offer equivalent results in patients with tremor; however, DBS offers greater flexibility in tremor control and a lower complication rate. Disadvantages include the cost of the equipment and the need for ongoing patient management.

▶ This important retrospective comparison study demonstrates that electrical stimulation and lesion–making at identical sites in the thalamus may achieve exactly the same result, being equally successful. Nevertheless, stimulation offers the patients an alternative to thalamotomy, with the advantage that tremor recurrence (23%) can be better controlled by stimulation parameter adjustment than by reoperation. The resulting reduction of contralateral rigidity was the same in both procedures, neither of them showing a striking effect on speech or gait. Nowadays, we are convinced that thalamic stimulation may be preferable to thalamic lesion, especially when treatment of both sides of the brain is necessary, because of the reversibility of its side effects.

R. Marino, Jr., M.D.

24 Neuro-Imaging

Magnetic Resonance Cisternography for Visualization of Intracisternal Fine Structures
Mamata Y, Muro I, Matsumae M, et al (Tokai Univ, Karagawa, Japan; Ikegami Gen Hosp, Ota-Ku, Tokyo)
J Neurosurg 88:670–678, 1998   24–1

Background.—Contrast-enhanced CT and intrathecal gas cisternography have been used to evaluate the subarachnoid cisterns. Now MRI can be used to visualize the cranial nerves and vascular structures in this location. A heavily T2-weighted turbo spin-echo MRI technique was used to assess normal fine structures and pathologic findings in the basal cisterns.

Methods.—Twenty healthy volunteers underwent MR cisternography, with the focus on the parasellar region in 10 participants and the posterior fossa in 10. The ability of the imaging technique to detect the cranial nerves was assessed. Forty-three selected patients were studied as well, including patients with tumors in the juxtasellar regions, cerebellopontine angle lesions, meningiomas, cerebral aneurysms, and facial spasms. Peripheral pulse gating was applied, optimized to reduce artifacts related to CSF flow.

Results.—Peripheral pulse gating with a time delay of 30% of the peripheral pulse gate interval was successful in minimizing the CSF flow artifacts. In all volunteers, the first through third cranial nerves and the seventh-eighth cranial nerve complex were clearly seen. The fifth nerve was visualized in 80% of patients and the sixth nerve in 50%; the fourth and ninth through twelfth nerves were more difficult to see. In the patients, MR cisternography could depict the intracisternal fine anatomy and enhance the contours of juxtacisternal lesions. The T2-weighted turbo spin-echo sequence could depict very small amounts of CSF between lesions and normal structures. Vascular compression was demonstrated in 13 of 13 patients with facial spasm by axial images and oblique coronal images in a plane parallel to the seventh-eighth nerve complex. In patients with pituitary adenomas, the scans clearly showed the tumor relationship to the optic nerve and other structures. Cerebral aneurysms and surrounding structures were also clearly seen.

Conclusions.—The use of MR cisternography to visualize the fine structures within the subarachnoid cisterns is described and illustrated. This technique appears useful for investigation of patients with neurovascular compression or tumors in this area. Imaging can be performed in a relatively short time and, when performed with peripheral pulse gating and a delay time of 30% of the peripheral pulse gate interval, can aid in surgical planning.

▶ The authors provide a detailed and instructive discussion of the application of MR cisternography (using a heavily T2-weighted turbo spin-echo sequence) to enable visualization of normal fine structures of cisternal anatomy, with particular attention to the structures of the basal and cerebellopontine angle cisterns. The authors review the application of this technique to individual cranial nerves from the first through the second cranial nerves, detailing advantages of the technique as well as difficulties. Special attention is given to dealing with CSF flow-related artifacts and to the application of peripheral pulse gating to reduce them. The article is recommended both as an introduction to the technical aspects of MR cisternography and as a review of pertinent anatomy and the methods for optimizing its demonstration. Selected pathologic examples are also presented.

The use of heavily T2-weighted imaging sequences to demonstrate in exquisite detail the anatomy of CSF-filled spaces, such as the cisterns, is a powerful technique which should see increasing application with more widespread availability of the required technology. This technique is increasingly employed in the detailed evaluation of inner-ear structures and internal auditory canal anatomy, and is the best available method for demonstrating the relationship between nerves and vessels in the cisternal spaces when investigating vascular compression. (As discussed by the authors, supplemental MR angiography may be required in such cases.)

Additionally, there has been good progress recently in applying a variant of this technique to myelography.

G. Pjura, M.D.

Use of a C-arm System to Generate True Three-dimensional Computed Rotational Angiograms: Preliminary In Vitro and In Vivo Results
Fahrig R, Fox AJ, Lownie S, et al (Univ of Western Ontario, London, Canada)
AJNR 18:1507–1514, 1997   24–2

Background.—Rotational angiography can provide limited three-dimensional (3-D) information about the cerebral vessels. The authors have developed a new technique, called computed rotational angiography, using a modified C-arm mounted radiographic image intensifier system to generate 3-D images during endovascular procedures. The projection data are reconstructed with CT, providing 3-D images with isotropic resolution. The quantitative data provided by the computed volume image offer greater spatial resolution than helical CT angiography. Preliminary evaluations of the computed rotational angiography technique are presented.

Methods.—The investigators used a modified clinical biplane angiographic system and a modified high-speed single-plane system. As the C-arm rotated around the object of interest, approximately 130 images were collected over the 200 degrees' rotation necessary for reconstruction of a 15 × 15 × 15 cm³ volume. Selective contrast injections were made during rotation of the C-arm. Image-based techniques were used to correct for distortion of the image intensifier and instability of the C-arm. Three-dimensional reconstructions were performed using an anesthetized, 20-kg pig and a human skull phantom to assess the impact of vessel pulsatility during data acquisition and in the presence of bone.

Results.—It took less than 5 seconds to collect an image sequence sufficient for 3-D reconstruction. Image intensifier distortion was corrected to 0.035 mm, and C-arm instability to 0.07 mm, below the level of a pixel. The system produced reconstructions of the intracranial vessels of the pig and the small, high-contrast structures of the skull with minimal artifacts.

Conclusions.—This article describes the development and initial evaluative studies of a true 3-D computed rotational angiography technique which uses a C-arm mounted radiographic image intensifier system. The findings suggest that data acquisition and reconstruction could be carried out during neuroendovascular procedures. With further development, computed rotational angiography could improve our understanding of the geometric, 3-D relationships between aneurysmal mouths and the adjacent branches.

▶ The authors provide a technically detailed discussion of a commercially available neuroangiography unit specially modified by its manufacturer to obtain 3-D angiographic images of diagnostic quality. The authors review pertinent technical considerations of hardware implementation, and results of both phantom and laboratory animal testing. The prototype system satisfies the principal acceptance criteria for intentional use, established by the authors at the outset, ie., near-real-time fluoroscopic capability and roadmapping, unobstructed patient access, and accurate 3-D anatomic information about vessel lumen, etc. The time currently required to generate the 3-D images (estimated at under 10 minutes using a workstation and hardware accelerator) is problematic but not insurmountable, given the rate of improvement in computer speed. The authors compare their technique with alternatives such as 3-D angiography, limited-view reconstruction algorithms, and conventional CT, citing in each case the advantages of true 3-D computed rotational angiography. Although the authors make a strong case for this particular approach in the field of neurointerventional angiography, cost of implementation and competition from developing alternative technologies, including hybrid CT-angiography suites, remain to be addressed.

G. Pjura, M.D.

Magnetic Resonance Myelography (MRM) as a Spinal Examination Technique

Ramsbacher J, Schilling AM, Wolf K-J, et al (Free Univ of Berlin)
Acta Neurochir (Wien) 139:1080–1084, 1997   24–3

Introduction.—The high proton fraction and very long relaxation time of cerebral spinal fluid can be imaged with a strongly T2-weighted measuring sequence on magnetic resonance myelography (MRM). The MRM approach is noninvasive and free of the side effects and complications from lumbar puncture and injection of contrast medium that can occur with conventional myelography. The diagnostic value and accuracy of MRM were compared with those of conventional myelography.

Methods.—Forty-one patients (24 women, 17 men) with radicular symptoms underwent both conventional lumbar myelography and MRM. Images were assessed by both a radiologist and a neurosurgeon.

Results.—Magnetic resonance myelography detected thecal indentation with amputation of a nerve root sheath in 35 patients and spinal stenosis in 6 patients. The results of MRM were the same as those of conventional myelography and coincided with intraoperative findings. A mean of 15 minutes was needed for measurement and calculation for MRM, compared with a mean of 29 minutes for conventional myelography.

Conclusion.—Magnetic resonance myelography had the same informational value as conventional myelography. It is fast, noninvasive, and requires neither contrast application nor radiation exposure. The results are stored on magnetic tape and may be reinspected from a different visual angle at any time.

▶ Magnetic resonance myelography has, for a variety of technical reasons, been difficult to implement, although it is conceptually very attractive, being a noninvasive method for obtaining the diagnostic information traditionally deferred to conventional contrast myelography, and not involving the potential side effects and complication inherent in puncture of the CSF space and injection of contrast media, nor requiring radiograph exposure. The authors report their success in overcoming these difficulties by using a state-of-the-art 1.5 T scanner and associated software to generate rotating projections of the CSF-filled spaces derived from sagittal and coronal acquisitions of strongly T2-weighted 3-D gradient echo thin slice sequences. The authors provide a reasonably complete description of their methodology and the results of a prospective comparative study of 41 patients who also underwent conventional lumbar myelography. The authors conclude that the sensitivity and specificity of the method are identical and indicate their intention to use MRM to replace conventional myography at their institution, with rare exceptions.

The enthusiasm expressed for the potential of this technique is warranted. However, as the authors indicate, successful implementation appears to be predicated upon state-of-the-art hardware and improved software, as well as upon adopting new assessment criteria which respect the physical differences between the 2 methodologies. Furthermore, MRM offers the unique potential of directly visualizing such causes of stenosis as a hypertrophic ligamentum flavum or a disc sequestrum. Magnetic resonance myelography should become more widely available as the technology of imaging advances and the subtleties of creating and interpreting reconstructed images of the CSF-filled spaces of the thecal sac and nerve root sheaths become more widely known and understood. Implementation of more sophisticated image reconstruction algorithms offering transparency and surface shading may advance this technique.

G. Pjura, M.D.

A Comparison of T2 and Gadolinium Enhanced MRI With CT Myelography in Cervical Radiculopathy
Bartlett RJV, Hill CR, Gardiner E (Hull Royal Infirm, UK; Univ of Hull, UK)
Br J Radiol 71:11–19, 1998   24–4

Introduction.—Cervical exit foramina are difficult to assess by MRI because of the smallness of the lesions and the presence of susceptibility and flow artifacts. In a prospective study, 20 patients with cervical radiculopathy were examined with 2 MRI strategies reported to be effective in assessing cervical exit foramina. Results were compared with those of CT myelography (CTM).

Methods.—Patients underwent CTM performed via the lumbar route, except 1 patient in whom the lateral cervical approach was required to obtain a good quality study. A 1.6 T Signa unit was used for MR scanning. The first MRI strategy used 3D T_2* images and the second gadolinium-enhanced 2D T_1 images. Axial scans covered the same anatomical region as the CT studies, providing 160 exit foramina for comparative analysis. Two experienced neuroradiologists independently viewed CTM studies in conjunction with plain radiographs and viewed each individual MR sequence without access to plain radiographs. An attempt was made to establish a gold standard or "best diagnosis" after all data were reviewed.

Results.—Gadolinium-enhanced images provided no benefit in the investigation of cervical exit foramina, a finding attributed to enhancement of herniated disk material and osteophytes adjacent to the neurocentral joint. The accuracy of 3D T_2* white CSF images was close to 90% for the diagnosis of foraminal encroachment.

Conclusion.—It is apparent that CTM can no longer be considered the gold standard for diagnosis of cervical radiculopathy. The recommended primary investigation for this condition is MRI including a 3D T_2* sequence. But when findings are at odds with clinical symptomatology, CTM is indicated. All gadolinium-enhanced sequences had very poor results.

▶ The authors compare the use of axial 3OT2* weighted images and gadolinium-enhanced 2OT1-weighted images with CT myelography and conclude that the T2* method is 90% accurate for the diagnosis of foraminal encroachment, but that, when findings are incompatible with clinical symptomatology, CT myelography is still indicated. This conclusion, that advances in MR myelography have yet to displace CT myelography as the final arbiter in clinical decision-making, is consistent with current practice and reflects the persistent technical difficulties in noninvasive evaluation of the cervical spine. The authors' discussion is instructive because it reviews these difficulties in some detail. The authors do not choose CT myelography as their "gold standard," but rather employ a form of consensus "best diagnosis," derived from both observers' review of all available imaging data. This decision probably reinforces the understanding that each modality contributes unique information based upon the underlying physics, and that, consequently, the specific pathology in a given situation (e.g., disk, osteophyte) may ultimately determine the most effective diagnostic approach.

G. Pjura, M.D.

Evaluation of the Post-operative Lumbar Spine With MR Imaging: The Role of Contrast Enhancement and Thickening in Nerve Roots
Grane P, Lindqvist M (Karolinska Hosp, Stockholm)
Acta Radiol 38:1035–1042, 1997   24–5

Introduction.—Patients who have undergone lumbar disk surgery frequently experience residual or recurrent clinical symptoms. To determine whether a postoperative change at the site of surgery is the actual cause of symptoms, MRI is usually performed both before and after contrast medium administration. Thickening in nerve roots and contrast enhancement in nerve roots have been noted recently at MRI. A study of 121 patients with postoperative symptoms in the lumbar spine examined the clinical significance of contrast enhancement and nerve-root thickening.

Methods.—All patients had symptoms after surgery for disk herniation at 1 or 2 of the 3 lowest lumbar levels. A total of 152 MR examinations were performed at a median of 18 months after surgery. Using nonaffected nerve roots as reference, focal nerve-root enhancement was identified visually. Intradural enhancement was quantified by pixel measurements that compared the affected nerve roots before and after contrast administration.

Results.—Twenty patients (16%) appeared to have intradural nerve-root enhancement, but true intradural nerve-root enhancement was present in only 12 (10%). The enhanced nerve roots increased at least 40% to 50% after contrast administration. In 7 of these 12 patients, enhancement findings confirmed clinical symptoms and associated pathological MR changes. An additional 26% of patients exhibited focal enhancement in the root sleeve, and 30% had nerve-root thickening. There was good correlation with clinical symptoms in 59% of patients with intradural enhancement, in 84% with focal enhancement, and in 89% with nerve-root thickening. In 86%, the combination of thickening and enhancement in the nerve root correlated with clinical symptoms.

Conclusion.—Although nerve-root enhancement at MRI is a useful indicator of symptomatic nerve-root compression in patients who have undergone lumbar spine surgery, several cautions should be noted: enhancement of an intradural nerve root needs to be confirmed by pixel measurements; in some cases apparent nerve-root enhancement may result from enhancement of radicular veins; enhanced nerve roots may be normal findings in the early postoperative (6 months) period; and enhancement is significant only when explained by causes such as compression of the nerve root by disk herniation, scar tissue, or osteophytes.

▶ The authors report their evaluation of 2 specific signs of lumbar nerve-root affection in the postoperative spine: nerve-root enhancement and nerve-root thickening. The authors employ both qualitative (visual) and quantitative (pixel measurement before and after contrast administration, with nonaffected roots at the same level as a reference) measures. Enhancement is a useful indicator of symptomatic nerve-root compression but cannot be used alone, and enhanced nerve roots may be a normal postoperative finding within 6 months of surgery. Nerve-root thickening did not correlate well with recurrent symptoms but may, in combination with other pathologic changes, strengthen the indication for repeat surgery. The authors' conclusions are consistent with other reports in the literature, and reflect the complexity and difficulty in evaluating the postoperative lumbar spine. The value of this article lies in its instructive review of the technical considerations and potentially misleading findings encountered in such evaluations, and in the authors' use of quantitative measures to assess both enhancement and thickening, an approach which reduces subjectivity, and may facilitate comparison of results among different researchers, if more widely applied.

G. Pjura, M.D.

Who Performs Neuroimaging? Results From the 1993 National Medicare Database
Rao VM, Levin DC, Spettell CM, et al (Thomas Jefferson Univ Hosp, Philadelphia; American College of Radiology, Reston, Va)
Radiology 204:443–445, 1997   24–6

Background.—More neuroimaging studies are being performed by neurologists and other nonradiologists. However, there are few data on exactly what proportion of such studies—particularly CT and MRI scans—are performed by nonradiologists. Medicare data were used to analyze the extent to which CT and MRI neuroimaging studies are performed by nonradiologists.

Methods and Results.—The 1993 Part B Medicare Annual Database was used to determine the number of CT and MRI scans of the brain, head and neck, and spine performed by radiologists and nonradiologists at hospitals, private offices, or imaging centers. The analysis included data on nearly 4 million CT and MRI studies billed to Medicare. Eighty-one percent of the scans were performed in hospitals; only 2% of these were read by nonradiologists. Nineteen percent of scans were performed at private offices or imaging centers; only 9% of these were interpreted by nonradiologists. Only 3% of scans were performed by nonradiologists, overall.

Conclusions.—Nonradiologists perform and interpret only a small percentage of the neuroimaging CT and MRI scans billed to Medicare. The data do not support claims that physicians from specialties other than radiology are playing a major role in neuroimaging studies.

▶ The authors state that their purpose is to determine the level of participation of nonradiologists in CT and MR imaging of the brain, head and neck, and spine at hospitals and at private offices and imaging centers in the United States. The authors conclude that the level of such participation "billed to Medicare" is minimal and had not changed significantly since a study of 1989. Although the Medicare database is attractive for such studies, because it is national in scope and readily obtained, it covers less than one third of all patients in the United States, as the authors acknowledge. Moreover, it is questionable at best to extrapolate directly from this rather uniquely defined segment of the patient population to the larger, more diverse population constituting the other two thirds of patients in the country. If, as the authors state, "radiologic procedures performed by nonradiologists are associated with both a higher use of imaging procedures and increased costs," there is a need for a more broadly based survey of the other two thirds of the patient population before potentially misleading conclusions regarding this matter are accepted.

G. Pjura, M.D.

Clinical Application of Functional Magnetic Resonance Imaging in Presurgical Identification of the Central Sulcus

Pujol J, Conesa G, Deus J, et al (Magnetic Resonance Ctr of Pedralbes, Barcelona; Univ of Barcelona)
J Neurosurg 88:863–869, 1998   24–7

Objective.—In patients undergoing neurosurgery to remove centrally located lesions, it is essential to identify the central sulcus as an anatomic and functional landmark. Functional MRI permits preoperative visualization of the central sulcus in relation to the surgical target. This study evaluated the clinical use of functional MRI for preoperative identification of the central sulcus.

Methods.—The analysis included 50 consecutive surgical patients with space-occupying lesions involving the central region of the brain: 31 men and 19 women, mean age 44. Each patient was examined with a 1.5 T MRI system, including a spoiled gradient recalled acquisition in the steady-state functional sequence and a cross-hand cancellation analysis method. The MRI data were used to create 3D models of each patient's head and brain, demonstrating the relative locations of the tumor and the eloquent cortex. The advantages and limitations of this MRI procedure for routine functional use were assessed.

Results.—The MRI studies identified a selective and reproducible focal activation, consistent with the probable location of the central sulcus, in 82% of patients. Intraoperative assessment by direct cortical stimulation was performed in 22 patients, and the results confirmed the functional MRI findings in each case. In the remaining 18% of patients, in whom the central sulcus could not be identified, the main cause was intrinsic damage to the primary sensorimotor region.

Conclusions.—In most cases, preoperative functional MRI is able to identify the central sulcus in patients with centrally located brain lesions. Some limitations of the technique are identified, including the inability of a single-section method to encompass a brain volume large enough to ensure inclusion of the eloquent cortex in patients with anatomic distortion. Further research is needed to optimize and validate an imaging protocol for routine use in surgical patients with centrally located space-occupying lesions.

▶ The authors evaluate the advantages and limitations of functional MRI in identifying the central sulcus.

The central sulcus is the major anatomical functional reference in neurosurgery, and its preoperative identification in relationship to the surgical target is particularly helpful in minimizing neurological deficits that could follow resection of centrally placed tumors in the posterior frontal or anterior parietal region.

The authors show that functional MRI will successfully identify the central sulcus in the majority of cases, although there was a substantial failure rate, 18% of the patients studied. The main clinical factor associated with poor functional results was the presence of a moderate-to-severe paresis in the involved hand, and it is in this situation that accurate identification is often necessary.

The authors used the technique to develop 3D models of the patient's head and brain, showing the relative positions of the tumor and the eloquent cortex. Functional and 3D MRI, together with other techniques such as magnetoencephalography, will provide important tools to assess surgical planning. The most relevant application of this study may be the optimization and validation of an imaging protocol sufficiently simple and rapid to be routinely applied in surgical candidates with centrally located lesions.

A.H. Kaye, M.D., M.B.B.S., F.R.A.C.S.

25 Pain Management

The Behavioural Response to Whiplash Injury
Gargan M, Bannister G, Main C, et al (Southmead Hosp, Bristol, England)
J Bone Joint Surg Br 79-B:523–526, 1997   25–1

Objective.—Because patients reporting chronic whiplash symptoms often do not have corroborative radiographic findings, some medical professionals attribute the syndrome to a psychological disorder. Results of a psychological test of the pre-existence and development of behavioral disorders after whiplash injury were compared with the incidence and severity of symptoms and physical signs.

Methods.—One week after injury and treatment, the symptoms and psychological test scores on the General Health Questionnaire (GHQ28) of 50 consecutive patients (24 males), aged 10 to 49, were evaluated. Patients were interviewed and tested again at 3 months and 2 years, and the range of neck motion was recorded. The severity of symptoms and test scores were compared statistically.

Results.—Although 3 patients were symptom-free at a mean of 5.5 days after the injuries occurred, all patients experienced discomfort at 3 months and 2 years. During this period, symptoms improved in 9 and worsened in 6. Of the 17 patients with severe symptoms at 2 years, most were female and most exhibited restricted neck movement at 3 months. At 1 week, GHQ28 scores were normal for all patients. The GHQ28 scores at 3 months and 2 years were significantly higher in patients with more severe symptoms at 2 years. The range of neck movement and GHQ28 scores at 3 months were predictive of clinical outcome at 2 years. The predictive accuracy was 76% for range of neck movement, 74% for GHQ28 scores, and 82% for both.

Conclusion.—Whiplash injury symptoms have both a physical and psychological component and are in place at 3 months. This psychological component can result in chronic symptoms unless measures are taken to influence the course of the syndrome within this period.

▶ Cervical sprain injuries result in pain from physical causes, and if the pain becomes chronic, it is often the principal reason for associated psychological problems of anxiety, depression, and irritability. A decrement in cognition may also develop because of deteriorating emotional status or medications.

Also, the negative social effects of unemployment and marital stress may ensue, exacerbating the depression and overall condition.

The authors suggest that the greatest potential for influencing the natural history of whiplash occurs within 3 months. Consequently, optimal management of these patients requires an early, comprehensive understanding of these factors and an effective multimodality approach to rehabilitation before the negative psychological effects become wrought beyond change.

S.R. Gibbs, M.A., M.D.

Fibre Type Characteristics of the Lumbar Paraspinal Muscles in Normal Healthy Subjects and in Patients With Low Back Pain
Mannion AF, Weber BR, Dvorak J, et al (Universität Zürich-Irchel, Switzerland)
J Orthop Res 15:881–887, 1997   25–2

Introduction.—There seems to be an association between low back pain and muscular insufficiency. Rehabilitation and functional restoration programs have focused on the attempted reversal of this condition, but first the specific physiologic or anatomical abnormality underlying the dysfunction must be identified. The decline in muscle performance with low back pain may result from associated modifications in the size and distribution of type of fibers of the paraspinal muscle fibers. Few previous studies have adequately compared the muscles of patients with low back pain with that of controls. The fiber type characteristics of the lumbar paraspinal muscles in patients with low back pain having posterior spinal surgery were compared with those of pain-free controls who were matched for gender, age, and size.

Methods.—Samples of lumbar paraspinal muscle were obtained during spinal surgery from 21 patients with low back pain and compared with the samples obtained by percutaneous biopsy from 21 control volunteers matched for gender, age, and body mass. To determine the characteristics of muscle fiber type, the samples were histochemically analyzed.

Results.—The muscles of patients had a significantly higher proportion of type-IIB (fast-twitch glycolytic) fibers than type-I (slow twitch oxidative) fibers, compared with those of the controls (Table 2). Between patients and controls, the mean size of a given fiber type did not differ. In the patients, the relative area of the muscle occupied by type-IIB fibers was higher and that of type-I fibers was lower when compared with the controls. Muscle samples with more than 1% type-IIC fibers were found in more patients than in controls. Abnormalities that could be described as pathologic were more marked in the patients than in the controls.

Conclusions.—A more glycolytic (faster) profile was found in the paraspinal muscles of patients with low back pain than in controls, which could be expected to render them less resistant to fatigue.

TABLE 2.—Erector Spinae Muscle Fiber Type Characteristics

	Men		Women	
	Patients	Controls	Patients	Controls
% fibre type				
I	51.0 ± 12.9*	66.1 ± 7.7	50.1 ± 7.7*	66.5 ± 12.0
IIA	24.0 ± 12.2	24.4 ± 4.2	17.3 ± 10.3	24.6 ± 7.3
IIB	23.4 ± 14.3*	7.9 ± 5.9	30.6 ± 11.8*	8.2 ± 6.6
IIC	1.6 ± 2.6	0.6 ± 1.0	2.0 ± 3.4	0.2 ± 1.2
Fibre diameter (μm)				
I	65.4 ± 10.4	62.5 ± 10.0	57.4 ± 12.4†	52.6 ± 4.6†
IIA	56.0 ± 8.5	59.4 ± 8.4	46.7 ± 16.3†	41.6 ± 4.7†
IIB	52.9 ± 10.3	55.9 ± 8.6	43.1 ± 19.0†	39.3 ± 6.4†
All fibres	58.5 ± 6.9	60.5 ± 8.8	50.1 ± 14.9†	47.9 ± 4.6†
Size I:II ratio‡	1.23 ± 0.28	1.08 ± 0.12	1.37 ± 0.31†	1.31 ± 0.22†
% fibre type area				
I	60.3 ± 12.1*	70.3 ± 6.6	64.5 ± 9.6*	77.1 ± 6.4
IIA	21.8 ± 12.8	22.9 ± 4.0	15.0 ± 10.2†	18.0 ± 5.2†
IIB	17.9 ± 11.7*	6.8 ± 4.3	20.5 ± 9.6*	4.9 ± 3.4

Note: Values are mean ± SD.

*$P < 0.05$, different from controls.

†$P < 0.05$, different from the men.

‡The ratio of the mean size of the type I fiber to the weighted mean size of the type II (IIA and IIB) fibers (i.e., weighted in relation to the proportion of each subtype). This was calculated for each biopsy sample.

(Courtesy of Mannion AF, Weber BR, Dvorak J, et al: Fibre type characteristics of the lumbar paraspinal muscles in normal healthy subjects and in patients with low back pain. *J Orthop Res* 15:881–887, 1997.)

▶ All muscles have varying percentages of fast- and slow-twitch fiber types, and the ratio of these fibers in any particular muscle depends upon its function. Phosphagen and glycogen–lactic acid energy systems are especially active in fast-twitch muscles requiring rapid releases of energy, whereas slow-twitch fibers are designed for endurance because they have a higher content of mitochondria and myoglobin for aerobic energy production. The erector spinae muscles provide tonic postural stabilization when individuals are upright; consequently a preponderance of type IIB (fast-twitch glycolytic) fibers seems maladaptive and likely to result in increased fatigability.

The authors were unable to determine whether this shift in fiber type precedes or follows the onset of low back pain. However, in either case, a shift toward type I (slow-twitch oxidative) fibers for improved endurance should, in part, be the aim of preoperative and postoperative physical therapy.

S.R. Gibbs, M.A., M.D.

Long-term Transcutaneous Electrical Nerve Stimulation (TENS) Use: Impact on Medication Utilization and Physical Therapy Costs

Chabal C, Fishbain DA, Weaver M, et al (Univ of Washington, Seattle; Univ of Miami, Miami Beach, Fla; Empi Inc, St Paul, Minn)
Clin J Pain 14:66–73, 1998   25–3

Background.—In transcutaneous electric nerve stimulation (TENS), low-voltage electrical current is used to activate large-diameter sensory fibers with the goal of reducing nociceptive input. This technique has been used in patients with a wide range of acute and chronic pain conditions. Studies have suggested that TENS may reduce the use of pain medications. However, there are few data on the impact of TENS on specific types or patterns of pain medication use or on the costs of medications or physical therapy used for pain. These issues were addressed in a study of the outcomes of long-term TENS for patients with chronic pain.

Methods.—The study comprised a random sample of 376 patients with chronic pain who had acquired an Epix XL TENS device. Telephone interviews were performed by an independent research company. The outcome variables assessed included changes in medication use, number of pain-related medications, and use of physical therapy/occupational therapy (PT/OT) services before and after TENS. The cost impact of TENS on medication and PT/OT use was also assessed.

Results.—The patients received TENS treatment for pain for a mean of 40 months. The use of several types of pain medications decreased after TENS, including opiate analgesics, tranquilizers, muscle relaxants, nonsteroidal anti-inflammatory drugs, and steroids. The mean number of pain-related medications taken decreased from 1.19 to 0.69. The number of patients using PT/OT decreased from 327 before TENS to 108 afterward. Cost simulations suggested significant savings for both medications and PT/OT—by up to 55% and 69%, respectively.

Conclusion.—Patients with chronic pain who receive long-term TENS treatment have significant reductions in their use of pain medication and PT/OT services. Substantial cost reductions are possible as well. These benefits of TENS are important to consider when creating a treatment plan for patients with chronic pain. Reductions in therapy and medication use, increased activities, and improved treatment satisfaction are likely to result in improved quality of life.

▶ Ever since the report by Melzack and Wall[1] on the gate theory of pain and the pioneering report by Wall and Sweet[2] on the temporary abolition of pain by electric nerve stimulation, TENS has been part of pain management. Although the technique is currently used as a stand-alone therapy, it was largely used as a screening technique for implantable neurostimulators in the 1960s.

Counterirritating sensory stimulation is not a new technique for alleviation of pain. Some of its oldest forms include rubbing, chaffing, and massaging. Other chemical, mechanical, and thermal forms include liniments, cupping, acupuncture, and moxa burning. Moreover, one ancient technique described a form of TENS—electroanalgesia performed with electric fish.[3]

Clearly, one does not have to be a clinical algologist to understand and apply this time-tested, safe, noninvasive, and relatively simple technique for treating postoperative and chronic pain. The authors provide an additional reason for using TENS—its documented effectiveness in reducing the cost of pain medication and PT/OT.

S.R. Gibbs, M.A., M.D.

References

1. Melzack R, Wall PD: Pain mechanisms: A new theory. *Science* 150:971–979, 1965.
2. Wall PD, Sweet WH: Temporary abolition of pain in man. *Science* 155:108–109, 1967.
3. Kane K, Taub A: A history of local electrical analgesia. *Pain* 1:125–138, 1975.

26 Pediatric Neurosurgery

Increased Hematocrit and Decreased Transfusion Requirements in Children Given Erythropoietin Before Undergoing Craniofacial Surgery
Helfaer MA, Carson BS, James CS, et al (Johns Hopkins Med Inst, Baltimore, Md)
J Neurosurg 88:704–708, 1998   26–1

Introduction.—Hematocrit levels increase and transfusion requirements are lessened when erythropoietin is given to premature infants in neonatal intensive care units. Erythropoietin administration in adults increases erythropoiesis and preoperative blood collection. If the response to exogenous erythropoietin were understood in infants, erythropoietin could be administered to infants before blood losses associated with craniofacial surgery become significant. The efficacy of preoperative erythropoietin administration was assessed in infants undergoing craniofacial surgery.

Methods.—Thirty infants undergoing craniofacial surgery were given subcutaneous erythropoietin 300 U/kg 3 times weekly for 3 weeks before surgery. Thirty matched control participants did not undergo erythropoietin therapy. Weekly complete blood counts including reticulocyte counts were measured, and blood transfusion requirements were noted.

Results.—Hematocrit levels increased from 35.4% to 43.3% during therapy in the erythropoietin treatment group. Baseline hematocrit levels obtained at the time of surgery were higher in the treatment group than in the control group (43.3% vs. 34.2%). During treatment, patients in the erythropoietin group had a significant rise in reticulocyte count from 1.7% to 6.9%, and a significant fall in the mean white blood cell count from $13.4 \times 10^3/mm^3$ to $10.3 \times 10^3/mm^3$. All patients in the control group required transfusions, compared with 64% of patients in the erythropoietin treatment group.

Conclusion.—Treatment with erythropoietin in otherwise healthy young children increases hematocrit levels and decreases transfusion requirements. This treatment has potential as a safe, cost-effective adjuvant to allogeneic blood transfusion and should be evaluated for other indications.

▶ Infants and children undergoing surgical correction of craniosynostosis are at risk for experiencing significant blood loss during these procedures. The goal of these authors was to determine the efficacy of administering erythropoietin to patients with craniosynostosis before the patients underwent craniofacial correction. The results indicate that it is safe to administer erythropoietin surgery. There is a significant increase in hematocrit levels from 35.4% to 43.3% after administration of erythropoietin at 300 U/kg 3 times per week for a total of 3 weeks. Although the authors state that there was a 64% decrease in transfusion rates, unfortunately the authors did not differentiate between surgical groups, i.e., between sagittal synostectomy and full cranial expansion. Nevertheless, it does appear that administration of erythropoietin to infants and young children before surgery elevates the hematocrit levels and decreases the need for blood transfusions in this patient population.

D.F. Jimenez, M.D.

Current Treatment of Brain Abscess in Patients With Congenital Cyanotic Heart Disease
Takeshita M, Kagawa M, Yato S, et al (Tokyo Women's Med College)
Neurosurgery 41:1270–1279, 1997   26–2

Introduction.—The combination of surgery and management of brain abscesses has dramatically reduced mortality rates from 60% to less than 10% with the advent of computed tomography. The risks of anesthesia and surgery increase in patients with brain abscess who have congenital cyanotic heart disease. Even in the computed tomography era, the mortality rate for cyanotic brain abscess is 13.3%. A retrospective review of patients with cyanotic heart disease and brain abscesses was conducted to define the role of managing these patients and determining the factors that influenced a poor outcome.

Methods.—Sixty two patients with cyanotic heart disease and abscesses were diagnosed by computed tomography. The following independent predictors of poor outcome were evaluated: number, size, location, computed tomographic classification, organism, type of abscess, convulsion, type of cyanotic heart disease, age distribution, immunocompromised status, intraventricular rupture of brain abscess, pretreatment neurological state, type of antibiotics and duration of administration, steroid medication, therapeutic modalities, aspiration with or without cerebrospinal fluid drainage, total extirpation after aspiration, or primary extirpation and medical treatment. Univariate and multivariate logistic regression analysis were conducted.

Results.—Patients with poor outcomes were older, had intraventricular rupture of brain abscess more frequently, and had a higher frequency of neurological deterioration than those with good outcomes. No other parameters had any statistically significant correlations between patients with good and poor outcomes. Poor outcome increased the relative risk of intraventricular rupture of brain abscess by a factor of 18.9, according to multiple logistic regression analysis. Positive immunocompromised states were seen among more patients with multiple abscesses than among those with a single abscess. Intraventricular rupture of brain abscess was more frequent in deeply-located abscesses and in those in the parieto-occipital region that ruptured into the occipital horn of the lateral ventricle in a short period.

Conclusion.—Intraventricular rupture of brain abscess strongly influences poor outcome in patients with cyanotic heart disease. Prevention and management of intraventricular rupture of brain abscess may be the key to decreasing poor outcomes. Abscesses should be managed by less invasive aspiration methods guided by computed tomography to reduce operative anesthetic risk in these patients. To decrease intracranial pressure and avoid intraventricular rupture of brain abscesses, those larger than 2 cm in diameter in deeply-located parieto-occipital regions should be aspirated immediately and repeated using computed tomography-guided methods. While evaluating intracranial pressure pathophysiology, intraventricular rupture of brain abscess should be aggressively treated by aspiration methods or coupled with the appropriate intravenous and intrathecal administration of antibiotics.

▶ Takeshita et al. provide us with a follow-up report of 62 patients with cyanotic heart disease and brain abscesses.

The authors demonstrate an increased rate of poor outcome associated with intraventricular abscess rupture. The conclusion is to identify abscess early and do our best to prevent abscess enlargement and ventricular rupture.

This retrospective study covers a period after the advent of CT, which corresponds to a significant decrease of mortality rate.

This very large experience is unique and can serve as a good point of reference in respect of its low morbidity rate.

Unfortunately, the very important heterogeneity of this series prevents the authors from obtaining statistically significant correlations between therapeutic parameters and outcome.

As the Pittsburgh team, we consider the highly recommended stereotactic biopsy and/or aspiration of all patients with suspected brain abscess regardless of size. As far as a specific antibiotherapy afterwards, aspiration is certainly the more effective way to avoid the use of some drugs with specific morbidity and mainly to prevent abscess enlargement and ventricular rupture.

J. Regis, M.D.

Outcome for Preterm Infants With Germinal Matrix Hemorrhage and Progressive Hydrocephalus

Levy ML, Masri LS, McComb JG (Univ of Southern California, Los Angeles)
Neurosurgery 41:1111–1118, 1997   26–3

Background.—There are questions about the benefits of early, aggressive management of progressive hydrocephalus in premature infants with intraventricular hemorrhage. Though outcome is related to the severity of hemorrhage, 75% of children with hemorrhage of any degree develop normally. The long-term outcomes of and outcome-associated factors in infants undergoing surgery for progressive hydrocephalus were analyzed.

Methods.—The study included 76 preterm infants with grade III or IV intracranial hemorrhage who underwent surgical repair of progressive hydrocephalus. Forty-one patients were long-term survivors. The following potential predictors of mortality, intellectual impairment, and motor deficit were evaluated: degree of prematurity, birth weight, sex, Apgar scores, extent of intracranial hemorrhage, seizures, age at initial placement of a ventricular catheter reservoir, need for conversion to a ventriculoperitoneal shunt, timing of the conversion, and number of shunt revisions.

Results.—On linear regression analysis, extent of intracranial hemorrhage was the strongest predictor of mortality, followed by number of shunt revisions and birth weight. The factors most strongly associated with motor outcome were grade of hemorrhage, birth weight, and seizures. On logistic regression analysis of the survivors, the main factor predicting cognitive outcome, motor function, and seizure activity was grade of hemorrhage. The major determinants of survival in a logistic model were grade of hemorrhage and more than 5 shunt revisions.

Conclusions.—Extent of intracranial hemorrhage is the major factor affecting outcome in preterm infants undergoing surgery for progressive hydrocephalus. The results suggest that long-term intellectual and motor outcomes of these patients are affected mainly by factors occurring before CSF removal or diversion to control hydrocephalus. Future outcome studies of intraventricular hemorrhage should include quantitative assessments of the extent of parenchymal hemorrhagic infarction.

▶ The results concerning mortality and quality of survival in this series of 76 children with intracerebral hemorrhage are no surprise and have already been published in the last decade. In the long-term survival group of 45 children, seizure activity, cognitive functions, and motor development correlate with the grade of hemorrhage. The poor prognosis in patients who had multiple shunt revisions was to be expected as well. But it is surprising that birth weight comes third in order of importance as a prognostic factor.

There are continuing dilemmas concerning the therapy for such patients. The authors suggest that in children with grade IV hemorrhage treatment should be withdrawn. Many neurosurgeons would object, but with the present therapeutical possibilities, this seems to be a difficult but logical decision. A long-term analysis may ease this dilemma.

B. Klun, M.D., Ph.D

The Incidence of Acute and Remote Seizures in Children With Intraventricular Hemorrhage
Strober JB, Bienkowski RS, Maytal J (Albert Einstein College of Medicine, New Hyde Park, New York)
Clin Pediatr (Phila) 36:643–648, 1997   26–4

Background.—The rate at which seizures occur as a complication of intraventricular hemorrhage (IVH) in premature infants is not known. The incidence of acute and remote seizures in infants with IVH and the seizures' association with hemorrhage grade were reported.

Methods and Findings.—The records of 103 infants were reviewed for the occurrence of acute and remote seizures as well as for morbidity and mortality. Mean gestational age was 29 weeks, with a range of 23–40 weeks. Grade 1 or 2 IVH developed in 50% of the infants, grade 3 in 18%, and grade 4 in 31%. Seventeen percent of the infants had acute seizures in the first month of life. Follow-up data were available on 61 infants surviving the neonatal period. Ten percent had remote seizures. Acute seizures were significantly more frequent in infants with grade 4 IVH than in those with grades 1 or 2 IVH. Remote seizures developed only in infants with grade 3 or 4 IVH. Among infants with grade 4 IVH, acute seizures were a significant risk factor for remote seizure development.

Conclusions.—In this cohort of neonates with IVH, the incidence of acute seizures was 17%. The current data suggest that antiepileptic drug treatment past the neonatal period should be reserved for patients with grade 4 IVH and a history of acute seizures.

▶ Seizures are a common complication after a brain hemorrhage. The authors selected a group of 103 neonates with intraventricular hemorrhage. As expected, the frequency of seizures correlates with the severity of bleeding. The percentage of acute seizures was 17% and 10% of the infants had remote seizures. These figures are high, probably because of the large number of newborns with grade 3 or 4 IVH. Remote seizures begin early. All but 1 infant had a history of acute seizures.

These data are quite important as a guideline for prophylactic antiepileptic therapy, a difficult choice at this age. The physician must weigh very carefully not only the probability of seizure recurrence, but the risk of prolonged antiepileptic therapy. The authors believe that the overall incidence of remote seizures is rather low and that long-term prophylactic therapy may not be justified, except in the high-risk group of patients with grade 4 IVH. This conclusion seems questionable because prophylactic antiepileptic drugs will not prevent the development of seizure focus or foci.

B. Klun, M.D., Ph.D.

Split Spinal Cord Malformations in Children

Erşahin Y, Mutluer S, Kocaman S, et al (Ege Univ, Izmir, Turkey)
J Neurosurg 88:57–65, 1998   26–5

Background.—Split spinal cord malformations (SSCMs) originate from the formation of an accessory neurenteric canal between the yolk sac and amnion, which subsequently forms an endomesenchymal tract that splits the notochord and neural plate. Two types have been defined: (1) type I, consisting of 2 hemicords, each within its own dural tube and separated by a dura-sheathed rigid median septum; and (2) type II, consisting of 2 hemicords housed in a single dural tube separated by a nonrigid, fibrous median septum. One patient series was analyzed.

Patients and Findings.—Seventy-four patients with SSCMs treated between 1980 and 1996 at 1 center were reviewed. Sixty-two percent were girls, aged less than 1 day to 12 years. Mean age of patients with neurologic deficits and orthopedic deformities was 43.2 months, significantly more than the mean age, 8.2 months of patients without deficits. Computerized tomography myelography was better than other radiologic methods at identifying SSCM type. Fifty-two patients had a single type I SSCM; 18 patients, a single type II SSCM; and 4, composite SSCMs. At least 1 associated spinal lesion that could result in spinal cord tethering was noted in 62 patients. Most patients remained stable after surgery, and clinical improvement was seen in 18 (Fig 2).

Conclusions.—This SSCM classification will clarify the current confusion in terminology. The radiologic method of choice for screening for SSCMs is MRI, although CT myelography is better than MRI at defining SSCM type.

▶ This article includes a very large number of children with split spinal cord, a condition otherwise seen only sporadically. Therefore, the question of some regional peculiarity should be raised. I believe the authors are right to propose replacing the confusing terms "diastematomyelia" and "diplomyelia" with the term "split spinal cord malformation." Magnetic resonance was the method of choice. However, the 2 tomography myelograms are very interesting.

The article suggests that surgery should be performed as soon as possible. This seems to be reasonable if there is a tethered cord, the only condition surgery could remove. This condition did exist in the majority of cases. However, most children had combined malformations (almost half had myelomeningocele) and already quite pronounced neurological signs (paraparesis in a third). There is no mention of a single child not having 1 of these conditions. Also missing are long-term results, and if the list of postoperative complications is complete, I am surprised that none of the children required a shunt, especially those children with myelomeningocele. It would be of interest to know how the authors managed the postoperative scolioses in already existing vertebral defects after obviously generous removal of vertebral arches. The authors certainly gained remarkable expe-

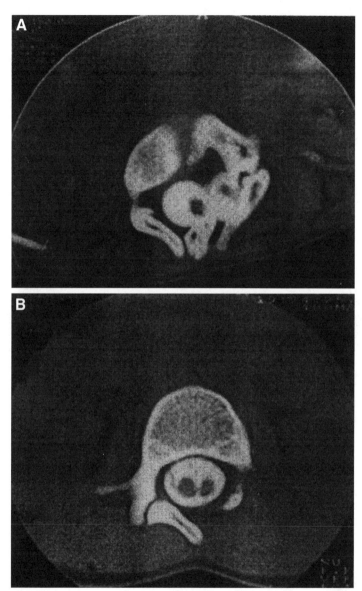

FIGURE 2.—Computerized tomography myelograms. **A,** Type I SSCM. Note the diagonal bone spur, two hemicords housed in two separate dural tubes, and bifid vertebra. **B,** Type II SSCM. Note two hemicords housed in a single dural tube. (Courtesy of Erşahin Y, Mutluer S, Kocaman S, et al: Split spinal cord malformations in children. *J Neurosurg* 88:57–65, 1998.)

rience with a disease which most neurosurgeons see only occasionally. However, congenital malformations of the nervous system in children are not a particularly rewarding area of neurosurgery.

B. Klun, M.D., Ph.D.

27 Peripheral Nerve Entrapment/Injury

Carpal Tunnel Syndrome

Predicting Acute Denervation in Carpal Tunnel Syndrome
Vennix MJ, Hirsh DD, Chiou-Tan FY, et al (Baylor College of Medicine, Houston)
Arch Phys Med Rehabil 78:306–312, 1998   27–1

Purpose.—Electrodiagnostic testing for carpal tunnel syndrome is painful for the patient, particularly during evaluation of the thenar eminence. If it were possible to predict the findings of denervation from the results of nerve conduction studies, it might be possible to avoid needle examination of the thenar muscle in many patients. This study sought to identify nerve conduction parameters that can predict the presence of acute denervation in carpal tunnel syndrome.

Methods.—The retrospective study included 1,590 consecutive patients at 2 electrodiagnostic laboratories with a diagnosis of median neuropathy. Needle electromyographic evidence of acute abductor pollicis brevis denervation was analyzed for its relationship to patient age and sex and to the results of nerve conduction studies, i.e., the sensory and motor latency and amplitude of the median nerve.

Results.—Predictors of denervation on logistic regression analysis were sex and median motor latency and amplitude. Ninety-five percent of all patients with denervation had a median motor amplitude of less than 7 mV. If this predictor had been used, it could have avoided needle examination of the abductor pollicis brevis for 52% of the patient population.

Conclusion.—In patients with suspected carpal tunnel syndrome, the motor amplitude of the median nerve can predict the presence of acute thenar muscle denervation. Consideration of this predictor has the potential to avoid a painful part of electrodiagnostic testing for more than half of patients. This is the first study to present guidelines to justify when abductor pollicis brevis examination is and is not necessary.

▶ This is an important report. The authors recognize a diminishing trend in denervation among patients with carpal tunnel syndrome and they attribute this to earlier diagnosis. Despite this trend, electromyographic studies are routinely performed as part of the electrodiagnostic evaluation for carpal tunnel syndrome. The authors have retrospectively determined nerve conduction parameters that will detect 95% of patients with motor denervation. As a result of the authors' findings, nearly half of all patients who undergo these evaluations could be safely spared the pain associated with needle electromyography of the hand. And, theoretically, this could produce a staggering cost savings.

S.R. Gibbs, M.A., M.D.

Ultrasound Treatment for Treating the Carpal Tunnel Syndrome: Randomised "Sham" Controlled Trial
Ebenbichler GR, Resch KL, Nicolakis P, et al (Univ of Vienna; Univ of Exeter, England)
BMJ 316:731–735, 1998   27–2

Background.—Ultrasound treatment has the potential to induce various types of biophysical effects within tissue. It has been suggested that ultrasound might help to enhance recovery from nerve compression, though few studies have tested ultrasound treatment for carpal tunnel syndrome under clinical conditions. This randomized, controlled trial assessed the efficacy of pulsed ultrasound for the treatment of idiopathic carpal tunnel syndrome.

Methods.—The double-blind trial included 45 patients with mild-to-moderate bilateral carpal tunnel syndrome, as demonstrated by electroneurographic studies. The patients received 20 sessions of active ultrasound treatment to 1 wrist and an identical-appearing sham treatment to the other. Ultrasound was delivered in 15-minute sessions at a frequency of 1 MHz, an intensity of 1.0 W/cm², and pulsed mode 1:4 using a 5 cm² transducer. Treatment was daily for the first week, then twice weekly for 5 weeks. The results between wrists were compared by subjective symptom ratings and by electroneurographic measures.

Results.—By both subjective and objective assessment, wrists receiving ultrasound treatment showed significantly greater improvement than those receiving the sham treatment. The improvements were sustained at 6 months follow-up. At 6 months, satisfactory improvement in symptoms was noted in 74% of ultrasound-treated wrists vs. 20% of placebo-treated wrists. Ultrasound also achieved significant and lasting changes in motor distal latency and the velocity of sensory nerve conduction.

Conclusions.—For patients with mild-to-moderate carpal tunnel syndrome, ultrasound therapy produces good short- to medium-term subjective and objective effects. The authors call for further study to confirm their results, to identify optimal treatment schedules, and to assess possible combinations of ultrasound with other nonsurgical treatments.

► Carpal tunnel syndrome is currently the most common type of peripheral nerve entrapment. Controversy exists regarding the best method of treatment of the syndrome. Conservative modalities are advocated initially and surgical release is recommended if conservative therapies are unsuccessful. These authors introduce the use of ultrasound to treat entrapment of the median nerve at the wrist. This article presents an excellent study design, adequate patient exclusion criteria, and sound statistical analysis. The authors theorize that ultrasound treatment with an intensity range of 0.5–2.0 W/cm^2 has the potential to induce biophysical effects within tissue that may lead to symptom relief. Forty-five patients with bilateral carpal tunnel syndrome were entered into this study. One wrist was used as experimental and the other wrist was used as a sham control. Results indicate that at 6 months there was a significant improvement in symptomatology of the wrist treated with ultrasound. Some of the drawbacks of the study include the lack of comparison with standard treatment methods (conservative or surgical), the lack of distinction between the severity of the carpal tunnel syndrome in the experimental and sham groups, and the short follow-up. It remains to be seen if ultrasound treatment is beneficial in the management of carpal tunnel syndrome.

D.F. Jimenez, M.D.

Carpal Tunnel Syndrome in the Mucopolysaccharidoses and Mucolipidoses

Haddad FS, Jones DHA, Vellodi A, et al (Hosp for Sick Children, London)
J Bone Joint Surg Br 79-B:576–582, 1997   27–3

Background.—Children with mucopolysaccharidosis or mucolipidosis experience progressive disability of the hand in relation to dysfunction of the median nerve. Bone marrow transplantation has significantly improved survival but does not seem to change the musculoskeletal symptoms. Some authors recommend decompression, but there is little objective information on cause, natural history, neurophysiology, or functional outcome after such surgery. The signs and symptoms of carpal tunnel syndrome are different in these children than in adults.

Methods.—Forty-eight consecutive children with mucopolysaccharidosis or mucolipidosis who required carpal tunnel decompression were evaluated. All patients were between ages 8 months and 16 years at the most recent review. Clinical, radiologic, and neurophysiologic assessments were performed. Symptoms, signs, radiologic, electrophysiologic and operative findings, histology, and upper limb function were analyzed.

Results.—At the time of surgery, the flexor retinaculum was thickened and a mass of white tenosynovium engulfed the flexor tendons. Most of the children had nerve constriction with a thickened epineurium. Functional improvement was seen soon after carpal tunnel decompression. Simultaneous tendon release also benefited some patients. Improved hand movement was maintained by regular physiotherapy.

Conclusions.—The standard protocol that the authors use for assessment, surgery, and follow-up of the effect of bone marrow transplantation, gene therapy, directed enzyme replacement, and other future treatments is described. The authors currently recommend early surgery to lower the risk of irreversible damage.

▶ As the title of this report reminds us, carpal tunnel syndrome may result from systemic, congenital diseases. A high index of suspicion for carpal tunnel syndrome is necessary in children with mucopolysaccharidosis and mucolipidosis, as the clinical changes are often very subtle. Classical signs and symptoms of carpal tunnel syndrome may be masked by other manifestations of these diseases. Diminution in fine motor skills, clumsiness, or alterations in grasp or playing pattern may be all that is revealed. This metabolic error, as the authors observed, results in bony dysplasia of the carpal tunnel and deposition of large amounts of glycosaminoglycan in the flexor retinaculum and the tenosynovium . The authors' data validate Fisher, Horner, and Wood's (1974) assertion that early carpal tunnel release will contribute to optimal limb function in these children.[1]

S.R. Gibbs, M.A., M.D.

Reference

1. Fisher RC, Horner RL, Wood VE: The hand in mucopolysaccharide disorders. *Clin Orthop* 104:191–199, 1974.

Endoscopic Treatment of Carpal Tunnel Syndrome: A Critical Review
Jimenez DF, Gibbs SR, Clapper AT (Univ of Missouri, Columbia)
J Neurosurg 88:817–826, 1998   27–4

Introduction.—Debate over the technique, results, and complications of endoscopic surgery for carpal tunnel syndrome (CTS) has appeared mainly in the orthopedic and plastic surgery literature, not in the neurosurgery literature. A critical review of current endoscopic procedures for the treatment of CTS was presented.

Findings.—The review covered 6 endoscopic techniques for carpal tunnel release reported from 1987 to 1997. These included the single-portal Okutsu, Agee and modified Agee, Menon, and Worseg Uni-Cut techniques and the dual portal Chow and Brown techniques. The Chow technique was the most frequently reported.

The articles included a total of 8.068 operations in 1,091 patients. The reported success rate was 96.5%, with a failure rate of 2.6%. For non-Workers' Compensation patients, the mean time to return to work was 17.8 days. The complication rate was 2.7%, with the most frequent complications being transient paresthesias of the ulnar and median nerves. Injuries to the superficial palmar arch, reflex sympathetic dystrophy, lacerations of the flexor tendon, and incomplete division of the transverse carpal ligament were reported as well. Comparative studies of endoscopic vs. open surgical repair suggested that the endoscopic procedures were associated with less pain and quicker return to work and activities of daily living.

Conclusion.—Endoscopic techniques for the treatment of carpal tunnel syndrome offer rates of success, complications, and failure, similar to those achieved with open techniques. The endoscopic techniques may reduce postoperative pain and tenderness while hastening return to work and activities of daily living. Neurosurgeons should be familiar with these endoscopic techniques, although the decision regarding technique depends on which technique the surgeon is most comfortable with. The authors currently perform the dual-portal Brown technique in carefully selected patients, while performing minimally open surgery in all others.

▶ Endoscopic techniques are preferred over conventional ones where access is required to lesions deep within a body cavity through a small entry. Carpal tunnel release (CTR) is performed through superficial, superimposed, and condensed layers of tissue. The lack of a clear difference in outcome between the open and endoscopic CTR (in prospective, controlled trials) and the steep learning curve of the latter make it difficult to determine which is the procedure of choice.

It would be helpful if we could compare the endoscopic CTR with the "best possible" open technique. The latter may involve MR localization of the transverse carpal ligament (TCL) followed by a precisely positioned 2–3 cm skin incision and a minimally invasive or microsurgical open CTR (with visual magnification through operating loops or microscope). Preoperative planning and choice of the most appropriate technique are likely to improve through modern MRI sequences (gradient echo or others). These provide high-resolution sections (less than 0.5 mm in thickness) and multidimensional spatial reconstruction of the carpal anatomy. They can be helpful in estimating size and location of the TCL; degree of flattening; and/or associated swelling of the median nerve, neuromas, tenosynovitis, and other pathological conditions.

Such studies may help us to develop objective criteria for endoscopic CTR. Until then, the minimally invasive open CTR (as described above) may represent a more widely applicable approach to ensure complete and safe incision of the TCL particularly in severe cases that satisfy any of the following criteria:

1. a history of hand trauma, previous surgery, or heavy occupational hand activity

2. "difficult" anatomy, i.e., tenosynovitis, very thick and/or wide TCL, heavy-built hand musculature, variations from normal bone anatomy

3. electromyography showing severe nerve compression with absent median sensory action potential or evidence of motor branch involvement with distal motor latency of more than 5 msec and denervation in the thenar muscle

4. MRI showing severe compression, i.e., a high "flattening ratio" and/or "swelling index" of the median nerve at the level of the hamate.

D.E. Sakas, M.D.

Miscellaneous

Ganglion Cyst Involvement of Peripheral Nerves

Harbaugh KS, Tiel RL, Kline DG (Brigham and Women's Hosp, Boston; Louisiana State Univ, New Orleans)
J Neurosurg 87:403–408, 1997   27–5

Background.—Ganglion cysts involving peripheral nerves have been described as having benign histologic appearance and favorable outcomes. However, they can also cause permanent neurologic deficits.

Methods.—Twenty-seven patients were treated surgically for ganglion cysts involving peripheral nerves at Louisiana State University Medical Center between 1968 and 1995. The 27 cysts involved nerves at 9 locations. The most common cysts, present in 52% of the patients, were cysts of the peroneal nerve. Eighty-three percent of the patients had motor deficits; 78% had pain; and 48% had sensory changes. Twenty-two percent had a history of acute trauma. The mean follow-up was 61 months.

Findings.—Only 58% of the patients had good motor recovery. Such recovery was related to the severity of the preoperative motor deficit. Eighty-nine percent of the patients had resolution or significant improvement of pain. Although none of the 5 patients had recurrences after repeat surgery, 4 patients (17%) had recurrences after the initial treatment. Overall, the mean time to recurrence was 16 months.

Conclusion.—Ganglion cysts involving peripheral nerves can be aggressive. Before surgery, patients should be counseled regarding the potential for limited motor recovery and the significant chance of recurrence.

▶ Given the authors' extensive experience with injuries, disease, and disorders of peripheral nerves, a larger series will likely only come from a collective, multi-institutional collaborative effort. Until then, this is the largest reported series of patients with this disorder, and it is the best information currently available regarding the diagnosis, treatment, and natural history of peripheral nerve ganglion cysts.

S.R. Gibbs, M.A., M.D.

Surgical Reconstruction of the Musculocutaneous Nerve in Traumatic Brachial Plexus Injuries

Samii M, Carvalho GA, Nikkhah G, et al (Nordstadt Med School, Hannover, Germany)
J Neurosurg 87:881–886, 1997   27–6

Background.—In patients with traumatic lesions of the brachial plexus, nerve structure disruption may occur at the level of the roots, trunk, cord, peripheral nerves, or in various combinations. This usually results in severely disabling symptoms and physical deficits. Surgical treatment to improve the restoration of function to part of the injured brachial plexus needs to be explored.

Methods.—Three hundred forty-five surgical reconstructions of the brachial plexus were done at the study institution in the past 16 years using nerve grafting or neurotization techniques. Graft placement between the C-5 and C-6 root and the musculocutaneous nerve was done to restore arm flexion in 65 patients. A subgroup of 54 patients was analyzed. The mean follow-up was 4.4 years.

Findings.—Sixty-one percent of the patients had reinnervation of the biceps. Results in patients with a preoperative delay of less than 7 months were significantly better than those with longer delays. Musculocutaneous nerve reinnervation was seen in 76% of patients undergoing surgery in the first 6 months after injury, in 60% of those with a 6- to 12-month delay, and in only 25% of those having surgery after 12 months. The root used for grafting the musculocutaneous nerve did not affect final outcome. Graft length was inversely related to postoperative outcome.

Conclusion.—Surgery should be done within 4 to 6 months after injury in patients without spontaneous reinnervation. Outcomes are unaffected by choice of donor nerve C-5 or C-6 but are affected by the intraoperative condition of the roots. Graft length will indirectly affect the final result, as it represents the extent of brachial plexus injury. Perfect coaptation with no tension at the nerve union site should always be attempted.

▶ This large retrospective case series underscores the importance of proceeding with nerve grafting or neurotization techniques within 6 months of the injury in patients with traumatic brachial plexus injuries who have failed development of spontaneous reinnervation.

S.R. Gibbs, M.A., M.D.

28 Spinal Disorders

Cervical Spine

Vertebral Artery Injury in C1–2 Transarticular Screw Fixation: Results of a Survey of the AANS/CNS Section on Disorders of the Spine and Peripheral Nerves
Wright NM, Lauryssen C (Washington Univ, St Louis)
J Neurosurg 88:634–640, 1998
28–1

Introduction.—Atlantoaxial complex instability is associated with unique problems in stabilization, largely related to the axial rotational capacity of the atlantoaxial complex. The C1-2 transarticular screw placement technique has become increasingly popular, although the anatomical variability of the atlantoaxial complex may limit its use. The course of the vertebral artery (VA) is a frequent limiting factor; however, few cases of vascular injury have been reported. Neurosurgeons were surveyed to assess the risk of VA injury with C1-2 transarticular screw placement.

Methods.—A questionnaire was sent to 847 members of the American Association of Neurological Surgeons/Congress of Neurological Surgeons Section on Disorders of the Spine and Peripheral Nerves. The surgeons were asked about the number of patients they treated with transarticular screws, the number of screws they placed, their experience with VA injury and resultant neurologic deficit, and their management of any known or suspected cases of VA injury.

Results.—The response rate was 25%. The 47% of respondents who had used C1-2 transarticular screws had placed a total of 2,492 screws in 1,318 patients. The surgeons were aware of VA injuries in 2.4% of patients and suspected VA injuries in another 1.7%. Of the total 54 patients with known or suspected VA injury, just 2 had neurologic deficits. One patient, with bilateral VA injury, died. When faced with an intraoperative VA injury, some surgeons placed the patient under observation whereas others performed immediate postoperative angiography for possible balloon occlusion. A number of other complications related to C1-2 screws were reported, including dural tears, screw fractures, screw breakout, fusion failure, infection, and suboccipital numbness.

Conclusion.—Based on this survey of neurosurgeons, the risk of VA injury associated with C1-2 transarticular screw fixation is 4.1% per patient or 2.2% per screw placed. The risk of neurologic deficit is much lower: 0.2% per patient or 0.1% per screw. The mortality rate is 0.1%.

▶ This important survey examined a number of issues related to VA injury in conjunction with C1-2 transarticular screw fixation. Over 200 surgeons participated in the survey, and I find it interesting that more than 50% of the respondents had not performed this procedure. Although these surgeons may provide thoughtful insight, their lack of experience with the operation should not be disregarded.

Thirteen hundred and eighteen patients were treated, and the risk of known VA injury in this survey was approximately 2.4% per patient. Vertebral artery injury was suspected, but not confirmed, at a rate of 1.7% per patient. This places the risk in the neighborhood of 4% per patient. Fortunately, the risk of neurologic injury as a result of placement of these screws was only 0.2% per patient. A single death was reported, resulting in a mortality rate of 0.1%. It is important to use these numbers to counsel patients concerning the true risks of this operative procedure.

I found the most interesting portion of the article to be that dealing with the choice of management of known or suspected VA injury. A number of respondents addressed this issue, and most of them stated that they would treat the patient with observation alone. I believe that this approach is fraught with potential complications. I favor immediate postoperative angiography. If there is partial disruption of the VA, the patient should be considered for an endovascular stenting procedure. If there is a marked disruption but the VA is still partially patent, I favor a trial balloon occlusion and, if this does not result in neurologic deficit, a balloon occlusion of the vessel. Such management would eliminate the risk of the development of dissection, pseudoaneurysm, or arteriovenous fistula.

This is an excellent means of obtaining an atlantoaxial fusion, but it does require experience, careful planning, and precise surgical technique. If 2 screws cannot be placed safely, only 1 should be positioned. The authors speculate that, at some point, frameless stereotactic systems will make the operation safer, but the accuracy of these devices is insufficient to reduce morbidity. I am also concerned that some surgeons will rely solely on the image-guided pictures to place screws, without personally verifying their trajectory with the exposed anatomical landmarks.

V.C. Traynelis, M.D.

Cervical Cord Neurapraxia: Classification, Pathomechanics, Morbidity, and Management Guidelines
Torg JS, Corcoran TA, Thibault LE, et al (Allegheny Univ for Health Sciences, Philadelphia; Hosp for Special Surgery, New York)
J Neurosurg 87:843–850, 1997   28–2

Background.—Cervical cord neurapraxia (CCN) is a distinct clinical condition characterized by narrowing of the anteroposterior diameter of the cervical canal. The typical patient is an athlete with an acute but transient neurologic episode of cervical cord origin. Symptoms include sensory changes, with or without motor changes, in both arms, both legs, both arms and legs, or the arm and leg on one side. The episodes can last from 15 minutes to 48 hours. The authors have reported the radiographic findings of CCN but not the MRI findings. A series of 100 cases of CCN were analyzed to develop a classification system, propose a new computerized measurement technique for MRI, and assess the relationship of the cervical cord to the canal.

Methods.—The patients were 109 males and 1 female, average age 21. All episodes of CCN occurred during participation in sports, with 87% being related to football. Follow-up data (average 3.3) were available for 105 patients. The clinical and imaging data were analyzed in detail to gain a clearer understanding of the condition, to assess the associated risk of permanent neurologic injury, to identify factors associated with recurrent episodes of CCN, and to propose clearer management guidelines. The MRI images were digitized to provide insight into the relationship of the spinal cord and intervertebral disk to the bony cervical canal.

Results.—The findings suggested that CCN was causally related to narrowing of the sagittal diameter of the cervical canal in the adult spine. There were no cases of permanent neurologic damage resulting from CCN. Sixty percent of the patients returned to sports competition, and none of these experienced any permanent morbidity. However, CCN recurred in 56% of the patients who returned to sports; the recurrence rate was particularly high for football players. Other factors related to recurrence risk were a smaller spinal canal–vertebral body ratio, a smaller disk-level canal diameter, and less space available for the spinal cord. The classification of the CCN episode and the imaging findings had no influence on the risk of recurrence.

Conclusion.—This experience shows that CCN is a transient neurologic condition. Athletes with uncomplicated CCN can return to competition with no increased risk for permanent neurologic damage. The occurrence of CCN appears to be related to congenital or degenerative narrowing of the sagittal diameter of the cervical canal. Most patients can return to their sport, although there is a high risk for recurrent CCN. This risk is strongly and inversely related to the sagittal canal diameter. Spinal canal measurements will be a useful aid to physicians counseling their patients as to future CCN risk.

▶ The authors answer an important question. Neurologists and neurosurgeons are often asked to evaluate and judge if and when an athlete who has sustained a cervical cord neuropraxia may return to sports, and with what risk? The authors' classification system and management guidelines should be useful in this circumstance, and, ideally, they may establish a treatment standard for this particular condition.

S.R. Gibbs, M.A., M.D.

Vertical Translocation: The Enigma of the Disappearing Atlantodens Interval in Patients With Myelopathy and Rheumatoid Arthritis. Part I. Clinical, Radiological, and Neuropathological Features

Casey ATH, Crockard HA, Geddes JF, et al (Natl Hosp for Neurology and Neurosurgery, London; London Hosp Med College)
J Neurosurg 87:856–862, 1997   28–3

Background.—Five percent to 34% of patients with rheumatoid arthritis have vertical translocation. The clinical and radiologic findings of vertical translocation in patients with myelopathy were reported.

Methods and Findings.—Of 186 patients with myelopathy, 116 (62%) had vertical translocation. Compared with atlantoaxial subluxation, vertical translocation occurred after a significantly longer period of disease. Clinically, translocation was characterized by a high cervical myelopathy with features of a cruciate paralysis, as noted in 35% of patients, compared with 26% exhibiting horizontal atlantoaxial subluxation. There were surprisingly few cranial nerve problems. Patients with vertical translocation had more severe neurologic deficits and lower survival rates. Radiology revealed vertical translocation to be secondary to lateral mass collapse and associated with a progressive reduction in the atlantodens interval and pannus. In 30% of the patients, the atlantodens interval was less than 5 mm.

Conclusion.—Vertical translocation, caused by lateral mass collapse, is associated with a progressive decline in the atlantodens interval and the degree of rheumatoid pannus. The degree of functional and neurologic impairment associated with vertical translocation is significantly greater than with horizontal atlantoaxial subluxation.

▶ This article details some of the outstanding experience of Dr. Crockard and his group in treating patients with craniovertebral junction abnormalities caused by rheumatoid arthritis. It is the first of a 2-part series dealing with this problem. One hundred eighty-six patients with myelopathy were prospectively studied. Although their myelopathy was attributed to either vertical translocation or C1-2 subluxation, I suspect that a number of these patients also had subaxial stenosis. In fact, it is stated that patients in both groups had radicular symptoms of 3 to 4 months duration. This would suggest that at least a portion of them had subaxial disease. This element is not truly controlled in the study and, therefore, may introduce bias. Survival is worse with vertical translation, but this may be caused by a number of factors such as the increased duration of rheumatoid arthritis and the increased severity of the myelopathy present.

In general, vertical translocation is believed to be caused by collapse of the lateral masses of C1. I was, therefore, surprised to note that only 24% of those patients with vertical translocation actually had lateral mass collapse. The state of the occipital condyle was not mentioned in the study, and I suspect that those without lateral mass collapse had translocation secondary to inflammatory changes occurring at the base of the skull itself.

The authors note for the first time that there is an inverse relationship between the atlantodental interval and the degree of vertical translocation. This is an extremely interesting finding and may be caused by a number of anatomical factors. The authors believe that this "fixed" situation makes the bony compression less "forgiving" and, therefore, responsible for the more advanced myelopathic state in the patients with vertical translocation. Myelopathy is often associated with a dynamic component. I think the dynamic factor came into play when the spine was flexed, resulting in stretching of the cord over the bony protuberance created by the vertical translocation.

V.C. Traynelis, M,D.

Vertical Translocation: Part II. Outcomes After Surgical Treatment of Rheumatoid Cervical Myelopathy
Casey ATH, Crockard HA, Stevens J (Natl Hosp for Neurology and Neurosurgery, London)
J Neurosurg 87:863–869, 1997   28–4

Objective.—A surgical approach to vertical translocation in patients with rheumatoid arthritis and the clinical and radiologic factors that influence outcome were described.

Methods.—One hundred sixteen patients (24 men), average age 62, who had rheumatoid cervical myelopathy and who underwent cervical spine surgery were observed prospectively. The Ranawat neurologic classification, the American Rheumatism Association functional grading system, the Stanford Health Activity Questionnaire disability index for rheumatoid arthritis, and the Myelopathy Disability Index were used to measure outcomes. Morbidity and mortality rates were calculated. Patients were observed for an average of 45.3 months.

Results.—Sixty-seven transoral decompressions were performed, and 33 patients received a bone graft. Nine patients required reoperation at an average of 16 months. There were 45 (39%) complications, including 23 respiratory, 12 cardiovascular, and 5 transoral, 1 posterior cervical wound infection, 3 meningitis infections, 11 gastrointestinal problems (peptic ulceration), and 5 pressure sores or decubitus ulcers. The 30-day mortality rate was 10.3%. There was improvement by at least 1 Ranawat class in 45% of the patients. Younger age and good preoperative muscle power were associated with good neurologic outcome. All scoring systems were significant predictors of outcome. Vertical translocation and spinal cord area were also significant predictors of outcome. Neither degree of transgression in the foramen nor anterior or posterior atlantodens interval was predictive of neurologic outcome.

Conclusion.—Preoperative neurologic function, spinal cord area, and degree of vertical translocation were predictive of neurologic outcome after surgical treatment of rheumatoid cervical myelopathy.

▶ This article follows the authors' previous work in which they prospectively examined the clinical, radiologic, and neuropathic features of patients with rheumatoid arthritis with myelopathy secondary to either vertical translocation or C1–C2 horizontal instability. This article focuses on the outcomes after surgery of those patients with vertical translocation. Although the data were collected prospectively, the surgical procedures were varied and, in fact, the authors state that surgery was influenced by "the available instrumentation and our own learning curve." This must produce irregularities within the data that could ultimately lead to bias. Nevertheless, the work provides us with insight, and several very important points are made.

In the authors' experience, their patients have severe neck pain on an average of 7.3 months before surgery. By history, symptoms consistent with myelopathy develop 5.5 months before surgery. It is clear from previous work and also from this report that the degree of myelopathy at the time of treatment is inversely related to a positive outcome. Therefore, I believe that this 2-month window is extremely important. I suggest that all patients with rheumatoid arthritis who begin to complain of neck pain need to be thoroughly examined and imaging studies of the craniovertebral junction should be obtained.

These authors are highly respected for their ability to manage patients with rheumatoid arthritis, and their experience with this patient population is extensive. Nevertheless, they use 2 methods that have not been widely adopted by others. The first is their limited use of preoperative traction. They note that other investigators have reported excellent results with the use of traction and that this treatment has saved many patients from an anterior decompression. Casey et al. claim to have had limited success in using traction, and it appears that they no longer use this treatment modality. Even more controversial is their failure to place bone grafts when performing dorsal occipitocervical fusions. These are done with instrumentation alone. The authors cite problems with morbidity in terms of harvesting graft as their reason for using instrumentation alone. Harvesting rib carries an extremely low morbidity rate, and this substance is perfect for use as an autograft in an occipitocervical fusion.

It is important to note that the morbidity and mortality involved with treating patients with rheumatoid arthritis and vertical translocation are high. The 30-day mortality rate is 10.3%. By 15 months, the mortality rate has risen to 25%. It appears from the Kaplan-Meier curve that survival levels off after that. Additionally, the morbidity rate approaches 40%. The authors advise that patients with rheumatoid vertical translocation who require surgical intervention be referred to surgeons experienced in performing such procedures. This advice should be taken seriously.

In patients who survived the treatment, 45% enjoyed an improved level of neurologic functioning, and 97% reported a decrease in pain. It is not clear how great the pain decrease was overall, but over half of the patients said that their pain had been diminished by 50% or more.

The only clinical predictor of outcome was the myelopathy disability index. The authors note that the degree of vertical translocation as measured by the Redlund-Johnell method was statistically significant in terms of outcome whereas that measured by the McRay method was not. They account for this discrepancy by stating that the Redlund-Johnell method more accurately assessed spinal cord compression. The amount of spinal canal compromise is important, and 1 way this is more accurately assessed with the Redlund-Johnell method is the fact that the tip of the odontoid is not used as a measurement. It is well known that the odontoid tip may be eroded and destroyed by the rheumatoid process and, therefore, its level of ascent is not truly indicative of the overall amount of settling that has taken place.

V.C. Traynelis, M.D.

Asymptomatic Grotesque Deformities of the Cervical Spine: An Occupational Hazard in Railway Porters
Kelkar P, O'Callaghan B, Lovblad K-O (Saint Joseph Health Ctrs, Chicago; Univ Hosp, Bern, Switzerland)
Spine 23:737–740, 1998   28–5

Introduction.—Acute and chronic injury to the spine result in persons having occupations requiring lifting and carrying. The most commonly involved segments are the thoracic and lumbar segments. The most common single cause of industrial accidents is careless manual load handling, ranging from 20% to 25% of reported accidents. Two patients with severe asymptomatic deformities of the cervical spine resulting from chronic low-grade occupational trauma are presented.

Methods.—Two patients in India, who were both railway porters, had occupational trauma causing spinal deformities in their thoracic and lumbar spines, and both patients had magnetic resonance imaging performed. The patients were age 39 and 40, and had kyphotic deformities of their cervical spines, with no neurologic symptoms. The patients had been railway porters for 25 years and had been carrying heavy loads on their heads.

Results.—There were advanced degenerative changes in the cervical spine, causing apparently normal cord signal intensity and obvious deformities. The patients had gross lordotic and kyphoscoliotic deformities of the cervical spine, with associated subluxation. No evidence of associated soft tissue masses in the prevertebral regions was seen.

Conclusion.—In industrialized countries, chronic, occupational, low-grade trauma of the cervical vertebral region is extremely unusual. This complication of an occupational exposure deserves attention as an unusual cause of cervical spinal deformity, in view of the increasing mobility of people in general and of the labor force in particular. The effects of chronic physical strain on the spine are similar to those of the aging process, with disk degeneration in the early stages and deformity of the bones in the advanced stages. When excessive loads are regularly carried, especially if carrying is begun at an early age, deformities usually develop.

▶ This unusual example of occupational trauma underscores the remarkable tolerance of the central nervous system for insidious deformity. These deformities, likely resulting from the summation of chronic heavy-axial loading insults, have caused the International Labor Organization to recommend a maximum permissible weight of 55 kg to be carried by an adult male, and a minimum age of 18 for employment as a manual laborer.[1]

S.R. Gibbs, M.A., M.D.

Reference

1. Parmeggiani L (ed): *Encyclopedia of Occupational Health and Safety*, volume 2, 3rd edition. Geneva, Switzerland: International Labour Organization, 1983: pp 1200–300.

Bisegmental Cervical Interbody Fusion Using Hydroxyapatite Implants: Surgical Results and Long-term Observation in 70 Cases
Kim P, Wakai S, Matsuo S, et al (Dokkyo Univ, Tochighi, Japan; Moriyama Hosp, Tokyo; Univ of Tokyo)
J Neurosurg 88:21–27, 1998   28–6

Introduction.—Various methods of grafting and fusion have been developed for anterior cervical spine fusion. Since 1991, the authors have used synthetic hydroxyapatite (HA), the main constituent of the naturally occurring bone matrix, as a substitute for autologous bone grafting in cervical interbody fusions. The design of the HA implants is reported, together with surgical techniques involved in their placement and with long-term outcome in 70 patients.

Methods.—The HA implants were made to be 30% porous; purity of the material is greater than 99%. In contrast to nonporous material, HA is amenable to cutting with a conventional high-speed drill. Implants are designed to provide maximum durability, biomechanical stability, and alignment preservation. Patients who received the implants ranged in age from 22 to 83 (mean 50.6). The most common underlying primary pathological conditions were spondylosis (31 cases) and disk extrusion (26 cases). Single interbody fusion was performed in 67 cases and fusion of 2 interspaces was performed in 3 cases. Patients were evaluated with imaging studies at 8 weeks, 6 months, 12 months, and annually thereafter. The mean follow-up was 37.1 months.

Results.—Surgery successfully achieved decompression and construction of the fusion mass, with no neurological deterioration related to the surgical procedure or to the HA implant. Stability of the graft was confirmed 8 weeks after surgery in all patients. Encasement of the implant and formation of union were seen at 6–12 months after surgery. Two patients treated early in the series required revision, and a third patient underwent a salvage operation. There were no signs of collapse or "sinking" of the vertebral body. Normal lordosis, if present before surgery, remained preserved in most cases through follow-up.

Conclusion.—Synthetic HA implants can safely achieve satisfactory interbody fusion in patients requiring anterior cervical spine fusion. The material is not amenable to absorption by the host cells, and the implant functions as the core for formation of the bone mass required to bear mechanical loads.

▶ The authors describe the design of hydroxyapatite implants for cervical interbody fusion, the surgical technique involved in their placement, and the results in 70 patients.

Although there is some debate as to whether a formal fusion is necessary after a simple discectomy, it is recognized that an anterior approach involving removal of a significant amount of vertebral bone to obtain adequate decompression will require a fusion. The problems associated with harvesting graft material from the iliac crest are well known, and patients often postoperatively find the graft site more troublesome than the condition for which they had surgery. Many types of graft material (artificial, allogeneic, and autograft) have been tried, but none has been ideal.

The authors mention the experimental studies that have shown the bioactive properties of hydroxyapatite, including the formation of direct bonding with bone. Unlike autogenic or allogeneic bone, hydroxyapatite undergoes little absorption and maintains its initial compressive strength.

This study of 70 patients does give some indication of the usefulness of hydroxyapatite, and the authors have described a simple technique for insertion of the graft.

The authors do not mention the cost of hydroxyapatite. It is possible that the hydroxyapatite implant will be of use in cervical spine surgery, and further studies are awaited with interest.

A.H. Kaye, M.D., M.B.B.S., F.R.A.C.S.

Anterior Interbody Fusion With the BAK-Cage in Cervical Spondylosis
Matge G (Centre Hospitalier, Luxembourg)
Acta Neurochir (Wien) 140:1–8, 1998   28–7

Objective.—For patients with degenerative conditions of the cervical spine and symptoms of radiculopathy or myelopathy, anterior cervical interbody fusion is the treatment of choice. The new autostabilizing interbody BAK-C cage can be implanted during anterior cervical surgery to stabilize the motion segment while permitting fusion to occur. This device produces good clinical results and fusion rates without the complications associated with autografting or allografting. A 2-year experience with the BAK-C for cervical spondylosis was reported.

Methods.—The BAK-C cage consists of a threaded, hollow, porous titanium-alloy cylinder and special instrumentation, including a bone-collecting reamer. Surgical site bone graft acts as osteoinductive material within the implant; the cage functions on the principle of distraction-compression using the tension forces of the annulus fibrosus. Biomechanical tests show improved stability with the BAK-C, while animal studies show good fusion.

The BAK-C cage was used in 101 levels in 80 patients: 72 with cervical radiculopathy and 8 with myelopathy. The indications were the same as for conventional anterior cervical interbody fusion, i.e., spinal degeneration. The most frequently operated levels were C5–C6 and C6–C7. The clinical results were evaluated using a 10-point analogue scale for neck and arm/shoulder pain, as well as neurologic examination. Dynamic x-rays, myelo-CT, and MRI were performed as well. The patients were followed up for 2–26 months.

Results.—The operative procedure provided excellent relief of neck and radicular pain. Neurologic recovery was significantly different for patients with radiculopathy vs. myelopathy—most of the former showed no deficit at 6 months, compared with only 1 of 8 patients in the latter group. The radiologic results were also good. There was 1 case of osteoporotic vertebral collapse requiring reoperation and additional anterior plate fixation. Otherwise, there were no problems with instability, cage migration, kyphosis, or pseudarthrosis. With proper technique—including correct distraction, symmetric endplate drilling, and lateral x-ray control—the complication rate was low.

Conclusions.—This experience demonstrates the safety of using the BAK-C to treat cervical spondylosis. This procedure provides immediate stability, good clinical results, a low complication rate, and minimal graft morbidity. The short-term results appear superior to those of the Cloward or Smith-Robinson procedure; the long-term results remain to be determined.

▶ This technique looks very promising because the implant device has been designed to overcome the shortcomings of the Cloward and Smith-Robinson techniques. The device is autostabilizing; consequently no additional internal fixation is necessary, and no external immobilization is necessary. The cage seems less subject to subsidence, and graft collapse is precluded because it is placed within the rigid cage. There is no graft site morbidity because this technique uses osteoinductive local autograft. Fusion rates at 6 and 12 months were quite good.

Postoperative imaging artifact from the titanium alloy is clearly and largely the disadvantage of this system of fusion. Also, I suspect that reoperative work, wherein a fusion cage has been placed, could be formidable unless an equally well-designed extraction technique is developed.

S.R. Gibbs, M.A., M.D.

Reduction Technique for Uni- and Biarticular Dislocations of the Lower Cervical Spine

Vital J-M, Gille O, Sénégas J, et al (Unité de Pathologie Rachidienne Tripode, Bordeaux, France)
Spine 23:949–955, 1998   28–8

Introduction.—Different centers vary significantly in their management of cervical dislocations. Points of disagreement include the maximum amount of traction used, the safety of closed manipulation with the patient under anesthesia, and the preferred surgical approach. The outcomes of a series of 168 consecutive cases managed with sequential use of these 3 techniques were reported.

Methods.—The study included 168 patients with dislocations of the lower cervical spine, C2-C3 to C7-T1. There were 77 unilateral and 91 bilateral dislocations. The initial attempt at treatment consisted of reduction by gradual traction, without the use of anesthesia. If this did not succeed, specific closed manipulations were performed with the patient under general anesthesia. Anterior surgical reduction was then performed if the 2 previous steps failed. Even if closed reduction was achieved, each patient underwent interbody fusion to address instability caused by ligamentous lesions.

Results.—The protocol was successful in 163 patients, the exceptions being 5 patients with longstanding unilateral dislocations. Among the patients with bilateral dislocations, the success rate was 43% with simple traction, 30% with closed manipulation with the patient under anesthesia, and 27% with anterior surgery. In cases of unilateral dislocation, the success rates were 23%, 36%, and 34%, respectively. Seven patients underwent repair of herniated disks causing neurologic signs during the anterior surgery. There were no instances of neurologic deterioration occurring during or immediately after the reduction protocol. Only 1 case required a posterior approach followed by anterior arthrodesis.

Conclusion.—Management of this reliable, sequential protocol for treating unilateral and bilateral dislocations of the lower cervical spine starts with rapidly progressive traction and is followed by 1 or 2 reduction attempts with the patient under anesthesia. If reduction is still not achieved, surgical reduction is performed through an anterior approach. The authors' experience shows a very high success rate, with no cases of neurologic deterioration after reduction. The anterior surgical approach permits the use of diskectomy and enlargement of interbody separation.

▶ This is a review of 168 consecutive patients with unilateral or bilateral cervical dislocations who were treated with a single standard treatment protocol. The protocol involved rapid cervical traction using cranial tongs up to a maximum of 18 kg for a C7-T1 dislocation. If reduction was not achieved, manipulation under anesthesia with fluoroscopic monitoring was attempted. If this was unsuccessful, the patients were reduced operatively. Even with successful closed reduction, all patients went to surgery for a fusion. The operation always consisted of an anterior diskectomy and then fusion with internal stabilization.

In general, the treatment protocol was well thought out and the results were excellent. Although most published surgical techniques for the reduction of dislocated cervical facets approach the problems through a posterior route, an anterior procedure is attractive for several reasons. First, and perhaps most important, patients do not have to be turned in the prone position while they are in a potentially unstable situation. Second, any herniated disk found at the time of surgery can be removed and, therefore, neural decompression is assured. Finally, there is excellent clinical and biomechanical evidence to suggest that placement of a graft and anterior instrumentation are adequate to maintain the reduction until osseous union takes place.

I am a little surprised that the authors had such a high success rate in obtaining reduction of their dislocations operatively. It may be difficult to realign all patients, particularly if facet fractures are present. For this reason, I believe that all patients should be evaluated preoperatively with a CT scan. Care must be taken in not overdistracting the injured segment and in placing a graft which is inadvertently large. Some distraction of the disk space is useful for opening the neural foramina, but overextending the interspace will limit the ability of the articular pillars to share some of the axial load, and the extra distraction, by itself, will upset the overall balance of the spine.

Finally, I would recommend that flexion/extension films always be taken with the fluoroscope in the operating room once the instrumentation is in place. This will allow the surgeon to be certain that the instrumentation is adequate and will verify the fact that there is not a previously undetected instability at another level.

V.C. Traynelis, M.D.

Thoracic Spine

Experience in the Surgical Management of 82 Symptomatic Herniated Thoracic Discs and Review of the Literature
Stillerman CB, Chen TC, Couldwell WT, et al (Univ of North Dakota, Minot; Univ of Southern California, Los Angeles)
J Neurosurg 88:623–633, 1998   28–9

Objective.—Only a small proportion of disk surgeries are for herniated thoracic disks. These herniations have historically been difficult to treat because of diagnostic delays, unclear indications, and debate about the surgical approach, among other issues. The authors analyze their experience with thoracic minidiskectomy, focusing on the presentations, surgical treatment, and patient outcomes.

Patients.—The experience included 71 patients operated on for 82 herniated thoracic disks over a 24-year period. There were 37 women and 34 men, mean age 48 years. Two thirds of the herniated disks were located from T8 to T11. Thirty-seven percent of patients had evidence of trauma. Seventy-six percent of patients complained of pain, either localized, axial, or radicular. Sixty-one percent had motor impairment, 58% had hyperreflexia and spasticity, 61% had sensory impairment, and 24% had bladder dysfunction. Myelograms, CT myelograms, or MRI scans were used to make the diagnosis. Ninety-four percent of disks were classified as having a centrolateral location, and 6% a lateral location. Sixty-five percent of patients showed evidence of calcification, and 7% were found at surgery to have intradural extension. Multiple herniations were present in 14% of patients.

Treatment and Outcomes.—A transthoracic surgical approach was used in 60% of patients, transfacet pedicle-sparing approach in 28%, a lateral extracavitary approach in 10%, and a transpedicular approach in 2%. After surgery, 87% of patients had improvement or elimination of pain. Hyperreflexia and spasticity were improved or eliminated in 95% of patients, sensory changes in 84%, bowel or bladder dysfunction in 76%, and motor impairment in 58%. The complication rate was 15%, including major complications in 3 patients. One patient died in the perioperative period of cardiopulmonary compromise, 1 had spinal instability requiring additional surgery, and 1 had increased severity of paraparesis.

Conclusions.—This experience, along with other recent reports, underscores the ongoing challenges of treating herniated thoracic disks. Complication rates have decreased compared with those of earlier series. However, it is still unclear which patients need surgery and which can be managed conservatively. All available surgical approaches carry a substantial potential for morbidity; minimally invasive alternatives are needed. The surgeon should be proficient in a number of surgical options, and thus able to tailor treatment to the individual patient.

▶ This is an important article. Classic writings on thoracic disk disease have stressed more anterior approaches and condemned nonoperative care as dangerous. This likely represents the well-discussed lack of clinical predictability with thoracic disk disease, the resultant advanced nature of the process at presentation, and the size of the lesion necessary to reach detection by early myelography alone.

The advent of modern studies, mainly MRI, and the rate at which these studies are ordered by various health care personnel (not necessarily physicians) have revealed the existence of the asymptomatic thoracic disk—a cohort, it seems, inappropriate for (prophylactic) surgery. The next big step, well-defined by this piece (though likely still quite controversial), is to recognize in prospect those minimally symptomatic or questionably symptomatic patients appropriate for nonoperative care and then choose the appropriate operative approach(es) for those few deemed surgical candidates. This article lends credence to intuition which has, until now, been poorly tested.

C.P. Bondurant, M.D.

Lumbar Spine

The Effect of Intraoperative Hip Position on Maintenance of Lumbar Lordosis: A Radiographic Study of Anesthetized Patients and Unanesthetized Volunteers on the Wilson Frame

Benfanti PL, Geissele AE (Dwight David Eisenhower Army Med Ctr, Fort Gordon, Ga)
Spine 22:2299–2303, 1997   28–10

Introduction.—In patients undergoing instrumented lumbar fusion, lordosis must be preserved to maintain normal sagittal alignment. Therefore the hips are usually extended on positioning devices, yet the true effects of this practice on lumbar lordosis are unknown. The specific intraoperative effects of differences in position are also uncertain. The effects of hip position on lordosis were studied in patients and volunteers in different positions on a Wilson frame.

Methods.—The study included 13 patients undergoing diskectomy or lumbar fusion, who were studied during anesthesia, and 14 unanesthetized volunteers. Lumbar spine radiographs were obtained with the patients in standing position and in lateral position with the hips extended and flexed on a Wilson frame. Comparable views were obtained in the volunteers. In each position, the investigators measured lumbar lordosis at L1 to S1 and intervertebral body angles. Changes in total and segmental lordosis between positions were assessed.

Results.—With the patients on the Wilson frame with the hips extended, 95% of preoperative standing lordosis was maintained. Seventy-four percent of lordosis was maintained with the hips in a mean of 33 degrees flexion. In the volunteer group on the Wilson frame, maintenance of standing lordosis was 98% with the hips extended and 86% with the hips flexed a mean of 28 degrees.

Conclusions.—In patients and volunteers alike, hip flexion significantly reduces lordosis. To optimize preservation of lordosis during lumbar fusion surgery, the patient should be positioned in maximal hip extension. With the Wilson frame, the lumbar sagittal contour can be adjusted to preserve or reduce lordosis. Other devices may affect lordosis differently.

▶ A variety of positioning devices have been designed for lumbar surgery, most of which allow the patient's abdomen to hang freely to prevent abdominal pressure from engorging Batson's epidural venous plexus. The Wilson frame is such a device. It is relatively inexpensive and is commonly used for lumbar surgery.

This report confirms the customary practice of positioning patients undergoing lumbar fusion in hip extension to maintain lumbar lordosis. More importantly, it quantitatively demonstrates that maximal hip extension is necessary to approximate normal standing lumbar lordosis.

In this era of internal spinal fusion devices, attention to maintaining normal sagittal alignment is especially important to prevent creating a conformation that may plague the patient with postoperative back pain. I suspect that operative positioning was relatively less important in the days of noninstrumented posterolateral onlay fusions because standing automatically restored lumbar lordosis.

S.R. Gibbs, M.A., M.D.

Outcome After Microdiscectomy: Results of a Prospective Single Institutional Study
Quigley MR, Bost J, Maroon JC, et al (Allegheny Univ, Philadelphia; Thomas Jefferson College of Medicine, Philadelphia)
Surg Neurol 49:263–268, 1998   28–11

Introduction.—Many patients undergo surgery for excision of a herniated intervertebral disk. However, reports vary substantially as to the success rate of this procedure, with prospective studies failing to confirm the excellent results of retrospective series. A prospective, single-center study of the outcomes of lumbar microdiskectomy was reported.

Methods.—The study included 295 men and 119 women, average age 42, undergoing first unilateral single-level microdiskectomy over a 16-month period. All operations were performed according to the same technique by 5 neurosurgeons. Symptoms had been present for a mean of 9 months; 31.56% of the patients were workers' compensation cases. Average hospital stay was 2 days. Outcomes were assessed by mail questionnaire or telephone interview. Treatment success was strictly defined by a combination of pain relief, work status, nonuse of narcotics, and patient satisfaction.

Results.—The overall surgical complication rate was 4%. The 6-month follow-up rate was 86%. By the study definition, microdiskectomy was successful in 74% of cases. Factors related to treatment success on multivariate logistic regression analysis were workers' compensation status and symptom duration longer than 6 months. Eighty-six percent of the patients who were not receiving workers' compensation and whose symptoms were of short duration had successful surgery, compared with 29% of those receiving workers' compensation who had symptoms of long duration.

Conclusions.—This prospective study shows that microdiskectomy is a safe procedure with minimal morbidity. The success rate is not as high as suggested by retrospective studies and is affected by workers' compensation status and duration of symptoms. This study identifies no technical or physical factors related to the success of surgery.

▶ Plaudits to the authors for this prospective work. This is one of very few prospective studies in spine surgery, and although it does not offer experienced spine surgeons any earthshaking findings, it does suggest that the success rate of lumbar microdiskectomy may not be quite as good as we had thought, based upon the reports of retrospective series. As usual, it is difficult to compare this study with others because there has not been a consistent definition of "success" or the criteria used to determine success after lumbar diskectomy.

The Joint Section on Disorders of the Spine and Peripheral Nerves of the American Association of Neurological Surgeons/Congress of Neurological Surgeons attempted to prospectively study lumbar diskectomy outcome, although only 740 patients were enrolled in the study and the follow-up at 1 year was less than 60%.[1] Perhaps it is time to try again, with a look at microdiskectomy bolstered by improved enrollment and follow-up.

S.R. Gibbs, M.A., M.D.

Reference

1. Abramovitz JN, Neff S: Lumbar disc surgery: Results of the prospective lumbar discectomy study of the Joint Section on Disorders of the Spine and Peripheral Nerves of the American Association of Neurological Surgeons and the Congress of Neurological Surgeons. *Neurosurgery* 29:301–308, 1991.

Lower Urinary Tract Symptoms in Lumbar Root Compression Syndromes: A Prospective Survey
Perner A, Andersen JT, Juhler M (Univ of Copenhagen)
Spine 22:2693–2697, 1997   28–12

Purpose.—When lower urinary tract symptoms (LUTS) develop in patients with lumbar root compression, they are usually considered a sign of cauda equina syndrome. However, this is a rather rare syndrome, whereas LUTS seem common among patients with uncomplicated disk herniation and spinal stenosis. The presence of LUTS in patients with uncomplicated lumbar root compression syndromes was prospectively determined.

Methods.—A total of 108 men undergoing surgery for lumbar disk herniation or spinal stenosis were studied. All were free of concurrent neurologic or urologic disease or previous spinal surgery. They were given a detailed questionnaire about their micturition, designed to evaluate the prevalence, nature, and severity of LUTS. The relationship between LUTS and age, pain, analgesic intake, and type and level of compression was assessed.

Findings.—Significant LUTS were present in 55% of patients, including 80% of those with spinal stenosis. The symptoms were irritative in 33 patients, obstructive in 36, and retentive in 23. Symptoms were severe in 24 patients. Patients with median compression had more symptoms than those with paramedian compression. The symptoms were unrelated to any of the other factors investigated.

Conclusions.—Men with lumbar root compression syndrome show a high prevalence of LUTS. The symptoms are of mixed type and are most frequent in patients with median root compression and spinal stenosis. More studies of LUTS in lumbar root compression syndromes are needed, including evaluation of their prevalence in female patients, their prognosis, and the incidence of monosymptomatic bladder dysfunction.

▶ Cauda equina syndrome, often from a massively prolapsed lumbar disk, is well known to cause "saddle anesthesia," lower extremity motor weakness, bilateral absence of Achilles reflex, low back pain with bilateral sciatica, and sexual and sphincter dysfunction. However, the effects of spinal stenosis, and lesser disk herniations on the genitourinary system have not been given much attention.

Somatic voluntary control descends through sacral roots 2–4, which may be variably affected along their course to the pelvic viscera. As the authors expected, I too would have expected more urinary retention symptoms. Instead the symptoms were mixed obstructive, retentive, and irritative symptoms. As the nerves of the lumbar and sacral roots are mixed nerves, the authors have offered an interesting, logical motor/somatosensory postulate for LUTS in patients with lumbosacral spondylosis:

Retention is a motor deficit symptom and equals paresis, urge symptoms are irritative sensory symptoms and equal paresthesias, and leg pain and loss of bladder sensation are sensory deficits and equal loss of sensation in dermatome. Urge incontinence and obstructive symptoms are irritative motor symptoms, the former with involvement of the nerve fibers to the muscle of the bladder and the latter with the involvement of nerve fibers to the sphincters.

This work raises our awareness of a higher prevalence of LUTS in patients with lumbar stenosis than with disk herniation, and significantly more LUTS in median vs. paramedian/lateral disk herniations.

S.R. Gibbs, M.A., M.D.

Accuracy of Using Computed Tomography to Identify Pedicle Screw Placement in Cadaveric Human Lumbar Spine
Yoo JU, Ghanayem A, Petersilge C, et al (Case Western Reserve Univ, Chicago; Loyola Univ of Chicago)
Spine 22:2668–2671, 1997   28–13

Introduction.—Spine surgery has come to rely on the use of the pedicle screw system to improve the success rate of posterolateral lumbar fusion, but a serious complication related to pedicle screw use is neurologic injury secondary to misplaced pedicle screws abutting or transecting a nerve root. Computed tomography has been used to rule out a causal relation between the placement of the pedicle screws and any neurologic complication, but the sensitivity or the specificity of using computed tomography imaging in identifying pedicle screw placement is still unknown. The sensitivity and specificity of predicting pedicle screw placement using the computed tomography scan was defined. To predict possible differences in identifying screw positions, both titanium and cobalt–chrome alloy screws were placed in matching locations.

Methods.—In 6 cadaveric human lumbar spine, cobalt–chrome and titanium alloy pedicle screws of identical size were placed. To allow complete visualization of the pedicle, wide laminectomy was performed. In each spine, there were 3 consecutive lumbar levels that were instrumented, resulting in 36 pedicle screw placements to identify. To identify the accuracy of screw placement within the pedicle, 4 orthopedic spine surgeons and a musculoskeletal radiologist read the imaged instrumented spines.

Results.—Cobalt–chrome screws had a sensitivity rate of 67±6% for identifying a misplaced screw compared with 86±5% for titanium screws. For cobalt–chrome screws, the specificity rate of radiographic diagnosis of misplaced pedicle screws was 66±10%; for titanium screws, it was 88±8%. For cobalt–chrome screws, the sensitivity rate of identifying screws placed correctly in the pedicle was 70±10%; for titanium screws, it was 89±8% (a statistically significant difference). For cobalt–chrome screws, the overall accuracy rate was 68±7%; for titanium screws, the overall accuracy was 87±3%.

Conclusion.—Inaccuracies in both clinical and research conditions can result from a reliance on the computed tomography scan data alone in determining accuracy of pedicle screws.

▶ Intraoperative x-ray fluoroscopy is mandatory in performing instrumentation on lumbar spine, but for further controls in our patient clinic basis, computed tomography (CT) has revealed the gold standard to assess good placement of screws. Instruments installed on the spine must be compatible with CT and Magnetic Resonance materials, some of them as good as titanium alloys. This article, sometimes quite obvious but not less useful, establishes real differences in terms of image evaluation between cobalt–chrome and titanium implants. The latter ones are clearly favored as less distorting devices, making them more accurate in their position into the pedicles. Clinical data are pointed out to stress the importance in prompt identification of a misplaced screw as a cause of postoperative pain and, which is crucial, its heralding role of consecutive more serious motor disturbances. The immediate conclusion—as the authors say—is that titanium implants could be more reliable in looking for better postoperative assessment than in waiting for further imaging techniques to obtain greater accuracy. My second point is to use 3D reconstructive CT techniques on both materials; perhaps, the former differences between them should be maintained in axial views. If it is demonstrated, titanium alloys could be ethically reputed as the material of choice to be implanted, to date, in human spine.

M.A. Perez-Espejo, M.D., Ph.D.

Vascular and Visceral Injuries Associated With Lumbar Disc Surgery: Medicolegal Implications

Goodkin R, Laska LL (Univ of Washington, Seattle; Tennessee State Univ, Nashville)
Surg Neurol 49:358–372, 1998   28–14

Introduction.—Perforation of the anterior annulus fibrosus/anterior longitudinal ligament with injury to the aorta, inferior vena cava, or iliac vessel is one complication encountered during removal of a herniated disc and frequently leads to death with an incidence as high as 17 per 10,000 patients. There are also visceral injuries to the bowel, ureters, bladder, and pancreas that have been reported. Patients who had injury to a major vessel or viscera during lumbar disc surgery and litigation resulted were reviewed to determine the medicolegal implications.

Methods.—There were 21 patients who had an injury to an intra-abdominal vessel or viscera. Litigation resulted with all patients and a settlement or verdict was rendered. The literature was reviewed to determine the medicolegal implications of symptomatic ventral perforations of the annulus fibrosus/anterior longitudinal ligament.

Results.—Eighteen patients had vascular injuries, and 3 had bowel injuries. There were 13 women, 3 men, and 5 patients of undisclosed gender. In 16 patients, the injury was repaired. It was unsuccessfully repaired in 2 patients. Three patients did not have a repair, and 2 of the 3 resulted in death. The outcome shows 12 patients alive, 7 patients who died, and 2 patients with an unknown outcome. Of the patients who had an injury to the aorta, 57% died. In 48% of the cases, the plaintiff was successful. Jury verdicts were rendered in 5 cases, and 5 had settlements achieved. The defense had a favorable outcome in 10 patients. A reviewing expert should concentrate on the management of the complication, weighing the significance and duration of the symptoms and signs of when a reasonable and prudent surgeon should become concerned.

Conclusion.—In most states, it is not considered below the standard of care to fail to counsel a patient about the possibility of a vascular or visceral injury secondary to a posterior approach for a lumbar discectomy; however, it may be better to inform the patient because of the nature of the potential consequences.

▶ The authors report 21 cases of lumbar disc surgery involving injury to a major vessel or viscera in which litigation resulted in a settlement or rendered verdict. On the basis of an analysis of the literature, they have concluded that these injuries probably are not the result of negligence, but rather the result of a number of *uncontrollable* (emphasis added) variables presenting to the surgeon at the time of surgery. These variables include those related to anatomy, position, and the instruments, all within the technical or judgmental control of the surgeon. Interestingly, they do not dwell on a most important variable, which is carelessness or inattention on the surgeon's part. With the previously recounted variables, so well enumerated in the article, it would appear the single most important contribution to these injuries is this last variable. Nevertheless, they are sound in their conclusion that the issue of standard of care should be most succinctly addressed during the diagnosis of the injury, as opposed to the technical cause of the injury. I certainly agree with their recommendation that the specific injuries should be discussed preoperatively with the patient, not only to make sure that the patient understands the gravity of the problem, with a 50% mortality, but also to reinforce in the surgeon's mind the possibility that these injuries may occur, thereby, hopefully, ensuring the surgeon's diligence.

C. Watts, M.D., J.D.

Degenerative Lumbar Spondylolisthesis With Spinal Stenosis: A Prospective, Randomized Study Comparing Decompressive Laminectomy and Arthrodesis With and Without Spinal Instrumentation

Fischgrund JS, Mackay M, Herkowitz HN, et al (William Beaumont Hosp, Royal Oak, Mich)
Spine 22:2807–2812, 1997   28–15

Objective.—Whether spinal instrumentation is beneficial in the operative management of patients with degenerative spondylolisthesis and spinal stenosis is controversial. A randomized prospective study was performed, involving patients with symptomatic spinal stenosis associated with degenerative lumbar spondylolisthesis to compare the results of decompression and arthrodesis alone with those of decompression and arthrodesis combined with instrumentation at the level of the arthrodesis.

Methods.—Patients, aged 53 to 86 (mean age, 66 years), were randomly assigned to 1 of 2 treatment groups: decompressive laminectomy and single level autogenous bilateral lateral intertransverse process arthrodesis or the same treatment but with transpedicular instrumentation. The former group comprised 6 men and 27 women; the latter, 7 men and 28 women. Patients were followed up for 2 years.

Results.—Patients in the instrumented group had 4 pedicle screws implanted. Clinical outcome was excellent or good in 78% of the instrumented group and in 85% of the noninstrumented group. There was no significant difference in results between the 2 groups. After surgery, leg and back pain were rated 0 (no pain) or 1 by significantly more (80% and 74%, respectively) of the instrumented group than of the noninstrumented group (64% and 58%, respectively). More patients in the noninstrumented group (75%) rated leg pain at 0 or 1 after surgery compared with the instrumented group (64%). Arthrodesis was significantly more successful in the instrumented group than in the noninstrumented group (82% versus 45%).

Conclusion.—Although the pedicle screws used in the instrumented group may have accounted for the significantly higher arthrodesis rate, there was no difference in back and leg pain between the instrumented and noninstrumented groups.

The Effect of Pedicle Screw Instrumentation on Functional Outcome and Fusion Rates in Posterolateral Lumbar Spinal Fusion: A Prospective, Randomized Clinical Study
Thomsen K, Christensen FB, Eiskjær SP, et al (Univ Hosps of Aarhus, Denmark; Holstebro Hosp, Denmark)
Spine 22:2813–2822, 1997   28–16

Introduction.—Surgery for spondylolisthetic or degenerative lumbar segmental instability is a common procedure, yet the indications, operative techniques, and outcome after lumbar fusion remain controversial. The effects of supplementary pedicle screw fixation (Cotrel-Dubousset) in posterolateral lumbar spinal fusion were evaluated.

Methods.—The 130 patients studied all had lumbar or lumbosacral instability and severe, chronic low back pain. Excluded were those with previous fusion, metabolic bone disease, or comorbidity. The decision to undertake fusion was made after clinical and neurologic examinations and a variety of imaging studies. Sixty-four patients were randomly assigned to Cotrel-Dubousset–supplemented fusion (CD group) and 66 to non-CD, posterolateral intertransverse fusion (non-CD group). Patients were followed up for 2 years for fusion quality and functional status.

Results.—Mean operative times were 212 minutes in the CD group and 127 minutes in the non-CD group. Mean perioperative blood loss was greater and duration of hospitalization longer in the CD group than in the non-CD group (1,639 mL vs. 1155 mL and 11.1 days vs. 8.9 days, respectively). Examination of plain radiographs showed no significant differences between instrumented and noninstrumented groups. Both groups reported significant improvements in functional outcome, as assessed by the Dallas Pain Questionnaire. Differences between groups were not significant, except that the CD group had significantly better functional outcome in relation to daily activities when neural decompression had been performed. Overall patient satisfaction was 82% in the CD group vs. 74% in the non-CD group, not a significant difference. Some instrumented patients (4.8%) had significant symptoms from misplacement of pedicle screws, and infections developed in 2 patients. Reoperations were required in 19% of CD vs. 6% of non-CD patients.

Conclusions.—The use of pedicle screw fixation in patients undergoing lumbar posterolateral fusion does not appear to be justified. Both functional outcome and fusion rate were comparable in the CD and non-CD groups, whereas instrumentation was associated with increased operation time, blood loss, and reoperation rates.

▶ The authors of each of these studies received the 1997 Volvo Award in Clinical Studies for their work.

These studies, contrary to popular opinion, suggest that segmental fusion does not improve clinical outcome for patients who have undergone posterior decompression for degenerative spondylolisthesis and spinal stenosis. Although there was a higher rate of fusion in the instrumented groups, the clinical outcomes were comparable. These findings are consistent with those reported by other spine surgeons,[1-3] and taken together, they effectively call into question the increasingly pervasive use of pedicle instrumentation for degenerative spondylolisthesis and spinal stenosis.

S.R. Gibbs, M.A., M.D.

References

1. Bridwell KH, Sedgewick TA, O'Brien MF, et al: The role of fusion and instrumentation in the treatment of degenerative spondylolisthesis with spinal stenosis. *J Spinal Disord* 6:461–472, 1993.
2. Herkowitz HN, Kurz LT: Degenerative lumbar spondylolisthesis with spinal stenosis. *J Bone Joint Surg [Am]* 73:802–807, 1991.
3. Zdeblick TA: A prospective, randomized study of lumbar fusion. *Spine* 18:983–991, 1993.

Freeze-dried Cortical Allograft in Posterior Spinal Arthrodesis: Use With Segmental Instrumentation for Idiopathic Adolescent Scoliosis
Stricker SJ, Sher JS (Univ of Miami, Fla)
Orthopedics 20:1039–1043, 1997   28–17

Introduction.—Freeze-dried bone allografts have many advantages when used in spinal arthrodesis, but questions remain regarding optimal harvesting technique, method of preparation, and the role of the immune response and histocompatibility during graft incorporation. In 32 patients with idiopathic adolescent scoliosis, the role of cortical bone implants was examined, and the efficacy of this material in posterior spinal arthrodesis was determined.

Methods.—Patients had a mean age of 11.3 years and an average preoperative Cobb angle of 54 degrees. There were 14 thoracic, 3 thoracolumbar, 2 lumbar, and 13 double-major curves. Freeze-dried, crushed cortical allograft bone chips were rehydrated, then placed along both lateral gutters. Procedures required an average of 4.5 hours to complete. Radiographs of the spine were obtained every 3–4 months during the first year, then semiannually. The average duration of follow-up was 34 months.

Results.—Patients without radiographic signs of pseudarthrosis and who were free of localized back pain or tenderness by 24 months postoperatively were considered to have successful spinal arthrodesis. The rate of incorporation of cortical allograft varied, but in all patients the allograft bone chips had completely disappeared radiographically by 9 months after surgery. One patient required revision of instrumentation at 1 month, and another had hardware removed at 15 months because of a late infection.

Conclusions.—In this group of patients, all with idiopathic adolescent scoliosis and treated by a single surgeon, the pseudarthrosis rate was presumed to be 0% with at least 2 years of follow-up. Freeze-dried, crushed cortical bone allograft, used in conjunction with stable spinal instrumentation, appears to yield an acceptable rate of arthrodesis. There were no significant complications related to incorporation or immunogenicity.

▶ Bony fusion or artificial ankylosis is the objective for long-term segmental stabilization in some spinal operations, although for some conditions, the clinical outcome does not seem to depend upon achieving fusion (Abstracts 28–15 and 28–16).

The authors have shared their particularly good experience achieving fusion with crushed, freeze-dried cortical allograft. Despite the enormous volume of spinal surgery performed to date, there is no definitive collective opinion or accord on which substrate, combination of substrates, and adjuncts are absolutely best for achieving spinal fusion.

S.R. Gibbs, M.A., M.D.

Spine Trauma

Causes and Costs of Spinal Cord Injury in the United States
DeVivo MJ (Univ of Alabama, Birmingham)
Spinal Cord 35:809–813, 1997   28–18

Objective.—About 10,000 people are hospitalized for spinal cord injury (SCI) each year. The costs associated with these injuries are very high and increasing rapidly. Accurate cost data are needed to ensure adequate funding, research, and medical management. This study examined the direct costs of SCI in the United States from a public health perspective.

Methods.—The cross-sectional multicenter study included a random sample of 508 patients treated in a model SCI care system 2–16 years previously and enrolled in the National Spinal Cord Injury Statistical Center database. A sample of 227 newly injured patients was assessed as well. During a 1-year study period, the investigators prospectively collected data on all charges for emergency medical services, hospitalizations, attendant care, equipment, supplies, medications, environmental modifications, physician and outpatient services, nursing homes, household assistance, vocational rehabilitation, and other direct costs. All values were reported in 1995 dollars.

Results.—Average charges during the first year and recurring annual charges were approximately $234,000 and $33,000, respectively, for patients injured in vehicle crashes; $218,000 and $17,000 for victims of violence; $296,000 and $27,000 for those injured in sports; $185,000 and $26,000 for those injured in falls; and $209,000 and $24,000 for those injured by other causes. Estimates calculated using various data sources, including survival statistics from the National Spinal Cord Injury Statistical Center, suggested average lifetime charges of $970,000 for patients injured in vehicle crashes, $613,000 for victims of violence, $951,000 for those injured in sports, $630,000 for those injured in falls, and $674,000 for those injured by other causes. Annual aggregate direct costs for the United States were estimated at $3.48 billion, $1.81 billion, $1.28 billion, $694 million, and $472 million, respectively.

Conclusions.—This study estimates the direct costs associated with spinal cord injury in the United States at $7.736 billion. These enormous costs underscore the need to develop effective primary prevention programs. The authors' data suggest that any intervention that can successfully prevent SCIs is highly likely to save money, even before the costs of lost productivity are considered.

▶ This report examines a random sample of 508 persons selected from the National Spinal Cord Injury Statistical Center database. The first year medical charges, as well as charges for treatment related to spinal cord injury for subsequent years, are estimated. It is interesting to note that the average lifetime charges per case vary by as much as 40%, depending on the cause of the injury. The reason for this variation is believed to be related to the severity of spinal cord injury as well as its level. Although one may argue with the author's methodology for determining costs, the estimated total annual aggregate of around $7.736 billion is staggering. It is also not tremendously out of line with data presented previously.

This cost places a significant burden on the already stressed Medicare system. Initially, only 5% of patients were covered by Medicare but within 5 years post injury, this number rose to 31%. This article lends economic support to the need for further research directed at preventing and treating these devastating injuries.

V.C. Traynelis, M.D.

Steroids and Gunshot Wounds to the Spine

Heary RF, Vaccaro AR, Mesa JJ, et al (Univ of Medicine and Dentistry of New Jersey, Newark; Thomas Jefferson Univ, Philadelphia; Rothman Inst, Philadelphia)
Neurosurgery 41:576–584, 1997   28–19

Background.—Neurologic benefits from "spinal cord injury" doses of methylprednisolone in patients with blunt spinal cord injuries have been reported. In the current study, the relative risk-to-benefit ratio of intravenous steroid treatment in patients with gunshot wounds to the spine was investigated.

Methods.—Two hundred fifty-four consecutive patients treated between 1979 and 1994 for gunshot wounds to C1–L1 and a spinal cord injury were included in the retrospective review. The patients had been given methylprednisolone, dexamethasone, or no steroid. Mean follow-up was 56.3 months.

Findings.—Neither methylprednisolone nor dexamethasone resulted in significant neurologic benefits. Both steroid groups had an increase in infectious complications, although the increase was not significant. However, significant increases were noted in gastrointestinal complications in the dexamethsaone group and in pancreatitis in the methylprednisolone group.

Conclusions.—Intravenous steroids were associated with no neurologic benefits in patients with gunshot wounds to the spine. Moreover, infectious and noninfectious complication rates were higher in the steroid groups than in the placebo group.

▶ This work deals to perfection in terms of methodology and philosophy of treatment of a large number of patients managed in a single reference institution. In fact, I agree with the authors that questions are more numerous than answers after the conclusions. In my opinion, axonal transport could be not totally absent or absolutely impaired after incomplete blunt spinal cord injury. This scenario marks a capital difference with the anatomical "transection" of the gunshot wounds to the spine. The neuroprotective effects of methylprednisolone can play a significant role on functional recovery at some extent if the pharmacological treatment is administered promptly and in adequate dosage. The real question in terms of recovery is which is the crucial "incomplete" amount of injury after a spinal cord that could be restored? Is it rational to expect the same beneficial effects of a particular neuroprotective drug acting mainly on secondary biochemical cascade after a penetrating spinal trauma in comparison with a blunt one? Experimental animal studies with grading model of penetrating spinal cord injuries using pre- and posttrauma pharmacological treatments, perhaps analyzing some electrophysiological (somatosensory evoked potentials) and the more important clinical (behavioral) tests, should be helpful to improve this devastating condition.

M.A. Perez-Espejo, M.D., Ph.D.

Associated Lumbosacral Junction Injuries (LSJIs) in Pelvic Fractures
Oransky M, Gasparini G (Catholic Univ, Rome)
J Orthop Trauma 11:509–512, 1997   28–20

Introduction.—Lumbosacral junction injuries (LSJIs) associated with unstable sacral fractures were first described and classified by Isler in 1990. These lesions were reported in 38% of vertically unstable sacral fractures and in 3.5% of the sacral fractures exhibiting rotary instability. A retrospective review of 89 patients with pelvic ring injuries was conducted to verify data from the previous study.

Methods.—Consecutive cases reviewed had been treated at the study institution between March 1985 and June 1993. Only those fractures with rotational or vertical instability were analyzed, for a total of 71 fractures. The sacrum was involved in 41% of the lateral compression fractures and in 65% of the vertically unstable fractures. Pelvic fractures were classified according to Tile's classification and LSJIs associated with pelvic ring fractures according to a modification of Isler's classification.

Results.—Thirteen patients were found to have LSJIs; 12 lesions were associated with vertically unstable fractures and 1 with a compression fracture. A facet fracture associated with a contralateral sacroiliac joint dislocation (an exception to the rule described by Isler) was identified in 1 patient. Three patients had lesions considered to be a new type of LSJI. These lesions were characterized by disruption of the annulus fibrosus associated with rising of the hemipelvis and inclination of the L5 body.

Conclusion.—Patients with transforaminal sacral fractures, especially when these fractures are displaced, should be examined by CT for lumbosacral junction injuries. The incidence of LSJIs may be underestimated because of the inability of current diagnostic techniques to achieve consistent detection.

▶ The authors of this prospective study share their experience of pelvic/sacral fractures and associated ligamentous and skeletal LSJIs. They advocate a high index of suspicion and CT evaluation of L5–S1 in patients with pelvic fractures, and especially in patients with transforaminal sacral fractures. Further, they suggest that LSJIs may be underdetected.

S.R. Gibbs, M.A., M.D.

Surgical Technique

Pars Interarticular Fenestration in the Treatment of Foraminal Lumbar Disc Herniation: A Further Surgical Approach

Di Lorenzo N, Porta F, Onnis G, et al (Univ of Cagliari, Italy)
Neurosurgery 42:87–90, 1998   28–21

Introduction.—When lumbar disk herniation occurs between the medial and the lateral margins of the pedicle, it is considered to be foraminal. To treat this subtype of disk herniation, several surgical procedures have been used, including hemi/interlaminectomy combined with partial or full facetectomy, and lateral fenestration and posterolateral exposure. The procedures can result in destruction, an increase in the risk of instability, and less exposure of medial foraminal abnormalities. A new surgical approach to foraminal disk herniation was proposed that spares the continuity and stability of the lumbar vertebrae, by limiting bone removal to a minimum. The procedure also adequately exposes the foraminal compartment medially and laterally, permitting optimal removal of the disk fragment.

Methods.—During a 3-year period, the procedure was performed in 28 patients. In 18 patients, the herniation was purely foraminal, and in 10 patients, it was mainly foraminal with a definite extraforaminal component. Only after 6 weeks of therapy with anti-inflammatory drugs and strict bed rest had proved to be ineffective was surgical treatment offered. The surgical technique involves unroofing the foraminal compartment by cutting an ovoid fenestration, with its major longitudinal axis at the level of the pars interarticularis, medially and slightly off-center under the lateral isthmic notch (i.e., below the pedicle projection). The foraminal root compressed by the herniated disk is exposed by this fenestration, allowing for easy removal.

Results.—All patients had successful treatment, with quick remission of pain and only mild postoperative discomfort. Within 10–30 days after the operation, all patients resumed their occupations, according to type of work. They were followed up for a mean of 24 months and had no return of pain.

Conclusions.—Pars interarticularis fenestration is advocated because it spares, with minimal bone removal, the facet joints and the anatomical continuity of the pars interarticularis. In addition, this procedure allows for the proper exposure of the foraminal compartment medially and laterally, permitting optimal removal of the disk herniation.

▶ Swift pain relief with minimal disruption of stabilizing structures is the objective of lumbar disk surgery. The authors report achieving this in patients, with foraminal zone herniations, through a creative pars fenestration technique without disrupting other posterior elements. This discreet technique seems best reserved for the rare patient that has a free fragment disk herniation, in the foraminal zone, without associated lateral recess or foraminal stenosis.

S.R. Gibbs, M.A., M.D.

Paraspinous Muscle Flaps
Manstein ME, Manstein CH, Manstein G (Albert Einstein Med Ctr, Philadelphia)
Ann Plast Surg 40:458–462, 1998   28–22

Introduction.—It can be difficult to achieve coverage of midline posterior wounds, particularly in patients with exposed spinal stabilization hardware. Latissimus dorsi muscle or musculocutaneous flaps are generally used to manage wounds involving the middle-to-upper thoracic spine. However, more complex solutions—including reversed latissimus dorsi flaps, free flaps, extended intercostal flaps, or fasciocutaneous rotation flaps—are needed for lower midline wounds, particularly those in the thoracolumbar region. An experience with the paraspinous muscle flaps for the coverage of difficult back wounds was reported.

Methods.—Paraspinous flaps were used to cover complex back wounds in 12 patients during a 10-year period. Eight patients had exposed Harrington spinal stabilization rods, 3 had CSF leaks, and 1 had exposed spinous processes. Five patients had wounds in the middle upper back, which were managed with both paraspinous muscle flaps and latissimus dorsi flaps; 7 patients had lower back wounds, which were managed with bilateral paraspinous flaps only.

Results.—At an average follow-up of 6 years, 11 patients had complete healing. None had recurrent infections. The complication rate was 41%. Four patients required postoperative aspiration of seromas, although all of these eventually resolved. All patients who were ambulatory preoperatively could walk postoperatively, including 5 patients with infected Harrington rods. The only failed repair was in the patient with recurrent CSF leak; this may have been related to failure to decompress CSF pressure when the dural defect was repaired.

Conclusions.—For complex back wounds, paraspinous muscle flaps provide good coverage with rapid elevation. No additional skin incisions are needed, and bilateral flaps can be placed through the same incision. Paraspinous muscle flaps will play an increasingly important role in covering exposed hardware, bone, or dura.

▶ The paraspinous muscles provide a well-vascularized muscle flap that will effectively cover most midline spinal defects. This anatomy is familiar to spinal surgeons, and the technique is straightforward and relatively simple.

S.R. Gibbs, M.A., M.D.

29 Stroke Prevention

Differences in Medical and Surgical Therapy for Stroke Prevention Between Leading Experts in North America and Western Europe
Masuhr F, Busch M, Einhäupl KM (Charité Med School, Berlin)
Stroke 29:339–345, 1998   29–1

Introduction.—Controversy exists in different areas of stroke prevention, particularly in regards to the optimal dose of aspirin to prescribe and the use of carotid endarterectomy in asymptomatic patients. The current management of stroke-prone patients by leading experts in Western Europe and North America was compared.

Methods.—A worldwide survey of 185 neurologists who are leading the discussions of stroke prevention practices was performed. The survey contained questions about oral anticoagulation, the use of antiplatelet agents, and the prevention of ischemic stroke. There were 73 neurologists

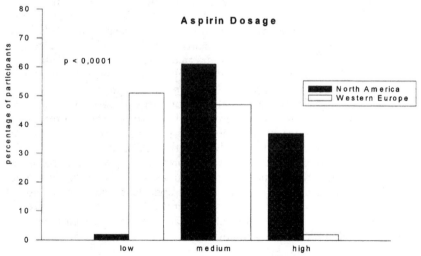

FIGURE 1.—Percentages of participants from North America and Western Europe reporting using low (30–175 mg), medium (200–400 mg), or high (500–1,300 mg) daily doses of aspirin for stroke prevention after previous atherothrombotic stroke or transient ischemic attack. (Courtesy of Masuhr F, Busch M, Einhäupl KM: Differences in medical and surgical therapy for stroke prevention between leading experts in North America and Western Europe. *Stroke* 29:339–345. Copyright 1998, American Heart Association. Reproduced with permission.)

TABLE.—Percentages of Participants Reporting Use of Warfarin and Aspirin in Patients With Nonvalvular Atrial Fibrillation

Patient's Age, y	Additional Risk Factors*	Cardioembolic Event	Warfarin		Aspirin		No Treatment		Warfarin+Aspirin	
			NA	WE	NA	WE	NA	WE	NA	WE
<60	No	No	21	26	54	43	23	31	2	...
60–75	No	No	65	62	33	34	...	3	2	...
<75	Yes	No	88	92	5	7	5	...	2	2
<75		Yes	95	96	2	3	...	...	2	2
>75	No	No	61	38	33	57	5	5	2	...
>75	Yes	No	74	66	19	32	5	...	2	2
>75		Yes	84	73	9	26	5	...	2	2

Note: NA indicates the percentage of participants from North America who reported using the respective treatment; WE, percentage of participants from Western Europe who reported using the respective treatment.
*Risk factors such as hypertension, diabetes, or cardiac disease.
(Courtesy of Masuhr F, Busch M, Einhäupl KM: Differences in medical and surgical therapy for stroke prevention between leading experts in North America and Western Europe. *Stroke* 29:339–345. Copyright 1998, American Heart Association. Reproduced with permission.)

from Western Europe and 48 from North America. The response rate was of more than 90%.

Results.—In patients at risk of atherothrombotic stroke, nearly all respondents reported prescribing aspirin, but 36% of American participants give aspirin doses of more than 500 mg daily, and 51% of European participants give aspirin doses of less than 200 mg daily (Fig 1). Ticlopidine was reported as the second choice by 86% of Americans vs. 59% of Europeans. Warfarin was used by 23% of European participants compared with 5% from North America. The use of anticoagulants in patients with atrial fibrillation increased in accordance with the patient's individual risk of stroke, but European respondents were less likely to use anticoagulants in patients older than 75 years than their North American counterparts (Table). European respondents reported relatively higher target international normalized ratio values. In patients with symptomatic carotid stenosis, nearly all participants recommended carotid endarterectomy. North Americans (48%) were more likely to recommend the use of carotid endarterectomy in asymptomatic patients than the Europeans (28%), particularly in patients with more than 95% stenosis.

Conclusions.—Leading experts from North American and Western Europe had significant differences in several areas of stroke prevention practices. Divergent results of trials from the 2 continents may partly explain these differences. In addition, in some areas of controversy, currently available trial data are not sufficient to reach an international consensus about optimal clinical management.

► Despite having access to the same published clinical studies, stroke experts from North America and Western Europe seem to have significantly different opinions about antithrombotic therapy, treatment of atrial fibrillation, and carotid vascular surgery for stroke prevention. It is clear that consensus on these issues does not evolve spontaneously. Perhaps it is time for a "consensus conference" and a dedicated effort to reach such.

S.R. Gibbs, M.A., M.D.

Helicobacter pylori Infection: A Risk Factor for Ischaemic Cerebrovascular Disease and Carotid Atheroma

Markus HS, Mendall MA (Inst of Psychiatry, London; Mayday Hosp Croydon and St George's Hosp, London)

J Neurol Neurosurg Psychiatry 64:104–107, 1998   29–2

Purpose.—Infection with *Helicobacter pylori* is strongly associated with duodenal and gastric ulcers and gastric cancer. Recent studies suggest that *H. pylori* infection may be associated with ischemic heart disease, independent of conventional risk factors. However, the potential mechanisms of this relationship are unknown. *Helicobacter pylori* infection was evaluated as a possible risk factor for ischemic cerebrovascular disease and carotid atheroma.

Methods.—A total of 238 patients with nonhemorrhagic stroke or transient ischemic attack and 119 controls were studied. The spouses of affected patients were used as controls to help control for socioeconomic status. Pathogenic mechanisms were evaluated to determine stroke subtype. Duplex ultrasound was used to estimate carotid atheroma load. Serologic studies for IgG antibodies to *H. pylori* were performed as well.

Results.—The rate of *H. pylori* seropositivity was 59% for cases vs. 45% for controls. Seropositivity for *H. pylori* was associated with a 1.78 odds ratio (OR) of cerebrovascular disease. This association remained significant even after controlling for socioeconomic status and other risk factors. The association was significant for large vessel disease (OR 2.58) and for lacunar stroke (OR 2.21), but not for stroke caused by cardioembolism or stroke of unknown cause (OR 1.16).

Patients who were seropositive for *H. pylori* had a mean carotid stenosis of 37%, compared with 28% for seronegative patients. About 60% of patients were seropositive, regardless of whether they had stroke or transient ischemic attack.

Conclusions.—Infection with *H. pylori* appears to be an independent risk factor for ischemic cerebrovascular disease. The mechanism of this relationship may involve increased atherosclerosis. If the link between *H. pylori* and cerebrovascular disease is confirmed, antibiotic therapy to eradicate the infection might reduce the risk of stroke and other vascular events.

▶ Increasingly, bacteria are being associated with diseases not formerly thought to be infectious diseases. For example, "nanobacteria" (measuring 200–500 nm), recently described in the July 7, 1998, *Proceedings of the National Academy of Sciences*, have been associated with calcium deposition and are now suspected to play a role in the formation of kidney stones.

Helicobacter pylori seropositivity seems to confer an independent incremental risk for symptomatic cerebrovascular disease. It has also been strongly associated with chronic active gastric inflammation, gastric cancer, and gastric and duodenal ulceration as well as ischemic heart disease. Because it can be readily detected and treated with antibiotics, I believe that a screening test for *H. pylori* will soon be available as part of most general health screening examinations.

S.R. Gibbs, M.A., M.D.

30 Miscellaneous

Lamotrigine (Lamictal) in Refractory Trigeminal Neuralgia: Results From a Double-blind Placebo Controlled Crossover Trial
Zakrzewska JM, Chaudhry Z, Nurmikko TJ, et al (Royal London School of Medicine and Dentistry; Eastman Dental Inst, London; Walton Centre for Neurology and Neurosurgery, Liverpool, England; et al)
Pain 73:223–230, 1997   30–1

Purpose.—Trigeminal neuralgia remains a therapeutic challenge: carbamazepine is the treatment of choice, but many patients cannot tolerate it because of CNS side effects. The new antiepileptic drug lamotrigine has potential for use in refractory trigeminal neuralgia, but has not been evaluated in a randomized, placebo-controlled trial until now.

Methods.—Fourteen patients with refractory trigeminal neuralgia participated in the trial at 3 centers. In crossover fashion, the patients took lamotrigine, 400 mg, and placebo for 2 weeks each, with an intervening 3-day washout period. During both arms, the patients continued to take a steady dose of carbamazepine or phenytoin. The study used a composite efficacy index, with superiority of 1 treatment over the other determined by a hierarchy of use of escape medication, total pain scores, and global evaluations.

Results.—Thirteen patients were eligible for inclusion in the composite efficacy index; 11 showed greater efficacy with lamotrigine than placebo. Lamotrigine also appeared superior on global evaluations. The adverse effects were mainly dose-dependent CNS effects. One patient had severe pain during placebo treatment, leading to withdrawal from the study.

Conclusions.—Lamotrigine appears to have useful antineuralgic properties. Its long-term effectiveness remains to be determined, though 9 of 14 patients in this study continued taking lamotrigine with benefit. The value of lamotrigine as a first-line therapy is limited because this drug must be introduced gradually.

▶ Although carbamazepine has long been the medical treatment of choice for trigeminal neuralgia, a substantial proportion of patients tolerate this drug poorly.[1] Lamotrigine, an antiepileptic agent, is believed to suppress the pathological release of glutamate, thereby providing an antinociceptive effect. It is generally very well tolerated in patients with epilepsy[2-4] and as the authors point out, it had no effect on hematological or biochemical indices and was not associated with increased hepatic enzyme concentrations and hyponatremia, which can be problematic with carbamazepine. Further, the authors noted that lamotrigine is only moderately bound to plasma proteins, consequently, its addition to a therapeutic regimen does not necessitate dose modifications of concomitant antiepileptic medications.

Lamotrigine appears to be an effective adjunct medication for patients with otherwise medically refractory trigeminal neuralgia. Its potential antinociceptive effect and its low incidence of untoward effects may hold some value in the management of other types of chronic pain.

S.R. Gibbs, M.A., M.D.

References

1. Patsalos PN: Medical management, in: Zakrzewska JM (ed.), *Trigeminal Neuralgia. A Practical Approach to Management, Major Problems in Neurology Series,* Vol. 28, WB Saunders, London, 1995, pp 80–107.
2. Betts T, Goodwin G, Withers RM et al: Human safety of lamotrigine. *Epilepsia* 32:S17–S21, 1991.
3. Steiner TJ and the North Thames Lamictal Study Group: Comparison of lamotrigine (Lamictal) and phenytoin monotherapy in newly diagnosed epilepsy. *Epilepsia* 35(7):61, 1994.
4. Brodie MJ, for UK Lamotrigine/Carbamazepine Monotherapy Trial Group: Double-blind comparison of lamotrigine and carbamazepine in newly diagnosed epilepsy. *Lancet* 345:476–479, 1995.

Risk Factors for Primary Central Nervous System Lymphoma: A Case-Control Study
Schiff D, Suman VJ, Yang P, et al (Mayo Clinic and Found, Rochester, Minn)
Cancer 82:975–982, 1998   30–2

Objective.—From the 1970s to the 1980s, the annual incidence of primary CNS lymphoma (PCNSL) has nearly tripled, from 2.7 to 30 cases per 10 million. This trend has been apparent in both immunocompetent and immunodeficient patients; the reasons for the increase among immunocompetent patients are unknown. Risk factors for PCNSL in apparently immunocompetent patients were analyzed.

Methods.—The case-control study included 109 nonimmunodeficient patients with PCNSL diagnosed between 1975 and 1994. The patients were 71 males and 38 females, all at least 13 years of age at diagnosis. Two groups of controls were studied as well: 101 patients with other types of cancer and 109 patients with other neurologic diseases. Potential risk factors included environmental exposures, personal history of diseases, drug exposure, medical intervention, and family history.

Results.—There was a significant association between PCNSL and lower education when cases were compared with cancer controls. This factor was not significant on comparison with neurologic controls. Patients with PCNSL were significantly less likely to have undergone tonsillectomy or to have used oral contraceptives than either control group.

There was no consistent relationship between PCNSL and the presence of autoimmune disorders or cardiovascular diseases. Risk of PCNSL was unaffected by farming or by personal or family history of cancer.

Conclusions.—Some possible risk factors for PCNSL are identified that warrant further study. History of tonsillectomy and oral contraceptive use appeared to reduce risk of PCNSL. It is hoped that the results will provide an impetus for further etiologic studies of PCNSL. The authors note the limitations of the study, given the referral nature of the case and control groups.

▶ The rising incidence of this disease can be attributed to, in part, the AIDS epidemic and the extensive use of immunosuppressive therapy.[1] A variety of other causative factors for PCNSL have come under scrutiny, especially in light of the rising incidence in nonimmunocompromised patients; however, the cause has remained enigmatic.

This entity should be strongly considered in the differential diagnosis of a hyperdense or isodense mass in the periventricular region, particularly involving the corpus callosum, thalamus, or basal ganglia. Computed tomography is very sensitive for PCNSL, with less than 5% of scans being falsely negative.[1]

Percival Bailey, a former editor of this YEAR BOOK, offered the first formal description of cerebral lymphoma in 1929,[1] and until recently, PCNSL has been considered a rare phenomenon. In 1992, a conservative estimate based upon the Surveillance, Epidemiology and End Result (SEER) program suggested that PCNSL represented up to 8% of all brain neoplasms.[1]

This work from the Mayo Clinic is the first published risk factor study of PCNSL in immunocompetent patients. Interestingly, tonsillectomy and use of oral contraceptives appeared to be independent "protective" factors for PCNSL.

S.R. Gibbs, M.A., M.D.

References

1. Kay AH, Laws ER Jr., (eds): *Brain Tumors*, Edinburgh, Churchill Livingstone, 1995.
2. Bailey P: Intracranial sarcomatous tumors of leptomeningeal origin. *Arch Surg* 18:1359–1402, 1929.

Depth of Insertion of a Lumbar Puncture Needle
Craig F, Stroobant J, Winrow A, et al (Children's Hosp, Lewisham, England; Kingston Gen Hosp, England; Central Middlesex Hosp, London)
Arch Dis Child 77:450, 1997   30–3

Background.—Knowing how far the needle should be inserted when performing lumbar puncture in children may reduce the number of unsuccessful attempts and bloody taps. The depth of lumbar-puncture needle insertion was documented.

Methods and Findings.—One hundred and seven children, aged 0.01–16 years, underwent lumbar puncture in the routine assessment of acute and chronic illnesses. The depth of needle insertion ranged from 0.5–6.5 cm. It was best correlated with the patient's height, the association being linear. The average insertion depth was 0.03 cm × height in centimeters.

Conclusions.—Height was found to be the best guide to minimum and maximum depths of needle insertion during lumbar puncture.

▶ Since the invention of the lumbar puncture by Quincke almost 100 years ago, the technical problems seem to be mastered and attention is now focused on more pragmatic questions, such as how to diminish discomfort to the patient and how to obtain samples not contaminated by blood. These should be achieved by the accurate position of the needle in the first attempt. This article gives very useful technical advice about how to evaluate the distance skin-subarachnoid space in children by simply measuring the length of the body and using a graph. It's surprising that nobody came across the idea before this. The method is obviously not applicable to adults, but should give an impetus to find similar parameters for that group of patients.

It is now up to the manufacturers to provide needles with a scale.

B. Klun, M.D., Ph.D.

Anatomic Position of the Asterion
Day JD, Tschabitscher M (Lahey Hitchcock Med Ctr, Burlington, Mass; Univ of Vienna)
Neurosurgery 42:198–199, 1998   30–4

Introduction.—For proper surgical planning and approach, surface anatomical landmarks are essential. In approaches to the posterior fossa and posterolateral cranial base, surface landmarks can be of help in locating the transverse-sigmoid sinus complex. A primary landmark in performing the combined petrosal approach to the cranial base may be the asterion—defined as the junction of the lambdoid, parietomastoid, and occipitomastoid sutures. The reliability and usefulness of the asterion as a surgical landmark for lateral cranial base approaches to the posterior fossa were determined.

Methods.—One hundred dried skulls were drilled at the asterion on each side. Recordings and determinations were taken of the position of the 2 mm drill hole on the inner surface of the skull.

Results.—In 32% of skulls, the asterion was located over the posterior fossa dura on the right, and in 25% on the left. The asterion was located over the transverse-sigmoid complex in 61% on the right and in 66% on the left. In 7%, the landmark was located above the transverse-sigmoid sinus complex on the right and in 9% on the left.

Conclusions.—The asterion is not a strictly reliable landmark for locating the underlying posterior fossa dura. Because it is often located directly over the transverse-sigmoid sinus complex, burr holes placed at the asterion may open the bone over the sinus, resulting in potential damage. The asterion may not be used as a safe reliable landmark, but it could be used to determine the underlying location of the transverse-sigmoid sinus junction.

▶ Although I know that the asterion has been described as a reference surface landmark for lateral posterior fossa exposures, I have always begun a lateral approach to the posterior fossa by placing the initial burr hole 1 cm inferior to a line drawn from the inion to the base of the mastoid process and 2 cm medial to the posterior edge of the mastoid process. This allows one to expand a single burr hole superiorly and laterally to reveal the transverse and sigmoid sinuses, respectively. Once this juncture is directly visualized, an inferomedial craniotomy or craniectomy can be performed without risk of sinus laceration.

With the advent and refinement of neuronavigational systems, operative planning by surface landmarks and corresponding measurements may ultimately become a lost skill, much in the way that pre-CT and pre-MRI radiographic interpretation skills have been lost.

S.R. Gibbs, M.A., M.D.

Risk Factors for Neurosurgical Site Infections After Craniotomy: A Prospective Multicenter Study of 2944 Patients
Korinek A-M, the French Study Group of Neurosurgical Infections, the SEHP, and the C-CLIN Paris-Nord (Pitié-Salpétrière Hosp, Paris)
Neurosurgery 41:1073–1081, 1997   30–5

Introduction.—Specific methods to prevent surgical site infections in patients having craniotomy might be feasible if infection risk was known and patients at risk could be identified. A multicenter prospective study to determine risk factors for neurosurgical site infections after craniotomy has not been performed. The National Nosocomial Infections Surveillance system score was developed to predict the risk of surgical patients acquiring surgical site infections after many types of operative procedures. Three risk factors were included in the score: an American Society of Anesthesiologists preoperative score of 3, 4, or 5; an operation classified as contaminated or dirty-infected; and an operation lasting more than t hours, with t depending on the specific procedure performed. The incidence of surgical site infections after craniotomy was ascertained. High-risk patients or procedures were identified, and the validity of the National Nosocomial Infections Surveillance system risk index in neurosurgical patients was assessed.

Methods.—During a 15-month period, a total of 2,944 adult patients undergoing craniotomy in 10 neurosurgical units were prospectively evaluated for development and risk factors of surgical site infections. They were followed up for at least 30 days. The Centers for Disease Control definitions for surgical site infections were used. Multivariate analyses were performed to include all significant risk factors of univariate analysis, and then only those known before surgery. Incidence was calculated per patient. In this population, the National Nosocomial Infections Surveillance system risk index was tested.

Results.—Of the 2,944 patients studied, 117 (4%) had surgical site infections; 30 had wound infections, 14 had bone flap osteitis, 56 had meningitis, and 17 had brain abscesses. Postoperative CSF leakage and subsequent operation were independent risk factors for surgical site infections. Emergency surgery, clean-contaminated and dirty surgery, an operative time longer than 4 hours, and recent neurosurgery were independent predictive risk factors. Lack of antibiotic prophylaxis was not a risk factor. The National Nosocomial Infections Surveillance system risk index effectively identified at-risk patients.

Conclusions.—Postoperative events are involved as independent risk factors for surgical site infections after craniotomy. In identifying at-risk patients, the National Nosocomial Infections Surveillance system risk index is effective.

▶ This is an important "benchmark" study because it is the first prospective, multicenter study of risk factors for surgical site infections (SSI) after craniotomy. Multivariate analysis revealed only 2 major independent risk factors for SSI—postoperative CSF leak and early subsequent operation. The authors report an overall SSI rate of 4% for craniotomy. Interestingly, the absence of antibiotic prophylaxis was not a risk factor for SSI.

Fastidious wound closure and hemostasis technique, as well as appropriate use of a wound drain and/or CSF diversion system, combined with close postoperative surveillance and early recognition of these factors will reduce SSI after craniotomy.

S.R. Gibbs, M.A., M.D.

Transverse Microincisions of the Outer Layer of the Dura Mater Combined With Foramen Magnum Decompression as Treatment for Syringomyelia With Chiari I Malformation
Gambardella G, Caruso G, Caffo M, et al (Univ of Messina, Italy)
Acta Neurochir (Wien) 140:134–139, 1998   30–6

Introduction.—The optimal surgical procedure for the treatment of syringomyelia associated with Chiari I malformation remains unclear. The goal of surgery is to restore the physiologic CSF dynamic at the craniovertebral junction. The results of a conservative surgical approach—foramen magnum decompression combined with transverse microincisions of the outer layer of the dura mater—were reported.

Methods.—The experience included 8 patients with syringomyelia and Chiari I malformation. There were 6 men and 2 women, with a mean age of 42 years. Five patients were initially seen with symptoms of paresthesias, hyporeflexia, and weakness and numbness of the upper extremities. Surgery, performed through an extradural approach, consisted of oblique transverse microincisions of the outer layer of the dura mater combined with decompression of the bony foramen magnum. This modified Isu technique sought to achieve an extradural correction of the CSF circulatory disturbance at the foramen magnum, avoiding inadvertent opening of the bulging inner dura mater. The patients were followed up for an average of 2 years.

Results.—Seven of the 8 patients showed significant improvement in neurologic signs and symptoms. Postoperative MRI, performed at 7 months, showed significantly reduced syrinx size in 7 patients. On T2-weighted scans, the cisterna magna was significantly expanded. One patient had progression of the neurologic deficit during follow-up.

Conclusions.—For patients with syringomyelia and Chiari I malformation, foramen magnum decompression combined with transverse microincisions of the outer layer of the dura mater appears to be a safe and effective form of surgery. This approach corrects the circulatory disturbance of the CSF dynamic while reducing the size of the syrinx. The result is a significant improvement in neurologic signs and symptoms. The conservative surgical approach avoids the complications of intradural approaches and syringosubarachnoid shunting.

▶ In 1993, Isu et al. proposed a technique for removing the outer layer of dura mater to correct the CSF circulatory disturbance seen in patients with Chiari I malformation and syringomyelia.[1] These authors report their success with a modification of Isu's technique, using oblique transverse incisions in the outer layer of the dura at the foramen magnum

This appears to be an effective treatment requiring less operative time, less risk of injury to neural and vascular structures, and less risk of postoperative CSF leak. However, the study population was small and the follow-up was just 2 years. It will be interesting to see long-term outcome data to compare with the traditional surgical technique for foramen magnum decompression and restoration of CSF circulation.

S.R. Gibbs, M.A., M.D.

Reference

1. Isu T, Sasaki H, Takamura H, et al: Foramen magnum decompression with removal of the outer layer of the dura as treatment for syringomyelia occurring with Chiari I malformation. *Neurosurgery* 33:845–850, 1993.

Subject Index

A

Author Index